Bearing Witness

Bearing Witness

Religious Meanings in Bioethics

COURTNEY S. CAMPBELL

CASCADE *Books* · Eugene, Oregon

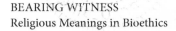

BEARING WITNESS
Religious Meanings in Bioethics

Cascade Books
An Imprint of Wipf and Stock Publishers
199 W. 8th Ave., Suite 3
Eugene, OR 97401

www.wipfandstock.com

PAPERBACK ISBN: 978-1-5326-6273-7
HARDCOVER ISBN: 978-1-5326-6274-4
EBOOK ISBN: 978-1-5326-6275-1

Cataloguing-in-Publication data:

Names: Campbell, Courtney S., 1956–, author.

Title: Bearing witness : religious meanings in bioethics. / Courtney S. Campbell.

Description: Eugene, OR : Pickwick Publications, 2019. | Includes bibliographical references and index.

Identifiers: ISBN 978-1-5326-6273-7 (paperback) | ISBN 978-1-5326-6274-4 (hardcover) | ISBN 978-1-5326-6275-1 (ebook)

Subjects: LCSH: Bioethics and professional ethics. | Bioethics. | Medical ethics—Religious ethics. | Bioethics—Religious aspects. | Bioethical issues.

Classification: R725.55 .C36 2019 (paperback) | R725.55 .C36 (ebook)

Manufactured in the U.S.A.   09/04/19

For Juliette, Jason, Scott, and Cassandra . . . for walking with me through the flowers, forests, and mountains.

Contents

Preface

I was nearing the end of a presentation and discussion on ethical issues at the end of life at an academic medical center when a thoughtful questioner laid down the "so what?" gauntlet to me: "I can see how your analysis would be interesting to scholars in your discipline, but what difference will this make in caring for patients?" Our conversation was a threshold moment for the development of this book. I have lived in the academic, pedagogical, professional, institutional, policy, and personal worlds of bioethics for the past three decades, and as fascinating as those conversations, classrooms, and conferences have been, I have always understood that *ideas matter* in the real world of experiences and decisions that all of us encounter in health and medical care. I have conceptualized my professional work to comprise a kind of calling to wrestle with difficult questions and concepts that inform and can transform persons, choices, and policy structures. I have wanted to affirm the authority of moral experience.

This vocational interpretation has underscored my interest in exploring the different implications of religion, and the study of religion, for the fields of bioethics and the health humanities. My argument in this book is that religious traditions are, among other things, communities of ongoing moral discourse and practice, and they are thereby essential rather than peripheral contexts for envisioning, interpreting, and enacting the ideas bioethics has affirmed as central to our common understandings of health and medicine. I make claims that religious traditions engage in "bearing witness" to various cultures of bioethics, insightful ways of constructing ideas that matter about the nature of the human person, the stories we tell in communities, the moral mission of medicine as a calling and vocation dedicated to healing, and our earnest quests for meaningfulness through the ordeals of suffering and mortality. Those are questions and ideas that matter to all of us, regardless of religious affiliation—or, increasingly in the United States, of no religious affiliation at all.

My introductory chapter, "Witnessing Meaning in Bioethics," identifies how ideas matter by beginning with a very personal account of a medical issue that confronted my mother and her three children and then explicates several meanings of bearing witness in medicine and bioethics: the person as an image-bearer of the divine (*imago Dei*), narrative meaning, a covenantal commitment of healing, and empathic presence in bearing burdens, including suffering, compassionate presence, encountering mortality, and prophetic and conscientious critique in public and professional life. It provides the intellectual and experiential infrastructure for the subsequent discussions. Chapter 2 presents an exposition of ways the relation between religion and bioethics has been constructed historically, including the recent postures of bioethical indifference and hostility to religion embedded in the culture wars. I start there because if I can't make a case for how religious traditions and discourse can make compelling contributions to bioethics, if religious concepts and ideas don't matter or are divorced from policy deliberations, there would not seem much point to further analysis.

Chapters 3 and 4 expand further on my fundamental metaphor of religious ethics as bearing witness. I address the theme of "bearing the image" of the person through an exposition of moral features of the *imago Dei*, which highlights concepts of agency, caring, covenant, creativity, embodiment, equality, gift, narrative, relationship, and stewardship. Chapter 4 addresses the moral witness of "bearing the story," using the New Testament parable of the Good Samaritan to illustrate how narratives and stories bear witness to questions of meaning in bioethics discourse. As the late physician-writer Paul Kalanithi articulated in his moving memoir *When Breath Becomes Air*, narratives provide "the richest material for moral reflection."[1] My analysis underscores how the story-borne witness opens up the kinds of questions that need to be asked in bioethical deliberations and manifests the potency of symbolic forms of rationality embedded in religious tradition.

Chapters 5 through 7 expand on the moral witness of "bearing burdens" by turning a moral focus to the professional commitments of medicine. My analysis takes seriously that medicine (and nursing) is a profession oriented by a commitment to *healing*. I seek to situate the ethics of medicine more as a professional art of healing that complements scientific and technical knowledge; more on transforming identities and less on transactional exchanges; and more about the meaning of medicine as a calling and vocation informed by covenant and less by contract. Healing integrally includes ways in which the human and professional community bears compassionate witness to suffering. My discussion of bearing witness to suffering emphasizes the multivalent nature of this existential experience: suffering is an evil that shatters a person's world and identity, and yet an ordeal that contains re-storying and transformative possibilities.

Chapters 8 and 9 situate the witness of the healer and of covenanted communities in bearing mortality and end-of-life experience with the dying patient. I explore the meaning of witness to both failures and possibilities about dying well. I also examine the ways physician aid-in-dying is assuming increasing appeal for dying patients,

---

1. Kalanithi, *When Breath Becomes Air*, 31.

their advocacy groups, and medical professionals, and is now reconstructed as medical aid in dying. I am both critical of conservative dismissals of physician-assisted dying and of philosophical and professional arguments that make hastening death a new end of medicine.

My discussion of ethical responsibilities regarding physician-assisted death marks a transition in argumentation from the personal, clinical, and professional to the public and civic cultures of bioethics. Chapters 10 and 11 examine how bioethics offers an illustrative window on the increasingly contested and complex public and professional influence of religious perspectives and symbols. I find it problematic for bioethics to be portrayed as a proxy for the wars of culture between political liberalism and conservative religion or for culture to be invoked as a hegemonic term that eclipses the social or public witness of religious traditions. These ongoing disputes indicate that both the culture and bioethics are increasingly under the sway of instrumental rationality and problem-solving to such an extent that religious discourse and tradition is supplanted in public and professional life, leaving some with recourse only to conscience-based objections.

In developing some of my interpretative analysis, arguments, and claims, I make recourse on occasion to the moral and communal resources of my own religious tradition, Latter-day Saint. A reliance on a rather distinctive set of sources, such as sacred writings considered heterodox at best, or heresy, by other Christian thinkers, or practices deemed offensive and outrageous by social commentators or philosophical writers, are nonetheless important for my own reflection on many bioethics issues. I am not aware, other than a few scattered articles of my own in bioethics publications,[2] of the presence of Latter-day Saint perspectives in academic bioethics. My interpretations will not always reflect the conventional wisdom of bioethics or of religious bioethics, as I have found myself often on the cusp of an insider-outsider dialectic in relation to many different professional cultures and moral communities. Still, I invite the reader to keep an open mind as I draw on diverse and resonant sources to explicate the meanings of bearing witness in bioethics.

2. Campbell, "Mormonism, Bioethics in," 2124–31.

Acknowledgments

Bearing Witness draws on my experience as an educator, a scholar and researcher, a participant in public-policy deliberations, a citizen, and a caregiver on some of the defining questions of human life and mortality. It is not, however, a solitary enterprise. As a scholar in the second generation of bioethics, I am the beneficiary of pioneers who initiated the field, a cohort of colleagues who have expanded and advanced the field, and of students who will become the professionals and policy-makers in a future of profound moral ambiguity. I want to acknowledge the invaluable teaching and mentoring I received from James F. Childress at the University of Virginia and from Daniel Callahan at the Hastings Center. They exemplified diverse methods of ethical inquiry while stressing that ethics begins by asking the *right* questions.

My work on this book, and in bioethics and the health humanities generally, has been cultivated by the critical and constructive insights of numerous colleagues. I am especially appreciative of the shaping comments from Andy Lustig at Davidson College, Richard Miller of the University of Chicago Divinity School, Tom Cole of the University of Texas Medical Branch in Houston, and Felicia Cohn, a bioethics consultant with Kaiser-Permanente in California.

An equally important set of teachers for me have been my students in bioethics and the medical humanities at Oregon State University. They bring their own distinctive experiences, questions, and aspirations to the texts we study, to the cases we analyze, and to the policies we critique. The commitments and ideals of my students about their prospective professional careers confer experiential credibility to my interpretations of medicine as a calling and vocation oriented by a responsibility of healing. Students shape the education of their professors in ways they cannot appreciate.

PART ONE

Bearing Witness

1

Witnessing Meaning in Bioethics

I was sitting on the floor in a darkened hospital room, writing by the illumination of lights from the nurses' station outside the room. New Age music emanated softly from a CD player on a chair. There was an unusual serenity and calmness present in that room, disrupted only by the ever-present beeping of the machines monitoring my mother's physiological status as she lay motionless in the hospital bed. The beeps and the statistical output from the data they relayed informed her professional caregivers, my siblings, and myself that my mother was still alive, despite her present condition of unconsciousness subsequent to a severe intracranial hemorrhage. Every two hours a nurse would enter the room, record the vital signs data, check the status of the fluids sustaining my mother's biological organism, and then leave us again to the shadows of the room, and of life itself.

I had felt quite helpless and very disempowered through this experience, sentiments in part attributable to what seemed to me to be a depersonalized medical staff trained to disclose as little information to myself and family members as was possible. An epistemic gulf lay between my experience of what was happening to my mother and the staff's experience of managing care for another patient in the ICU. My siblings and I were empowered through an advance directive to act as proxy for medical decisions on my mother's behalf. Short conversations between the staff and family members had addressed more or less successfully proxy consent for necessary interventions to reduce the swelling in the brain and the administration of medications. My siblings and I were acknowledged as not only stakeholders but also decision-makers in important aspects of our mother's care and treatment; we were consulted in treatment decisions, rather than having treatment determined exclusively by specialists in neurology and cardiology.

Still, as I sat alone in that darkened room at the end of each day at what might be the end of a life, I experienced something missing from a discourse largely directed by matters of medical assessment, institutional protocol, and legal procedure. We had the requisite procedural documents, and had received information about my mother's prognosis subsequent to the intracranial hemorrhage, as well as recommendations regarding the medical evaluation of risks and benefits of possible surgical interventions. However, we were ultimately up against one of the boundaries of human existence, an identity-defining and identity-expressing question about the meaning of mortality that cannot be readily reduced to the interplay of medical beneficence and legally-sanctioned consent processes, and no professional was willing to acknowledge this. I felt somewhat like the protagonist in Tolstoy's classic novella, *The Death of Ivan Ilyich*, who grows increasingly frustrated and resentful as his physicians debate the biological causes of his condition and neglect what was the only question for Ilyich, "the real question of life or death."[1]

As family and professional staff deliberated on several alternatives over the space of some weeks, including "wait and see" if my mother would regain consciousness, additional medical interventions to stabilize her regulating bodily systems, or perhaps discontinuation of treatment, a chasm of discursive dissonance opened up between the practical decision to be made and its existential meaning. If it came to a choice about invasive surgical procedures or discontinuing treatment (and it was yet too soon to know), what decision should be made? This is a question that medicine does not know how to answer, and neither does the culture as a whole.[2] The silence on how persons ought to exercise the choices they have been empowered to make by legal statute and by bioethical reasoning is deafening. This question cannot be answered without incorporating some profound value convictions and assumptions about the purpose of life and the meanings of mortality.

What the hospital physicians referred to as my mother's "stuporous" condition continued for weeks; some treatment decisions became necessary, and my siblings and I experienced disagreements amongst ourselves and with members of the medical staff. The familial disagreements occurred because we situated our mother's current condition somewhat differently within the context of her prior life history, her spiritual and relational values, anticipated prospects for recovery and recuperation, and our own concerns about the burdens of anticipated caregiving on family members. Our disagreements with the physicians occurred because they did not have experience with my mother as a person outside the context of the hospital setting. She was, for them, yet another stroke victim who deserved the kind of care, treatment, and professional attention any stroke patient should receive. The medical and nursing staff members were professional, and carried out their responsibilities efficiently and with the technical skills of their diverse expertise. They were not, however, healers, and it

1. Tolstoy, *Death of Ivan Ilyich*, 113.
2. Gawande, *Being Mortal*, 149–90.

seemed to me that it was precisely a commitment to healing that was missing in the circumstances.

Personally, if it came to it, I was inclined to have treatment discontinued rather than have a further surgical intervention undertaken. Although the specialists could not make a confident prognosis until (or if) my mother revived to consciousness, they had raised the prospect that, as things stood, in an unconsciousness stupor of this duration, the effects of the stroke on my mother's physical, cognitive, and relational capacities were quite likely to be very significant. Even were surgery successful, they anticipated she would have some permanent paralysis, loss of mobility, compromised memory, and speaking difficulty. These impairments would not mean her condition would be incompatible with a life of some duration, but cumulatively they could entail a compromised quality of life for a woman who had been quite independent. I questioned whether this would be a life my mother would desire. This was a perspective that my brother and sister, the other proxies, did not share with me. At a deeper psychological level that I really didn't wish to explore with myself, let alone my siblings, I envisioned that an impaired life for my mother would also entail an impaired relationship between my mother and I. Existentially, I had little doubt that my mother had fulfilled whatever calling or purpose brought meaning for her mortal life, and I felt it important to honor her convictions that her spiritual self would continue to exist, learn, and progress in an afterlife.

My concern here is not with assessing or justifying the rightness of the decisions made: my mother recovered without surgical intervention, a testimony to the resiliency of the body, and she lived semi-independently with impairments less severe than anticipated for over fourteen years. She and I experienced a different kind of relationship that required some adaptations, but I was certainly appreciative of this outcome. Physicians and proxies alike experienced their fallibility and their finitude. My central point is that the decisions and choices required in this setting were not solely matters of medical judgment: such decisions cannot even be made without incorporating some values, commitments, and convictions. We cannot live in the contemporary biomedical world by the formalistic procedures of medicine, institutions, and law alone. The chasm I experienced in the hospital between the practical necessity of making some decisions and the meanings of those decisions needed bridging. Perhaps it was not surprising that I remained troubled by how it was possible in the twenty-first century that what Tolstoy refers to as the "awesome act" of dying[3] could be rationalized through the pedestrian procedures of family consults, consent documents, and advance directives.

The academic field of bioethics has been very adept and successful in critiquing reductionism in biomedical research and practice, in which the totality and mystery of a person is ultimately reduced to their genetic traits. Yet, bioethical methods engage in their own form of reductionism by making the disembodied will and choice the

3. Tolstoy, *Death of Ivan Ilyich*, 104.

threshold determinant for moral reasoning: bioethics offers moral analysis shorn from substantive convictions about who we are, how we should live, why we suffer, or the meanings of mortality. In my own writings and methods in bioethics, I have wanted to explore connections between our actions, our reasons for them, and the profound questions of meaning and purpose that we live with and through. I simply do not find it plausible to engage in deliberation over the moral choices confronting, for example, the professional caregivers for a person whose body is harrowed by a disease without first situating the person within a narrative history and relational contexts comprised in part by her values and worldviews.

The study of religious experience, as well as many of the humanities disciplines, inescapably evokes an encounter with the ultimate questions of the human condition, such as our origins and identity, our nature and destiny as persons, the purpose(s) to our ordeals with pain, suffering, and diminishment, and our experience of mortality. Having the courage to explore these kinds of questions is itself a necessary feature for living an examined life, and that exploration can in turn generate profound philosophical and theological speculative insights. But I have found myself unwilling to leave such issues metaphorically "up in the air." Our identities and ideas, our worldviews, and our questions matter to who we are and how we ought to live; the moral issues embedded in medical decision-making and in bioethical inquiry provide a very practical context within which diverse responses to these questions are enacted in ways that make enormous differences in the way that people live, die, and make sense and meaning of their experience. I have been "drawn into" bioethics because it displays a remarkable synergy of the theoretical and speculative with the practical and concrete. *Ideas matter* in bioethics.

Who Is Bioethics For? Cultures of Bioethics

No person has mortal immunity from the defining experiences of a human life, such as embodiment, parenting, relationships, disease, suffering, and dying. These are some of the givens of our existence, even if, as the pioneering bioethicist Paul Ramsey once sardonically asserted, "the purpose of modern medicine is to relieve the human condition of the human condition."[4] A bioethics of meaning requires attentiveness not only to the physical, emotional, relational, and spiritual ordeals that comprise the human condition, but also to the awe inspired by the presence of the human person who reposes their trust and places their life literally in the caring hands of strangers in medicine. This presents a fundamental question: Who is bioethics for?

The answer to that question is much more complex than may first appear. Many conflicts over the values, methods, and procedures of bioethics are attributable to attempts to address very diverse audiences. I resist the proposition that bioethics is of,

---

4. Ramsey, "Ethics and Chronic Illness."

by, and for the professional academy. Rather, I propose that patients and their experience are at the core of bioethical practice, inquiry, and reflection that is carried out by various forms of intermediate moral communities: health care professions, religious communities, civic cultures, academic discourse, and bioethics pedagogy.

The practical nature of bioethical inquiry is clearly undertaken *for patients*, and not only in the sense that clarity about the moral dimensions of medicine will effectuate better care. The power wielded by health care professionals and institutional cultures of care make advocacy for patient self-determination a bioethical imperative. From its inception, bioethics has rightly promoted respect for patient self-determination and borne witness against various forms of moral authoritarianism and paternalism. Patients and their families are increasingly the beneficiaries of education in bioethics and the medical humanities directed to clinicians, nurses, and other health care professionals provided in institutional and professional settings. Bioethics is also for, even when it critiques, *clinical professions and institutionalized contexts of care*, particularly as reflected in burgeoning programs in clinical ethics, ethics committees, and ethics consultation.

As illustrated by the preceding narrative of my mother's liminal status, patients do not show up in hospital beds as cases for presentation on rounds. Patients are members of and are shaped by a range of intermediate communities, including families, friendships, and various forms of identity-expressing association. The necessary focus of bioethics on the dyadic physician-patient relationship often neglects these intermediate communities that provide the fabric and texture of everyday life. Among the most significant of such communities for purposes of my discussion are *morally-formative religious communities*. Moral reflection on the framing questions of bioethics engages the implications of different technological advances, such as reproductive, regenerative, or life-extending technologies, within the contexts of the convictions and belief-systems of these communities. Ecclesiastical representatives of faith traditions may be called to consult in deliberations of moral choice for a patient within the tradition in an institutionalized forum such as an ethics committee or ethics consult. Occasionally, scholars of particular faith communities are invited to articulate the relevance of ethical values and commitments of their tradition for public policy deliberations, including the extent of the tradition's commitment to the autonomy of the medical profession, scientific freedom, and respect for religious liberty. I affirm the necessity of reciprocity of literacy: Bioethical literacy should be a feature of religious communities of moral discourse, and religious literacy should be a feature of pluralistic bioethics discourse.

Insofar as bioethical issues such as parenting and family formation, research advancement, rationing of medical resources, and end-of-life care surface in realms of decision-making regarding freedom and fairness in a well-ordered society, bioethical discussion is increasingly incorporated in the cultures of *citizenship and civic life*, especially as mediated through *public policy* and *legal regulation*. Numerous public commissions, at federal, state, and regional levels, have been established for purposes of policy regulation about matters of life and death, genetic technologies, and perennial issues of oversight of biomedical research by institutions and researchers. The public presence of bioethical inquiry can be traced through the influential, sometimes transformational, cases adjudicated through various legal systems. These forms of public bioethics both reflect and manifest accountability for civic responsibility in a pluralistic democratic society.

While bioethics has long aspired to be a model of interdisciplinary academic inquiry,[5] over the last three decades bioethics has undergone processes of professionalization and developed its own academic professional cultures, methods, and organizations. Some of these academic cultures give primacy to scholarship in certain disciplines, such as medicine, philosophy, and law, while neglecting others, such as the social sciences or theology and religious studies.[6] At its best, bioethics is for *scholars in diverse professions* shaped not only by the critical methods particular to their own disciplinary fields, but also by commitments to cross-professional discourse. In the wake of the culture wars that have recently permeated bioethics, my analysis emphasizes common characteristics of ethical reasoning and modes of critical inquiry necessary for complementing the science of medicine with the art of healing.

As an educator, I find that almost all of my students find bioethics as engaging intellectually as the science courses mandatory for many of them to prepare for medical or nursing school. I challenge my students to think critically about the role of bioethics courses in an undergraduate education, and to examine the various critiques offered of bioethics classes, including that bioethical inquiry pursues unanswerable questions, provides no definitive answers, is driven by theory with minimal practical import, creates confusion about moral responsibilities, and more broadly presents obstacles to medical progress and technological advances. Those are serious pedagogical questions that require a partnership in learning between students and between students and educators. While bioethics is certainly for the current and rising generations of *students,* the professional academic cultures of bioethics should provide for students something more than engaging educational courses, and in particular, mentoring of the *next generation of scholars, medical professionals, and citizens* who will wrestle with issues my generation will bequeath to them in such realms as gene editing, resource allocation, and death with dignity advocacy. The academy must take seriously its responsibilities not only to future generations, but to these current generations of future scholars and citizens who will confront enormously complicated and perplexing questions of practice, policy, and theory.

I have participated in all these forums and cultures of bioethical deliberation, and the ethical reflection contained in this book is informed by these experiences. A principal aim of my scholarship is comprised of infusing these diverse cultures of

5. Callahan, "Bioethics as a Discipline," 66–73.
6. Evans, *History and Future of Bioethics*, 3–72.

bioethics with the inescapability of the human quest for meaning. As will become evident, I raise particular questions about the presence and absence of religious voices and convictions in the pedagogical, professional, and policy cultures of bioethical deliberations.

Bearing Witness

One of the pioneering scholars of bioethics, William F. May, observed that persons who situate themselves in applied ethics sometimes are perceived to have a particularly odd vocational responsibility: claiming expertise neither in theory nor praxis, "they carry water from wells they have not dug to fight fires they cannot find."[7] This perception of losing one's way can be reinforced when a scholar such as myself is influenced and informed by religious commitments, and for whom community wells of moral discourse contain ideas shaped by faith perspectives. To extend May's analogy, the wells of moral wisdom drawn on by the religious bioethicist are different than those used by secular colleagues, and may sometimes be deemed noxious or flammable themselves; alternatively, by the time the religious contribution arrives at the situation of moral perplexity, the fire is out and the smoke is gone.

There is a valid point to such critiques, particularly when matters of public policy are at the forefront of bioethics deliberation. However, insofar as bioethics is not merely a matter of institutional or policy expediency but permeates the various cultures delineated here, a discourse of meaning, responsibility, and integrity must suffuse bioethical inquiry and instantiate understandings of the world, nature, and medicine in relation to human experience. A bioethics of meaning and integrity recognizes that ideas matter, that understandings of the ultimate questions of the human condition are embedded in, and enacted through, moral choices in medicine, and that the victim of stroke in the hospital bed is not merely another patient, but an embodied witness to a moral reality that defies diminishment to the effective and efficient. Bioethics is about more than firefighting; religious convictions bear witness to the human challenge to live through the ordeals and fiery trials of the human condition. I wish to briefly identify some substantive convictions that shape my approach to the methods and moral morasses of bioethics as displayed in the subsequent chapters.

In particular, I seek to develop the significance of religious meanings for the cultures of bioethics through the concepts of "witnessing" and "bearing witness." These metaphors are not isolated from professional caregiving: I have listened to many a caregiver, especially in the context of end-of-life settings, express their identity and their commitment to be a witness of and for the patient and the family. Physicians David Rosenthal and Abraham Verghese emphasize that, at the core of the medical vocation, the cultivation of meaning is intertwined with the physician's responsibility

---

7. May, "Corrective Vision," 2.

as witness. They encourage professional colleagues to "recall the original purpose of physicians' work: to witness others' suffering and provide comfort and care. That remains the privilege at the heart of the medical profession."[8] The professional enactment of witness is clearly an ethical commitment through which the caregiver expresses their ongoing presence to the patient and the family, their commitment to non-abandonment no matter the patient's ordeal, and their honor and respect for the patient's intrinsic humanity and dignity.

My explication of an ethic of bearing witness incorporates insights not only from professional constructions of medicine, but also the moral resources of religious community and nonreligious interpretations found in law and in caregiver-patient interactions. In my own religious tradition, a person who makes a public profession of those convictions and values that bestow their life experience with meaning and purpose frames this affirmation with (variations of) phrasing of "I bear witness that . . ." or "I testify that . . ." The initiating ritual of baptism in the tradition symbolizes a religious commitment to "stand as witnesses of God" that is inseparable from ethical responsibilities of presence and solidarity to the needy, afflicted, and vulnerable: "to bear one another's burdens . . . to mourn with those that mourn . . . and comfort those that stand in need of comfort."[9] The title of this book, *Bearing Witness*, thereby aims to foreground the role of religious values, worldviews, and the human quest for meaning embedded in bioethics. I want to briefly highlight ten features of an ethic of bearing witness shaped by a religious context: relationship and community; answering; narrative; re-storying; truthfulness and integrity; vulnerability; non-abandonment; solidarity; fair procedures; and prophetic critique.

The social context for an ecclesiastical declaration of witness is morally significant. The bearing of witness is a matter of public discourse; the intelligibility of such an action presupposes the moral realities of *community and relationship*. A moral community functions as an audience of accountability towards whom the moral agent has a responsibility for *answering*. Though the experience to which a person bears witness may be deeply personal and intimate, the public bearing of witness transforms the private and invites the community into a shared, common narrative. A practice of witness in the ecclesiastic context is thus an ethical act because of its profound influence in community formation and identity. The possibility of bearing witness implies that relationship and community are inherent to moral life, and, ultimately, the witness is borne not solely by the solitary individual, but as a shared narrative through the lives of a moral community.

It is also morally instructive that the witness in the ecclesiastic setting is conveyed commonly through a *narrative* or story: storytelling is a primary, though not exclusive, mode for bearing witness. Forms of narrative and story are especially important in religious communities as ways to sustain and interpret the ongoing life and values

8. Rosenthal and Verghese, "Physician's Work," 1815.

9. Mosiah 18:8–10.

of the community and to present a moral identity to others outside the particular community; the community itself is an embodied witness of a living story of truthfulness and meaning. The bearing of witness as communal narrative becomes a shared project in the creation and development of meaning. This necessarily means that the narrative construction of a moral community may invite what I call *re-storying* when the community and its integrity require restoration.

The community as a participatory audience to witness-bearing extends and engages in certain moral assumptions regarding *truthfulness*, *honesty*, and *integrity*: the person bearing witness is presumed by the community to articulate truths they know through the moral authority of personal experience. A witness or attestation of certain commitments and values presumes both the morally good character of the person bearing witness and the ethically right action of honesty and veracity. An ethic of bearing witness encompasses communal responsibilities for answering, speaking truthfully, and living with integrity. Truthful dialogue in community, courage and honesty in communicating to those with social, professional, or ecclesiastical power, and public accountability for enacting values are thereby necessary ethical presuppositions of bearing witness.

These assumptions of the community are not invariably valid; hence, the religious traditions of witness have established procedural safeguards to assure the integrity and authenticity of a witness. These include requesting corroborating stories that are framed as a "law of witnesses" as well as delineating prohibitions against the bearing of a "false witness" against a neighbor because it violates the community-constituting relationship.[10] The moral character of the community ultimately reflects the moral integrity of its shaping narratives, its witnesses, and the moral character of its procedures.

As public declaration of the personal and private, the ecclesiastical bearing of witness exposes the agent's experience of *vulnerability* to the community. This has two meaningful ethical implications. First, vulnerability presumes a profound expression of *trust* by the moral agent in the community, especially trust in the community's own commitment of *non-abandonment*. Secondly, like many other experiences preceded and modified by the language of "bearing" (such as bearing children, bearing burdens, bearing grief), the activity of witness is an ordeal for the moral agent: It is not an easy or readily undertaken activity. The vulnerability manifested in bearing witness invites an opportunity for community expression of *solidarity*. The invitation to solidarity is expressed in a common plea in everyday discourse, "bear with me." An ethic of bearing witness is thereby in part comprised of an embedded reciprocity of vulnerability and non-abandonment, as well as trust and solidarity.

The appeals of the witness also manifest an important claim about experience as both an epistemic and ethical authority. The wisdom of tradition, the lessons of history, the narratives of others, even the sermons of Scripture, however influential,

10. Marrott, "Witnesses," 1569–70.

are ultimately insufficient attestations of religious and moral convictions: an ethic of bearing witness reflects the responsibility and authority of moral agency. For the narrative to form, transform, and empower the community, it must first be owned by the witness. The bearing of witness will often come less in the form of discursive argument and more through a matter of storytelling and exemplification, of living out the story.

These aspects of an ethic of bearing witness in an ecclesiastic setting can be augmented and expanded by insights embedded in legal contexts. The experience of witnessing is initially comprised primarily of "seeing" or "observing," that is, a person may have witnessed a traffic accident or overheard some conversation. The witness assumes importance because, at least at some level, there is some dispute or uncertainty about what actually happened, and the witness is presumed to possess *special or distinctive knowledge* that is generally unrecognized or is not part of common public awareness. The witness then is relied on to bring insight and clarity into what may be epistemic confusion.

In giving their firsthand account, whether reporting the story as they observed it or assuming the more formal responsibility of assuming the witness stand in a courtroom setting, the witness not only gives public disclosure to what may have been solitary knowledge, but also presumes or expresses confidence in *fair procedures* for adjudicating conflicting claims to further the institutional and societal ends of achieving justice. The procedures established for discernment of "the whole truth" in the legal context would lose their intelligibility without a commitment to a moral infrastructure comprised of fairness, equal treatment, and justice. This is not to imply that the process invariably leads to a just outcome: undoubtedly, miscarriages of justice occur. Nonetheless, bearing witness in both the ecclesiastical and legal settings attests to trust and confidence in a fair process of answering and accountability.

The report or legal testimony of the witness is often sought to provide different insight or knowledge in circumstances of uncertainty. The story of the witness can confirm and validate prior understandings or a broader background narrative about the matter in dispute. This is the point of a law of witnesses as not only a religious precept but as a matter of legal governance: various stories should confirm, corroborate, and verify.

However, it is important not to neglect the quite distinct contrary possibility of a witness: rather than being confirmatory, the bearing of witness can instead signify a rupture. The bearing of witness may disrupt, subvert, and require a re-storying by the community in order to restore justice and integrity. A critical, subversive prospect is necessarily inherent in the practice of bearing witness. When this disruptive witness occurs within a legal proceeding, it may overturn conventional expectations; when the subversive witness manifests in a religious or cultural setting, the ethic of bearing witness becomes *prophetic*. Bearing witness is thus suffused with moral meaning because a commitment to the right and the good can necessitate the enunciation of unsettling and inconvenient truths. The witness is thereby not simply a problem-solver, but can also be a problem-creator.

The community of medicine as embodied in commitments of its professional caregivers exemplifies the kind of reciprocity of witness reflected in the idea of solidarity in the religious community. The defining work of the profession consists of a witness of compassionate presence, caring, and non-abandonment in the midst of a patient's vulnerability, illness, and suffering. This is what hospice workers have in mind when they portray their care for dying patients primarily as a matter of "witness." This is what author Jo McElroy Senecal has in mind as she bears witness to the dying of her father and to young children in hospitals: "when they are too sick to get out of bed and their breath is ragged and their hands are starting to curl into their palms, they are the sacred vulnerable and it is up to the ones standing to take good care."[11] A witness to persons as sacred vulnerable beings does not involve settling a dispute or conflict, as in the legal context, but rather is embodied in the faithful presence of community to the dying person. The embodied presence of caring commitment symbolizes to the patient that illness does not displace a person from the human community.

An authentic ethic of witness is at once articulated, embodied, and enacted. Among the primary virtues and values of the healing professions are those of sympathy, empathy, and compassion, which are often enacted in the shared bearing of burdens with patients and families, including the ordeals of illness, disease, suffering, dying, and death. These communities of care manifest themselves as distinctively healing professions through their commitments of presence, non-abandonment, and care. Bearing witness within the health professions encompasses patience ("bear with me"), shared vulnerability ("bear up"), and mutuality in the sharing of burdens.

The patient's experience of vulnerability provides a context for the witness of disruptive declaration. As suggested by medical sociologist Arthur Frank, a patient bearing the embodied burdens of illness and affliction may communicate the moral realities of their illness experience as an act of witnessing: "I will tell you not what you want to hear, but what I know to be true because I have lived it."[12] The patient as witness is not presenting pleasing rhetoric for professional and public consumption, but rather speaking truth from a place of experiential vulnerability and nobility refined through adversity.

The moral authority of the experience of the patient provides an existential depth to witnessing. In the legal setting, the expertise of the observational witness resides in the assumption that we must first see in order to acquire knowledge, but the moral authority of a patient as witness about the existential condition of disease or suffering stems from the view that often we must first be a particular kind of person, or embody a particular experience, in order to see well. An observational witness knows about an

---

11. Senecal, "Bearing Witness," para. 14.

12. Frank, *Wounded Storyteller*, 63.

experience, but the embodied witness of patients (or a moral community of believers) knows the experience because they have lived it.

As attested by these religious, legal, and professional traditions, an ethic of witness can sometimes move towards resolving a dispute, but it is often directed toward creating conflict, challenging conventional consensus, or disrupting the status quo. Bearing witness both attests to formative values and moral commitments and against other interpretations. In the biblical traditions as well as my own faith tradition, the unsettling character of witness is a prophetic responsibility: the prophetic witness provides a different vision or way of seeing the world, and bearing witness is often assumed by a prophetic figure or narrative.

The prophetic witness is especially socially meaningful when certain persons or communities experience conditions such as disease, poverty, or oppression that deprive them of bearing their own witness, or when that witness is not heard or listened to by those in power in the society or institution. The prophetic witness then speaks truth as critique to power, one directed against broader social patterns of moral hypocrisy and neglect of a society's most vulnerable persons. The bearing of prophetic witness is indicative that the moral community, the profession, or the society has betrayed its core values and constitutive story. The prophetic witness calls on the community to remember, to recollect itself and tell again the story of why and how it came into being. The prophet, as an embodied witness of moral memory, reminds the community of its constitutive, community-forming values and gifts. Furthermore, the prophetic voice, figure, or community understands that an ethic of bearing witness is a risk-filled activity: the Greek root for our words "witness" or "testimony" is *martus*, from which we also derive the sobering word "martyr."[13]

The foregoing exposition provides a distinctive orientation to an ethic of bearing witness. The ethic will be rooted in diverse experiences of moral communities, relationships, and cultures. The ethic will often assume the form of narrative and re-storying as a complement to the philosophical discourse of moral argumentation. Within this narrative and relationally-oriented ethic, certain substantive values emerge to provide moral identity, including integrity as both wholeness and as honesty, non-abandonment, compassionate presence, solidarity, and commitments to both procedural fairness and societal justice. An ethic of bearing witness also calls on persons to assume moral agency and manifest patterns of answering and public accountability for their reasoning, decision-making, and actions. A necessary aspect of the ethic is that of a prophetic voice that bears witness of injustice and serves as the moral memory for a religious, legal, or professional community.

My formulation of a witness metaphor and ethics as an organizing theme of religious meaning in bioethics is representative of symbolic rationality. In his sociological interpretations of the secular and bureaucratized modern world, Max Weber

---

13. Miller, "Some Observations," 55–71.

proposed two principal accounts of rationality.[14] Weber designated purpose-rational or goal-rational (*zweckrational*) conduct as a manner of action that relies on instrumentalist reasoning to determine the most efficient and effective means to achieve a particular end. The concern of instrumentalist rationality is achieving a goal: it thereby has some affinities with utilitarian ethical reasoning. Weber perceived that instrumentalist rationality would predominate under the sway of modern secular and bureaucratic rationalization, especially as displayed in patterns of political, economic, scientific, and technological authority.

Contemporary health care, as well as certain cultures of bioethics, rely in necessary and important ways on goal-rational conduct and instrumentalist patterns of rationality. In settings of policy-making, institutional oversight, and legal regulation in health care, it is an indispensable form of reasoning. However, it cannot be the exclusive reasoning pattern as it divests means, which may manifest as actions, values, or persons, of intrinsic or inherent value, or reduces these merely to instrumental value. Under the influence of the instrumentalist rationality of a market-based, consumer-oriented medicine, critical moral relationships (such as the physician-patient relationship, the profession-society interaction, or the religious community-society relationship) may be reduced to a transactional relationship in which goods are exchanged for mutual advantage.

However important instrumental and transaction values are in some of the specific cultures of bioethics, I do not want to endorse a totalizing of moral life to a quest for efficiency and effectiveness. The alternative mode of conduct and reasoning described by Weber, more frequently associated with religious forms of relationship and authority, though gradually being displaced by the rationalization of the world in a secular image, is value-rational (*wertrational*) conduct that manifests symbolic rationality. The focus of this mode of conduct and form of reasoning is on the values, virtues, sentiments, and symbols that are resistant to means-to-ends instrumentalization. As Weber articulated the point, value-rational conduct pertains to "the conscious faith in the absolute worth of the conduct as such, independent of any aim, and measured by some such standard as ethics, aesthetics, or religion."[15]

In the paradigm of symbolic rationality, ends are not viewed as fixed or immutable, but can be discovered or recovered. The virtues, identities, and symbols embedded in symbolic rationality do not focus on achieving goals, but rather on expressing values. A symbol such as the concept of life as a gift expresses a different way of understanding and being in the world, and ultimately witnesses to a larger framework of narrative meanings. The core differentiation between instrumental and symbolic rationality can be illustrated through a soteriological distinction regarding the relationship of faith or belief and works or actions. On the instrumentalist account, good works or acts are a means to achieve the goal of salvation, while on the symbolic account, good works

14. Rheinstein, *Max Weber on Law*, 1.
15. Rheinstein, *Max Weber on Law*, 1.

witness to and express values of salvation, such as gratitude for divine grace. Value-rational conduct and symbolic rationality thereby expand the scope of relationships from the transactional to the transformational as new identities and patterns of life are interpreted, revised, re-storied, adopted, and discarded.

My emphasis on the meaning and ethics of bearing witness, as well as the substantive forms that bearing witness may take in health care, has more affinities with the Weberian interpretation of value-rational conduct and symbolic rationality, and critiques an exclusive reliance on instrumental rationality. I focus on an expressive ethics through modes of witness, values, symbols, narratives, and practices whose content and meaning cannot be reduced to efficiency and effectiveness. Various symbolic constructions of the person as bearing the image of the divine or of the nature of embodiment set constraints on instrumentalized efficiency and effectiveness. I am more critical of bioethical positions that either dismiss or neglect symbolic forms of valuing, whether these emerge in medicine, in law and public policy, or in professionalized cultures of bioethics. Religiously-informed narratives, concepts, symbols and rituals are complex and potent ways of bearing witness that "resist tidy philosophical analysis."[16]

My contention throughout the book is that an essential role of religious approaches to bioethics is to bear witness to ways of seeing the world, of expressing and enacting values and practices, and of offering modes of constructing meaning, to those oriented to secular bioethics, to a secular and commodified medicine and health care industry, and to a liberal, democratic society organized according to secular principles and instrumentalizing institutions. Moral vision is integrally connected to moral action in medicine and in the world. This critical role of an ethic of bearing witness may be conveyed in seven distinctive ways, beginning with the personal and experiential, expanding to the relational, communal, and professional, and ultimately encompassing the public, social, and civic, thus attending to the various cultures of bioethics. The meaning and ethics of witnessing I will articulate includes bearing witness to (1) the profound dignity of the person; (2) the moral expression and power of narrative and story; (3) the substantive, and not merely procedural, value of relationship, especially resonant with professional images of the physician as healer who shares in and bears the burdens of illness with a patient; (4) the presence of meaning and the meaning of presence in the midst of a person's ordeal of suffering; (5) the significance of death as a teacher of wisdom about how to live; (6) the role of religious voices as connected critics in the professional and public cultures of bioethics; and (7) conscientious convictions that present a prophetic witness to those in professional, political, and economic power, as well as in bioethical power. I will briefly develop these seven themes as a prelude for the chapters to follow.

16. Childress, "Religion, Theology, and Bioethics," 56.

Bearing the Image: Witnessing the Person

A shared conviction of the Abrahamic traditions is that human beings bear the image or signs of the divine in their essential character. This understanding is historically referred to as the image of God or *imago Dei*. The meanings of this concept have made for substantial theological debate, but at minimum it invokes a symbol of the dignity of the human person and witnesses to human nature and possibilities. Persons have inherent value and resist the reductionism of the ethics of instrumentalized rationality. Insofar as all human beings are marked with the handiwork of the divine, the *imago Dei* provides grounding for commitment to the equality of persons and their dignity in that equality. In all our relationships, including those in the context of medicine, moral agents have a responsibility to bear witness to the image of the sacred embodied in other persons.

The *imago Dei* is the primary concept of theological anthropology that informs the ethical perspectives presented in this book. While certainly not unique to my scholarship, my interpretations of its meanings and implications display differences from other accounts. My exposition focuses on a coherent cluster of eight interrelated characteristics—creativity, narrative, embodiment, relationality, giftedness, covenant, stewardship, and agency—that mark human beings as bearers of the *imago Dei*. I contend that the moral responsibilities embedded in this symbol cultivate an ethic structured around features of gift-responsiveness-responsibility-transformation.

The first four characteristics of the *imago Dei*—creativity, narrative, embodiment, and relationality—articulate pre-moral convictions and background beliefs that influence assessments about (a) the framing or envisioning of a question or problem as an ethical consideration, (b) the applicability of the principles and norms of ethics to the issue, and (c) judgments about obligatory, permissible, prohibited, or supererogatory courses of action in a concrete circumstance of moral choice. These convictions comprise central aspects of the moral vision or problem-seeing and problem-creating elements that necessarily precede problem-solving in my moral analysis. The four features of the *imago Dei* with more direct normative implications—gift, covenant, stewardship, and agency—reflect a moral reality characterized more by existential responsiveness to giftedness than by legalistic obedience to command or compliance with tradition.

My interpretation of the *imago Dei* places significant emphasis on understanding that corporeality and embodied life is essential to our personal identity and integrity. I affirm a view of the body as a temple or tabernacle that bears witness to the inscriptions or marks of the divine in the human person; the body is not extraneous and dispensable, the body is not a prison of the self, a commodity, or a disposable property. In this respect, the fundamental dispositions generated by moral witness of the body are those of awe and wonder at both its intricacies and its mysteries. These dispositions of the relevance and moral meaning of embodiment provide a moral presumption of caring for the living body in its organic unity and totality.

When the biological organism falters, the body experiences disease; the force of the moral presumption is diminished as medicine necessarily objectifies the body in order to treat the person. Encountering the body in medical care, as patient as well as by physician, opens to inescapable engagement with the profound reality of the person. Our awareness of our body, our body-consciousness, is seldom more manifest than when we experience disease and sickness as patients and require medical ministrations. The illness experience accompanied by pain and deprivation transports us out of our mental reflective lives and rams us directly into our embodiment. Pain is the witness the body bears to illness.

The various scientific, philosophical, and religious traditions that separate self from body, and treat the body as contingent rather than intrinsic to personhood, lose the significance of embodiment for moral life and contribute to a perpetual objectification of the body as specimen for analysis.[17] Paul Ramsey's critique that Christian ethical approaches "fly too high" above the grounded Hebraic and Jewish understanding of the wisdom of the body[18] has contemporary relevance for medicine's reductionistic propensity to disorganize the body and diminish its moral witness. It is ethically problematic for scholars to generate formative moral principles for medicine in the context of a moral anthropology that affirms an independent, disembodied will or mind—that is, an entity of which we have no experience. The ethical principle of respect for autonomy conceptually needs to reflect respect for the embodied wholeness of the person.

Bearing the Story: The Moral Witness of Narrative

My mother had a medical history as a patient that was familiar to her physicians, but she also had a story about her person, her identity, and her constitutive life values with which they were unfamiliar. In focusing on the needs of the patient, medicine and bioethics can lose the person. The self as storyteller is embedded in the concept of *imago Dei*. Stories bestow and transform identity, bring strangers into community, and invite dialogue on the experience of the human condition. There is a profound intertwining between restoring health and a sense of self in the wake of serious illness and finding a different story or re-storying. An essential characteristic of an ethic of witness is an authentic narration of a formative story that carries meaning.

The most meaningful account of the Christian witness of neighbor love is the exposition of Jesus through the parable of the Good Samaritan. The story discloses the exemplification of enacting love, care, compassion, and mercy. As important, the story is framed within a context of a prophetic witness against ethnic exclusivity,

17. Meilaender, *Body, Soul, and Bioethics*, 37–88.

18. Ramsey, *Patient as Person*, 187.

pretentious power, and institutionalized indifference to the vulnerable. The Samaritan as social outcast bears witness to the moral memory of the community: the community is called by the story to accountability about its ways of being and ways of living by remembering its formative norms and precepts, including care for strangers. The moral audiences of the parable—historical, professional, and contemporary—are invited to engage in re-storying of their lives embedded in the concluding admonition of Jesus to "do likewise" as the Samaritan.[19]

This is an especially relevant story for medicine and bioethics. As bioethicist Albert Jonsen recounts, a principle of assistance embedded in the Samaritan parable complements a Hippocratic principle of competence in modern medical culture. Still, Jonsen's own formulation of how a Samaritan would be challenged to respond to a contemporary bioethics-type of triage problem misses the central point of the parable for bioethics. The narrative bears witness against the moral hypocrisy of persons in power who could have prevented a triage issue from arising.

In general, moral principles or norms are embedded in and illuminated by narratives. Prior to engaging in moral reasoning to solve a moral problem, stories, analogies, images, and metaphors aid interpreting situations requiring moral deliberation so we see the moral questions in the first place. Moral perception is a matter of corrected vision or knowledgeable re-visioning of the world,[20] and it is fundamentally prior to the problem-solving processes of moral deliberation. The moral power of bearing witness bespeaks the necessity of cultivating imaginative capacities, moral vision, and the virtue of empathy as formed through attentiveness to the witness of narrative, story, and metaphor.

Beyond stories and parables, numerous extended imaginative examples and moral mythologies are invoked in bioethics discussions that range beyond the immediate clinical setting of a moral issue and stimulate discourse on the broad social implications of decision-making that impinges on the human condition. As we commemorate the two-hundredth anniversary of Mary Shelley's novel *Frankenstein: The Modern Prometheus,* it is worth remembering that Willard Gaylin, a pioneer of bioethics in virtue of his cofounding of the Hastings Center, situated both the opportunities and the prospective perils of emerging medical technologies in the 1970s through what he designated as "the Frankenstein factor."[21] The appropriation of the Frankenstein mythology, centered on the rebellion of the created organism against the creator, continues to have moral influence in public discourse about genetic modification, gene-editing methods, synthetic biology, and on humanistic understandings of identity. As with the biblical parable, this moral mythology stimulates the moral imagination, offers penetrating moral vision, and conveys moral meaning, even though it is not dispositive of specific moral actions.

19. Luke 10:37.
20. May, *Physician's Covenant*, 1–5.
21. Gaylin, "Frankenstein Factor," 665–67.

The emergence of new technologies that have transformed moral choices in such areas as life beginnings, genetics, regenerative and transplantation medicine, and life endings, commonly generates uncertainty and even apprehension about their immediate uses and long-term implications. Often, in engaging in predictive bioethics, moral wisdom is discerned by looking backwards to anticipatory moral mythologies and narratives. In a liberal pluralist society that is agnostic about the human good, though we may not have a substantive account of human flourishing to guide decisions and policy, we are much clearer about what we want to avoid. This clarity is shaped both by historical experience and by parabolic or mythic meanings exemplified in bioethically-relevant literature on the human condition.

Narratives, stories, moral mythologies, and parables presuppose a moral community with whom the story is shared and so bear witness of a shared quest for meaning and purpose. The stories also witness to the necessity of awe and wonder in the presence of mystery as a source for moral direction. It is not necessary for a narrative to be "true" for its meaning to bear truthfulness about the kinds of questions we need to ask. The pretensions of scientific post-modernity may tempt us to believe we have advanced past the point of requiring instructive parables or myths; the temptation is deconstructed when recalling the embedded myth of progress in the scientific enterprise and by remembering just how much of contemporary bioethics has been influenced by mythic or fictional accounts of the origins of social morality, such as the philosophical fictions of the state of nature or of the veil of ignorance. Bearing the story in an ethic of witness keeps us grounded in our embodied experience as storytellers, helps us see and imaginatively envision, and gives context for why we understand certain matters as moral problems in need of resolution.

Bearing the Burdens: The Physician as Healer

The emerging bioethics movement of the mid-seventies understood advocacy of patient rights to self-determination, informed consent, reproduction, bodily integrity, and privacy as central to ethical medical practice. This meant philosophically and conceptually supplanting a model of medical care shaped by formative narratives and metaphors of paternalism, an imaginative construction of physician as father or as parent. Medical paternalism presumed that the physician's technical knowledge, skills, and expertise were complemented by authority for decision-making in the moral realm of medicine as well. Constructing the physician-patient relationship in terms of parent and child effected a morally problematic generalization of professional expertise from the factual to the ethical.[22] Normatively, reposing authority for moral decision-making in the physician is a moral insult to patients with full decision-making capacity.

22. Veatch, *Hippocratic, Religious, and Secular*, 26.

The prevalent language in contemporary medicine that emphasizes the physician as provider symbolizes an important shift from the paternalist perspective in that the physician's responsibility of caring is effectuated through communication skills: information disclosure comprises the moral medium of the physician's relationship with the patient such that a patient is empowered to make an informed judgment about their medical care and treatment alternatives.[23] The principle of respect for patient autonomy is an indispensable feature of the moral landscape of medicine, while the patient's values and preferences direct the physician's commitment of beneficence, the primary ethic embedded in the paternalistic understanding. The provider model shifts moral authority from physician to patient and gives moral primacy to self-determination.

The moral questions embedded within a provider model of medicine include affirming instrumental rationality in the relationship of physician and patient. A provider-consumer medical relationship changes out the familial metaphors of paternalism for an economic set of metaphors to help construct what is at stake in health care interactions; in the moral foreground are not only information, but also efficiency, health care costs, and embedded lack of trust. As the moral logic of instrumental rationality prevails, medicine increasingly becomes merely the technical means to meeting patient goals; however, as patient ends supplant the ends of medicine, the identity and integrity of what makes medicine a profession, and a healing profession, can be compromised. Insofar as contemporary medical practice participates in and mimics the broader context of the marketplace in which it is inescapably intertwined, relationships in medicine become reducible to transactional interactions between self-interested moral strangers. The moral character of the relationship shifts from familial caring and beneficence to a market ethos of *caveat emptor* or "buyer beware" in which consumer choice prevails, but trust is effectively displaced by effectiveness and efficiency.

At a broader societal level, the provider-consumer relationship is situated within an underlying narrative of health care as an industry, health care insurance as a venue of marketplace exchange, and medical care as a commodity or private good accessible to persons with the financial means to pay. While medical paternalism implied an excess of power and moral authority on the part of physicians, the provider-consumer model morally disempowers physicians and their profession, while conferring some moral authority to patients about decisions pertinent to their health. However, substantial control over the relationship and the social expression of medicine is reposed in nonmedical authorities, including insurers and regulators, in a business or industry narrative.

In many respects, my interactions with the physicians and specialists treating my mother's condition following her stroke manifested a provider or technician understanding of the physician (and of other professionals, such as nurses and rehabilitation

23. Emanuel and Emanuel, "Four Models," 2221–25.

therapists). They were scientifically-informed, proficient in technical skill, and efficient in application. I emphasize that these professionals were treating my mother's condition, rather than caring for my mother. However, physicians who attentively listen to the narratives and ordeals of their patients, and who compassionately and empathetically bear with their patients the burdens of their diseases, are more than providers with technical expertise. They bear witness to patients and to the society that medicine is a moral profession oriented by a commitment to healing, and that physicians who care for and take care of patients ideally aspire to be healers.

Physicians and physician organizations are cognizant of the healing legacy of medicine. A thoughtful statement of principles of medical professionalism for the twenty-first century asserts that members of the profession in every culture "share the role of the healer."[24] As articulated in the professional principles and responsibilities of this "physician's charter," the concept of healing is presented as entirely compatible with scientific medicine, advancements in knowledge, and core ethical principles, and encompasses the responsibility of a physician to be an advocate for social justice in the realm of health care. The vocation of healing bears witness against a provider and market account of medicine. The primary commitments of the healing ethic of medicine are enacted through care, trust, empathy, and presence to the patient and a promise of non-abandonment. Furthermore, the physician is a witness of a social justice commitment that illness or disease does not separate the person from the human community; patients will not be abandoned to the vagaries of a market society.

In the religious interpretation of bearing witness, healing requires relationships and responsibilities comprising a covenant. This covenantal character means that medicine is more than an occupation, a career, or even a profession; it embodies a sense of vocation and calling. Physicians are not only "on call" for a rotation or shift, but are "called to" a way of being in the world. The covenantal relational model witnesses to an emphasis on gift-based transformational relationships and critiques the transactional exchanges of law and the market. The moral excellence of healing embedded in the covenantal relationship can take medicine away from depersonalization and distrust and towards relationships that express empathy, compassion, and presence, and foster integrity-bearing institutions.

Bearing the Unbearable: Suffering

Physicians, nurses, and other health care professionals have received through their professional education and experience the knowledge and skills by which the physical and emotional burdens of patients can be shared, alleviated, and overcome. These responsibilities are embedded in professional commitments to alleviate pain and mitigate physical suffering inherent to the organizing purposes of the healing professions.

24. ABIM Foundation et al., "Medical Professionalism," 244.

However, some burdens are really not susceptible to the manipulations and aspirations of professionalism; they are not puzzles to be solved as much as ordeals that are lived through.

Suffering refers to an assault on, or threat to, the integrity and identity of the self that is substantially beyond the person's control. At an intensely personal level, my mother's self-understanding, physical being in the world, her relationships, and her voice were all irretrievably altered by the assault inflicted by her stroke. In the realm of bioethics, a groundbreaking video, "Please Let Me Die," depicting the experience of burn patient Dax Cowart,[25] portrays how the healing professions must minister to bodies deconstructed and disfigured by pain and suffering, even as the embodied person experiences an unmaking of their world, the loss of voice, self-identity, world-orientation, and meaning. Few experiences are more difficult to bear, let alone bear witness of, than the ordeals of patient suffering.

The perceived loss of a future entails that suffering is identity-transforming and even identity-deforming. Yet, as physician-writer Eric Cassell has insightfully claimed, influenced by the reductionist methods of its underlying scientific and research foundations, contemporary medicine has little room for, or even a comprehension of, a conception of suffering.[26] The medicalization of suffering, by which suffering is reduced to a form of pain susceptible to medical treatment, is one of the central category mistakes of the contemporary philosophy of medicine. Medical discourse and bioethical literature that routinely use the terms "pain" and "suffering" interchangeably without remainder reinforces the medicalization mistake.

Suffering would seem to be a central organizing experience in medical and bioethics discourse. The Latin root for patient is *pati*, which means the "one that suffers" or "undergoes." Yet, under the medicalization model, suffering is typically an extreme point on the continuum of pain. Professionals have at least some ways to assess pain, including relying on patient subjective experience: who hasn't been asked by some physician or assistant at some point, "On a scale of 1–10, how is your pain?" Biomedical research has developed increasingly rigorous methods for determining the efficacy of treatments for pain.

It is disrespectful to patients and their experience, however, when all suffering is conceptualized as physical pain and falls under the interpretative sway of medicalization. Following her stroke, my mother seldom complained of pain, but her suffering in body, voice, relationship, and identity was almost unbearable. Suffering and pain can clearly overlap, but it is also the case that patients can experience pain without suffering (which the medicalized construal of suffering can acknowledge) and can experience suffering without being in pain, which the model cannot account for. The ordeal of patient suffering has much to teach caregivers, professionals, and bioethics about both the goals and the limits of medicine.

25. Kliever, *Dax's Case*, 1–22.
26. Cassell, *Nature of Suffering*, v.

The in-breaking of the arbitrary and abusive into the domain of the creative and nurturing is at the core of the biblical narrative of Job; this in-breaking represents what Max Weber referred to as the "ethical irrationality" of the world.[27] I do not wish to discount the experience of the ethically irrational; the authentic voice of human suffering demands attentiveness to such a construction of human experience. Furthermore, as voiced by Dr. Rieux, the physician-witness of Albert Camus's *The Plague*, the medical imperative is to relieve suffering rather than praise it.[28] Nevertheless, the compassionate response to suffering requires first acknowledging the ordeal of the patient, whose self, identity, and world are at stake, and the responsiveness of the community to bear witness through presence, compassion, non-abandonment, and narrative re-storying.

In the face of threats or assaults to self-identity and integrity, an insistent human need is to make sense of the experience or seek for some reason for the ordeal. Patients and their families seek a coherent understanding of what is transpiring medically and existentially so that a person who is suffering can, with communal presence, hold their world together or remake it with integrity in the face of moral dilemmas, existential ordeals, or world-shattering losses. A compelling (though oft-criticized) feature of the Christian narrative is its resources—personal, communal, soteriological—for meaning-making in the experience of suffering. The narrative assures both that suffering is an ineliminable feature of the human condition and that, as such, all of us will feel the wintry chill of suffering, abandonment, and isolation; it does not guarantee success in making meaning or finding a reason for the ordeal. This response may be what Tolstoy's character Ivan Ilyich learned when he queried his soul about the "why?" to his unrelenting suffering: "there is no why."[29] A person who expresses trust in creative, nurturing and sustaining powers can experience suffering as profound betrayal and even abandonment to the arbitrary and abusive. However, an absence of response to the question of meaning does not entail that there is no meaning to compassionate presence. The presence of meaning may be found through the meaning of a presence that witnesses to a suffering self that they remain in relationship with caring community.

My interpretation on suffering thus conflicts with the medicalization ideologies of contemporary medicine and bioethics, which seem to have appropriated the utilitarian view of John Stuart Mill that suffering is an evil towards which we should devote our full energies to eradicate.[30] Though suffering is an ineliminable feature of the shared human condition, I do not dispute that suffering can be a condition deemed worse than death, or an experience that prompts a yearning for death. I do question the instrumental rationality underlying views in bioethics and medicine that, when

27. Weber, "Politics as a Vocation," 122.

28. Camus, *Plague*, 126.

29. Tolstoy, *Death of Ivan Ilyich*, 100.

30. Mill, "Utilitarianism," 23.

it is not possible to alleviate suffering, ethics requires directly ending the life of the person who suffers, such as in practices of physician-assisted death or physician administered euthanasia. It is a failure of moral imagination and moral responsibility to end suffering by ending life. I take particular issue with constructs in contemporary medicine and bioethics that equate suffering with pain and then deny meaning to suffering. The compassionate witness of presence may not be the final response, but it is where healing humanly commits us to begin.

Bearing the Burden of Mortality

In *The Plague*, Dr. Rieux gives voice to the provocative observation that "the orders of the world are shaped by death."[31] Death's ordering or organizing of the world of medicine can be discerned through the pervasive use of military and war metaphors that depict an understanding of a basic goal of medicine: to prolong life and defeat (or at least defer) death to a later point in the lifespan. In general, death is constructed as an enemy of medicine.

The experiences of my mother in an emergency room and subsequently for several weeks in intensive care are illustrative of many of the perplexities and dilemmas embedded in contemporary medicine's encounter with death. Among many physician-writers who have recently taken up medicine's responsibilities in the encounter with mortality, I have found the most compelling articulation of these perplexities in Atul Gawande's book *Being Mortal*.[32] As both a physician and as a son, Gawande found himself very ill-prepared to help his patients as well as his father work through the decisions and experiences encountered in relation to impending death; very immediate practical concerns about whether to seek out aggressive treatment or forego treatment are shadowed by a deeper question about the responsibilities of medicine when it is no longer possible to save life.

Medicine has become very adept in using various technological advances to delay or postpone death; however, the successes of medicine in extending life can lead to profoundly diminished quality of life, an expanded duration of the dying process, and wrenching decisions such as when to cease life-sustaining treatments. As Gawande contends, since there is always "something else" that medical expertise can try, physicians treating a seriously ill patient with increasingly invasive procedures may find it difficult to differentiate when a patient has entered the circumstances of irreversibly dying that call for palliative and comfort care rather than life extension. Patients and their families, empowered by bioethical advocacy of patient rights, have expectations that what treatment is available, whether by established or innovative protocols, will be tried, even though most medical interventions in the last few months of life have

---

31. Camus, *Plague*, 128.
32. Gawande, *Being Mortal*.

negligible medical benefit for the patient. A technological imperative can supplant ethical imperatives.

While initiatives emphasizing physician communication with patients and families about the prospects of dying have emerged, these remain conversations that many professionals find difficult, or seek to evade. Alternatively, some studies indicate that physicians significantly inflate the prospects of effective medical intervention, instilling potentially misleading hopes in patients and their families about "beating the odds,"[33] a very striking probabilistic metaphor for a medical culture that aspires to the definitiveness of scientific inquiry. Physicians, patients, and families are reluctant to give up or let go, leading to lower rates of utilization of palliative care and hospice programs, and often a less than desirable duration of the dying experience.

In many respects, the hardest bioethical and professional choices come after a person is determined to be irreversibly dying. An increasing number of patients in an increasing number of states[34] may request physician assistance in dying, which designates a process by which a physician prescribes a lethal dose of medication to a terminally ill patient. The patient may or may not ingest the medication prior to their death. This practice is justified primarily in the name of advancing patient self-determination, and secondarily as a form of relieving patient suffering; legalization advocacy has, however, paid negligible attention to its impact on the calling and integrity of medicine as a profession devoted to healing. The advocacy of physician-assisted dying is the exemplary case of the prevalence of instrumental rationality in the cultures of medicine and bioethics.

Hospice professionals relate that they understand their roles in caring for the dying as "witnessing" and "companionship." The burden of bearing and experiencing mortality can be best carried by the patient in company with a witnessing presence of a caring community, caregivers and professionals who exemplify a covenantal character of being with the dying person. The very different philosophy of care and understanding of death that underlies hospice practice can engender narratives of healing even in the midst of suffering and dying.

Connected Criticism: Religious Witness in Public Bioethics

A defining feature of the political and societal cultures of the United States is openness, at least in principle, to a non-preferential plurality of religious traditions. Alexis de Tocqueville found this vibrant flourishing of different religiosities one of the more remarkable characteristics of the American experiment with democracy.[35]

---

33. Gawande, *Being Mortal*, 170–72; cf. Jennings, *Frontline*.

34. As of this writing, seven states—Oregon, Washington, Montana, Vermont, California, Colorado, and Hawai'i—and the District of Columbia have legalized physician-assisted dying.

35. De Tocqueville, *Democracy in America*, 287–301.

It is also clear that the beliefs and/or practices of certain communities, traditions, or religious adherents can run contrary, even to the point of death, to received medical wisdom and professional recommendations. Numerous recent examples of this can be cited, such as judicial decisions dealing with religious objections to mandated contraception coverage, parental refusals of vaccinations, parental avoidance of medical treatment for their seriously ill children, requests for life-prolongation when medical judgment believes continuation of such treatment would be futile, and religious-based objections to neurological criteria for death. Some physicians, nurses, and pharmacists cite religious values to both explain and justify their refusal to provide certain medical treatments requested by patients, such as reproductive technologies, emergency contraception, sterilization, abortion, or prescriptions to hasten death. These conflicts are situated within the bioethical equivalent of an ongoing "culture war" about the place of religion in professional and public life.[36]

Roland Bainton, a scholar of the history of Christianity, once ironically observed, "War is much more humane when God is kept out of it."[37] Given the cultural polarization embedded in and precipitated by these issues, scholars in bioethics have similarly deliberated on whether ethical discourse about emerging medical technologies or evolving professional practices in the professional and policy cultures of bioethics would be more humane, civil, and professional were religion "kept out." During a break at a scholarly conference on methods in bioethics some years ago, I was engaged in conversation with two prominent scholars, one of whom strenuously objected to the presence of a conservative Christian as a community member on a hospital ethics committee at his institution. The first scholar indicated that the Christian participant customarily responded to an ethics case or issue before the committee by quoting from Psalms or a New Testament story, much to the great annoyance of other committee members. The scholar questioned whether persons of pronounced religious commitment should be excluded from such a semi-public forum as they contributed little of substance and often presented obstacles to committee deliberation; the appeals to Psalms illustrated the construct of "religion as a conversation stopper" delineated by philosopher Richard Rorty.[38] The scholar's conversation partner, whose own bioethics method was informed almost exclusively by analytic philosophy, replied that "it was wonderful" that committee members received a reminder that other persons, who perhaps would have to live or die based on the committee's deliberations, did not share the medicalized mindset of the committee; the presence of a true believer was illustrative of resiliency in a moral community and of the cross-disciplinary character of bioethics inquiry.

Public, professional, or institutional cultures of bioethics discourse should be widely accessible to persons of religious commitments, to persons who believe religion

36. Charo, "Celestial Fire of Conscience," 2471–73.

37. Bainton, *Christian Attitudes*, 49.

38. Rorty, *Philosophy and Social Hope*, 168–74.

is a profiteering charade, and to persons who believe religion, for better or worse, is an inescapable influence for most patients and for many citizens. The scope of the bioethical principle of respect for autonomy encompasses not merely self-determination of those patients who talk like bioethicists, but also patients oriented by membership in religious communities with different moral vocabularies. When inevitable conflicts emerge between the diverse domains of religion, medicine, and law, we should welcome the poetic or prophetic witness of the Psalms, but ultimately be guided by values consonant with public reason-giving. Indeed, even Rorty acknowledged the relevance of the Psalms in public moral discourse about health care.[39] Having graduated from the University of Virginia, I have always admired the affirmation of Thomas Jefferson in the founding of that first public university: "For here we are not afraid to follow truth no matter where it may lead, nor to tolerate any error so long as reason is left free to combat it."[40]

Intellectual patterns in bioethics nonetheless reflect tendencies to marginalize religion, obscure its distinctiveness if not eclipse it altogether, or relegate it to the private realms of life, such as personal commitment, families, insular faith communities, perhaps some caregiving relationships, or religious-affiliated health care institutions. One of the more jolting experiences in my professional career occurred when I was invited to be a member of a task force convened by the American Academy of Sciences and the Institute for Civil Society to deliberate and make recommendations on the ethical and policy questions generated by the then-emerging research on embryonic stem cells. The task force included participants from numerous scientific, social scientific, medical, and research professions, the corporate pharmacological industry, and a few academicians with backgrounds in normative ethics, public policy, and science policy. Two persons who represented conservative religious perspectives on the issue, from the then-National Conference of Catholic Bishops (now United States Conference of Catholic Bishops) and the Ethics and Life Commission of the Southern Baptist Convention, were also members of the task force.

At the conclusion of the initial meeting, I was invited by the chairpersons to compose and circulate prior to the second meeting a brief exposition of some of the religious argumentation on embryonic stem cell research, as informed by a consultative process with the NCCB and the SBC representatives. Perhaps I was deemed the safe scholar of academic religious studies who could be counted on to respectfully acknowledge (different) religious ethical views on the questions and also affirm that, when it came to matters of scientific policy and public policy, the argumentation needed to be framed in a common, secular discourse. At least, that's what I understood my responsibility to be, and I carried out my research, consulted the task force colleagues, and composed my interpretative overview with those objectives in mind. My essay went into some detail on the religious convictions of traditions like Roman

39. Rorty, "Religion in the Public Square," 142–43.
40. Jefferson, "Follow Truth (Quotation)," para. 5.

Catholicism and the Southern Baptist Convention that led to their opposition to embryonic stem cell research, but also explored convictions of other traditions, such as Judaism, Protestant Christianity, and Islam, that supported such research, and even offered arguments for federal funding. My purposes were to be informative, interpretative, and to provide academic balance on an excessively contested topic.

It may have been the best paper I ever wrote that never was discussed, let alone never was published. As I attended the second meeting, I found, much to my bewilderment, that my paper had not only not been distributed to the other participants on the task force, it had been essentially rewritten. The chairpersons had asked another participant with a background in secular normative ethics to rewrite the section I had composed on religious views. This ethicist had begun with some introductory remarks from my discarded paper on the complexity of the stem cell research issue for many religious traditions, and then channeled the metaphor and methodology of the "veil of ignorance" from philosopher John Rawls to articulate a conclusion that there was a negligible role for religious values in matters of public policy. The "religion" paper distributed to task force participants actually had nothing of substance about religious values or reasoning, but simply excised the religious content of my analysis entirely and supplanted it with the philosophic fictional procedure of the veil of ignorance; religious reasoning was portrayed as encapsulated within the traditions of liberal political philosophy and the ethics of social contract. In short, the task force need not be concerned with a religious stop to the conversation. With religious considerations no longer a possible obstacle to consensus, it then became possible for the task force to compose a report advocating both research and public funding on embryonic stem cells.[41]

This was my first experience with what were soon designated the "bioethics culture wars" and it left a very bitter taste. It is one thing to disagree or argue against an ethical position, it is another to treat it with such intellectual indifference that the argument isn't even raised. I could not help but reflect on my experience some two years previously when I was invited to prepare a commissioned paper for President Clinton's National Bioethics Advisory Commission (NBAC) on religious themes pertaining to the ethics of human reproductive cloning. In all the public manifestations that I witnessed, the NBAC was appreciative of the ethical insights on human cloning from public testimony of scholars of various religious traditions. There seemed to be compelling policy reasons for NBAC to receive the witness of the moral wisdom of these various traditions,[42] many of whom had (along with various scientists) given consideration to issues of human cloning decades preceding the scientific breakthrough of somatic cell nuclear transfer methods. There was no feature of the disrespectful and patronizing indifference I was to encounter two years later. However,

---

41. Chapman et al., *Stem Cell Research.*
42. Childress, "Challenges of Public Ethics," 9–11.

in the concluding chapter of the Commission's published report,[43] which involved a series of ethical, policy, and educational recommendations, the witness of the religious traditions became entirely invisible. Religious values were subsumed under the language of "cultural" traditions and values. To borrow a phrase from philosopher William James, culture was invoked as the public moral equivalent of religious ethics without remainder.

I found it extremely troubling in both circumstances that religious considerations should be so readily dispensed with, treated with indifference, or effaced for the purposes of scientific literacy, policy consensus, and ethical discourse. The exclusion of religious perspectives violated argumentative tenets of philosophical charity and intellectual humility. I could not help but experience marginalization and an emerging identity as an outsider to the actual world of professional and public bioethics cultures, and I was no longer sure I wanted to participate in that exclusivist discussion. Perhaps I had been naive to anticipate that academic balance and ethical integrity would prevail even on highly politicized questions. Still, the posture of indifference and intellectual arrogance and a practice of suppression of religious ethical reasoning within a secularizing bioethics and policy culture reflected a dissipating historical consciousness. There was inescapable irony in the fact that religious communities and teachings provided both initiative and indispensable leadership in the era of civil rights, which had the residual effect of advancing the cause of patient rights and self-determination in the formative years of bioethics.

Those events were influential in moving my ethical reflection to embody a more prophetic voice. While that may seem an appropriate discourse for the moral outsider, in fact, as philosopher Michael Walzer has argued drawing on Jewish tradition, the prophetic exemplar is seldom removed from a community and tradition. Rather, the prophet is an "insider" whose witness should resonate with communities that remain attentive to their formative and constitutive values. The public credibility and resonance of a prophetic witness presupposes some shared or common values. The prophetic witness is necessarily socially situated, and the prophetic moral epistemology is better understood as that of a "connected critic" than that of outsider.[44] My analysis of bearing witness will challenge the too-hasty stereotypes and generalizations that emerge from some of the difficult controversies in bioethics. In particular, I challenge the embedded policy conviction that all religious viewpoints are necessarily divisive, obstructionist, and conversation stoppers. I critique the intellectual pretension that bioethics is necessarily more humane and humanizing when God and religion are, in Bainton's words, "left out" of bioethics discourse or are subordinated to the hegemony of culture.

---

43. National Bioethics Advisory Commission, *Cloning Human Beings*, 103–6.
44. Walzer, *Interpretation and Social Criticism*, 30–34.

Prophetic Critique and Conscience

The thesis of the moral equivalence of culture and religion is indefensible as it does not permit religious traditions to differentiate themselves from the varieties of bioethics culture I delineated previously nor to provide cultural critiques. The neo-Orthodox theologian H. Richard Niebuhr insightfully demonstrated how various Christian communities have historically presented religious identity in relation to the broader society, as characterized through five interrelated patterns: critique, accommodation, hierarchy, dialectical tension, and transformation.[45] The Abrahamic religious traditions of Judaism, Christianity, and Islam each display prophetic figures who criticize customs and practices that deviate from values the society claims to espouse. The core problems that are catalysts for these prophetic witnesses are those of idolatry; the human tendency to absolutize the finite, material, and temporal; and moral hypocrisy. A central consequence of misplaced valuation is neglect of the poor, vulnerable, and voiceless, and oppression of the stranger, who is not considered to possess equal standing in the society. Prophetic criticism by connected critics that the ethical integrity of society has been compromised calls society to attend to its formative values and recalls prior affirmations of these values.

Since its inception, bioethics has been concerned with disparities in power, particularly as displayed in the relationship between physician and patient. While dyadic disparities are not to be neglected, it is no less important to address disparities that occur in institutional settings and public or social contexts. The inexcusable disparities in access to health care, in which social neglect of the vulnerable and voiceless is most palpably and tragically experienced, reflect matters of social and economic power and its inequitable distribution. These experiences evoke a prophetic witness to the constituent values of moral community embedded in a social contract model of governance and a witness against the instrumental values that allow for indifference to the health status of the vulnerable, the oppressed, and the stranger. This makes the commitment of the medical profession to be advocates of social justice in health care delivery all the more compelling and potent.

A voice of moral critique may also emerge in the conscientious witness of professionals who say "no" to participation in certain legal practices of the profession on grounds of conscience, as well as parents who say "no" to medicine even if it means foregoing treatment that would have saved the life of their infant or child or prevented a serious disease. The religious-based conscientious objector to or within medicine is not a prophetic witness for societal or professional restoration and re-storying; the claim is more modest and personal: "My convictions do not allow me to participate. My self will be violated if I engage in this action."

A moral presumption of respect for and tolerance of claims of religious difference is compatible with the values of society, a profession, and a bioethics oriented by

45. Niebuhr, *Christ and Culture*, 1–44.

moral pluralism and grounded in the formative values that James Madison referred to as "the sacred rights of conscience."[46] A claim of conscience must be distinguished from a call for a war on the culture, or on the cultures of medicine and bioethics. In addressing religious-based objections by professionals to legal medical services or religious-based avoidance of medicine by parents for their seriously ill children, a crucial consideration is the insider-outsider situatedness of the objector. My interpretation of both the religious traditions of liberty and the cultural landscape of pluralism supports religious-based conscientious objection of medical professionals in limited circumstances, but provides no grounds for religious-based exemptions of parents who avoid necessary medical care for their seriously ill children.[47] There are alternative ways to meet both the medical needs of the patient and the conscience-based needs of the objector, whereas parental avoidance of care can be an irrevocable and irreversible decision that makes the child a martyr for the beliefs of the parents.

It is not my view that accounts of bioethics rooted in philosophical traditions or traditions of political liberalism are ethically sufficient and all-encompassing. On (many) occasions when secular and religious traditions come to similar conclusions on a bioethics issue, religious communities can bear witness to this congruence of conclusions, even if the methods or values appealed to in reaching those conclusions differ. Moreover, in a polity governed by procedures of democratic pluralism, inclusionary processes for bioethical deliberation require the participation of religious communities, who assume responsibilities of integrity and truthful witness to their own formative values. Participating in deliberative processes that welcome religious voices bears witness to the values of trust, community, and fair procedures that can ensure that bioethics does not become narrowly closed-in or constrained, even if in certain settings of shared public space, language, positions, and modes of discourse differ.

The Journey Ahead

As is evident from this introduction, I do not understand bioethics to be solely an enterprise by, of, and for academic professionals. My objective in this book is not merely to talk about bearing witness, but also to engage in bearing witness. This means I will draw on numerous kinds of sources both within and outside of academic bioethics writing. My claims about the relevance of religious commitments for interpreting the human condition require drawing on a full range of humanities scholarship and experience. This begins with an interpretive exposition of witnessing how the bioethical problematic with religion is constructed.

---

46. Madison, "Proclamation," 459.
47. Campbell, "What More," 1–25.

2

Witnessing Bioethics

Religion and Cultural Criticism

Even though it is not yet fifty years old, the field of bioethics has experienced such significantly different interpretations over its origins that some scholars have used the language of "myth" to portray the divergent accounts. These differences can be attributed to several factors, including the nature of the scope of inquiry denominated by the phrase "bioethics" as well as its orienting questions, institutional considerations and affiliations, and the different narrators of the history and stories of origins. It is not my purpose here to provide a master narrative of bioethical inquiry; as indicated in the introductory chapter, I am particularly open to the concept of a variety of cultures of bioethics that have perhaps their own idiosyncratic influences and histories. I do think it is important to have some kind of consensus about the concept of bioethics, and so, for my purposes, I will understand bioethics to be comprised of critical inquiry about ethical issues in medicine (and other healing professions), the biological and life sciences, and medical and biotechnologies. The critical, reflective nature of this ethical inquiry may occur in diverse settings, from a clinic to a classroom, from a community to a broader culture, from an individual to an institution, and from a profession to a policy context. I also understand bioethics as necessarily a multi-disciplinary enterprise; while much of its locus of intellectual moral gravity may be embedded in professional academic settings, it is often the praxis of bioethics in its clinical, communal, institutional, and policy cultures that provides a catalyst for new questions as well as occasional resolutions. In this respect, I do not see the different cultures or the different disciplines that are manifest in bioethical inquiry as necessarily in a kind of conflict over jurisdictional authority over the field.[1] I have imbibed

---

1. Evans, *History and Future of Bioethics*, 3–32.

enough of the moral wisdom of my faith tradition to affirm that understandings, insights, truths, and meanings can best be found in openness to diverse experiences, narratives, and patterns of thought.

The critical academic study of religion, as well as religious thought and religious experience manifested in the ethics of historical faith communities and traditions, can make meaningful and substantive contributions to bioethical inquiry. There are, however, important objections that have been raised against this type of a claim, some of which stem from the dispute over origins stories or myths of bioethics, and some of which are reflected in more recent advocacy of indifference or hostility to religion in bioethics that grow out of the culture wars in bioethics.[2] Such argumentation necessarily raises a critical challenge to the core premise upon which my interpretation of religious ethics as bearing witness is based. In this chapter, then, I analyze some of the competing histories and critique some of the adversarial objections to a religious presence in bioethical inquiry.

Myths of Origins

There are many ways to tell the histories of bioethics and its cultures. I understand bioethics to have emerged as a response to a convergence of professional, political, social, and academic movements that stem from quite diverse and yet thematically-related sources. As is often the case with an innovative initiative, its nature, development, and scope is not recognized by participants, but only becomes clearer in retrospect. There is a layering, texturing, and interweaving of persons, institutions, and highly visible professional and public events that help mark the evolution of professional ethics in medicine into a field of bioethics. Here I present an overview of some of the principal developments without claiming one particular root or causal origin. The different narratives of the origin of bioethics generate different interpretations of the roles and influence of religious thought, experience, and communities.

The Research Catalyst: Bioethics as Crisis-response

One context for the emergence of bioethics concerned protections of vulnerable human subjects in research studies. Abuses in American research received prominent exposure in the mid-1960s through publications of physician Henry Beecher.[3] Within a few years, public revelations of the Tuskegee syphilis study would call into question the integrity and the ethical standards of medical research. Lurking in recent historical memory were the various atrocities carried out by German researchers in the context of the Holocaust. This history of abuses in medical research, the ongoing ex-

2. Murphy, "Irreligious Bioethics," 3–12.
3. Beecher, "Ethics and Clinical Research," 1354–60.

ploitation of vulnerable persons who became victims offered on the altar of scientific progress, and an absence of professional and public accountability, provided a legacy of injustice and indignity that could not be ignored within the research and medical professions and by policymakers. The necessity for establishing a set of criteria and procedures for the ethical conduct of research emerged quickly on the intellectual and policy agenda of bioethics and fostered a perception of bioethics as a crisis-response mode of inquiry.

The National Commission for the Protection of Human Subjects of Biomedical and Behavioral Research was established by the National Research Act of 1974 and provided professional visibility and a public profile for ethical reflection on medicine that was both remarkable and unprecedented. The National Commission ultimately developed and published *The Belmont Report*, the policy document that sociologist John Evans designates as "the origin of the profession [of bioethics]."[4] The formulation of three basic principles for the conduct of research—respect for persons, beneficence, and justice—in *The Belmont Report* shaped the intellectual architecture of bioethics. Even if subsequent bioethics scholarship were to disagree with a principles-based model of ethics, it is not possible to understand the origins and history of the field without acknowledging its formative intellectual architecture.

The existence of the National Commission itself provides an illustration of contested terrain over the significance of religion in bioethical reflection, at least with respect to the academic and policy cultures. Bioethics scholarship offers conflicting narratives regarding the role of religion prior to, during, and subsequent to the work and reports of this Commission. As will be discussed in a subsequent chapter, the sociological narrative Evans presents of a theological retreat from bioethics is exemplified in the work of the Commission and *The Belmont Report*. In striking contrast, LeRoy Walters references the background disciplinary training of commissioners and the overall composition of the Commission as part of his evidence for "the dominant role of religious ethics" in the origins of bioethics.[5]

My purpose of analyzing the religious problematic of bioethics is more constructively advanced through an essay published by one of the staff philosophers of the Commission, Stephen Toulmin, which subtly and indirectly raises the question of the significance of religion, at least in this particular policy culture of bioethics. In "The Tyranny of Principles," Toulmin claims to provide an interpretative account of the processes of ethical reasoning present in this first bioethics commission. As is evident from the title of his article, Toulmin takes issue with the construction of the Commission's moral reasoning as a matter of "appeals to [abstract] principles"—such as respect for persons, beneficence, and justice—which were then applied or integrated with the ethical problems embedded in human research to generate specific

4. Evans, *History and Future of Bioethics*, 42.
5. Walters, "Religion and the Renaissance," 14.

conclusions and recommendations.[6] Toulmin maintained that the process of reaching consensus among members of the Commission was rather different than this applied ethics and principle-oriented account. In Toulmin's observation, the Commission obtained general agreement about the ethics specific to particular cases: "[the commissioners] came close to agreement even about quite detailed recommendations—at least as for so long as their discussions proceeded taxonomically, taking one difficult class of cases at a time and comparing it in detail with other clearer and easier classes of cases."[7]

By contrast, recourse to various principles to justify the conclusions was, Toulmin contends, a retrospective exercise that reflected an experience of "Babel"; that is, a metaphor drawn from the biblical narrative for moral confusion and chaos rather than consensual agreement. Toulmin asserts that the "appeal to principles" functioned "not to give particular ethical judgments a more solid foundation, but rather to square the collective ethical conclusions of the Commission as a whole with each individual commissioner's other *non*ethical commitments."[8] Toulmin constructs the Commission's deliberative processes as empirical evidence for the method of casuistry for which he and Albert Jonsen subsequently developed a historical exposition and contemporary defense as a contrasting model to principle-based bioethics.[9]

Subsequent scholarship on the work of the Commission has challenged Toulmin's account and presented alternative understandings for the composition of *The Belmont Report* and its construction according to principles.[10] The methodology issue is of relevance for illustrating at least one account of how religious values and religious ethics are construed as functioning in the bioethics policy culture. Toulmin's central contention is that there was no direct connection between ethical principles enunciated by various members of the commission and the conclusions that the entire Commission endorsed. Instead, ethical principles on Toulmin's narrative, including those of *The Belmont Report*, are connected with worldviews, especially including religious worldviews about which there is no agreement: "Such principles serve less as foundations, adding intellectual strength or force to particular moral opinions, than they do as corridors or curtain walls linking the moral perceptions of all reflective human beings, with other, more general positions—theological, philosophical, ideological, or *Weltanschaulich*."[11]

The metaphor of "corridors" of ethical reasoning is elegantly articulated, but embedded in it is a very striking conclusion: If principles are tyrannical and really unnecessary for moral deliberation to obtain agreement about specific cases, it follows

6. Toulmin, "Tyranny of Principles," 32.

7. Toulmin, "Tyranny of Principles," 31.

8. Toulmin, "Tyranny of Principles," 32.

9. Jonsen and Toulmin, *Abuse of Casuistry*, 279–332.

10. Beauchamp, "Origins and Evolution," 12–26.

11. Toulmin, "Tyranny of Principles," 32.

there is also no reason to incorporate the content-full worldviews, including those of a religious nature, to which the principles are linked. This implies that in any bioethics culture in which reasoning proceeds more casuistically, such as in hospital ethics committees, bioethical deliberations will have more clarity and integrity without explicit appeals to concepts, principles, or values embedded in religious worldviews or theological frameworks.

Playing God: The Technological Catalyst

A second influence inextricably bound up with the origins of bioethics was the emergence of new technologies that challenged previously held conventions about reproduction and fertility, understandings of life and determinations of death, and life extension and prolongation. Questions about meaning and ultimacy are embedded in appropriation and application of various technologies of life beginnings or life endings. The technological context of bioethics presents some different insights about the role of religious thought, experience, and community in bioethical deliberation. An early watershed event that bioethics historian Albert Jonsen identifies as a "birth of bioethics"[12] concerned the deliberative processes of a lay committee on the rationing of a scarce technological resource, the newly developed kidney dialysis machine, or artificial kidney. This formative narrative in which medical professionals expressly sought to evade "playing God" was related in an article by journalist Shana Alexander.[13]

Alexander took special note of the fact that the King County (Seattle) medical society had turned over responsibility for life-and-death decisions to a committee drawn from the public. The import of this unprecedented delegation was not lost on several members of the committee who emphasized the necessity of protecting the medical community. One committee member asserted: "The purpose of our committee is to protect the medical men from [these] highly emotional situations," and this was likewise echoed by other members who portrayed the committee as "a buffer for the medical profession."[14] Alexander's own rendition of this process presented a related but different lesson: the delegation of responsibility implied a principle of solidarity in sharing burdens of decision-making about life and death, including a more collectivist approach to what she specifies as "playing God." The formation of the committee from the public "meant acceptance of the principle that all segments of society, not just the medical fraternity, should share the burden of choice as to which patients to treat and which to let die. Otherwise society would be forcing the doctors alone to play God."[15]

12. Jonsen, *Birth of Bioethics*, 211–17.

13. Alexander, "They Decide Who Lives," 102–25.

14. Alexander, "They Decide Who Lives," 117.

15. Alexander, "They Decide Who Lives," 124.

This initial delineation of the concept of "playing God"—that is, decision-making by a professionally-authorized committee of human beings about the continued life or the inevitable death of other humans—is portrayed by Alexander as an inescapable part of the professional, moral, and even religious terrain of modern medicine. "Playing God" at least in this institutional culture of bioethics was not a moral limit to avoid crossing. The question as it presented itself to Alexander, and to the committee members, was whether physicians would have to assume this responsibility in solitude or whether the community on whose behalf physicians had undertaken their calling would collaborate in sharing the burden of decision. However, a shared burden of "playing God" doesn't mean the burden can be entirely evaded.

Alexander's interpretation of the committee process is framed through the playing God metaphor. She situated the enormous scope of responsibility assumed by the committee through a Hebrew poem, known within Judaism as *Unetaneh Tokef*, from which she quoted the following: "Who shall live and who shall die; who shall attain the measure of man's days and who shall not attain it; who shall be at ease and who shall be afflicted."[16] In Jewish liturgy, the entire poem is voiced congregationally at a climactic moment during Rosh Hashanah and Yom Kippur worship. Alexander thereby situated the task of the committee members within a context of divine judgment and human finitude and fragility. The resonance of the ethical determination within a religious context is inescapable.

Alexander did not develop her interpretation beyond the immediate issue, but several features of her analysis remain influential for understandings of a religious presence in bioethics.

1. Medical developments and technologies place immense powers of life creation, manipulation, and extension, including divine-like powers to design miraculous machines, into the hands of the medical profession.

2. The professional community embraces these technologically-mediated powers as a way to enhance the efficacy of their medical ministrations, but may shrink from the accompanying responsibility of determining their use, especially in circumstances of scarcity. While God's providential care may make the rain fall on everyone in an indiscriminate manner, the profession is not so fortunate (or powerful), and finitude may require rationing of a scarce resource.

3. In the context of professional reticence, the human burden of responsibility for enacting what the *Unetaneh Tokef* liturgy designates as a divine role of determining "who shall live and who shall die" is shared with, and delegated to, the public that medicine seeks to serve through a committee process. It may often be unclear whether the lay community is representative of the community; indeed, Alexander misrepresented the Seattle composition of the committee as a microcosm of the public. In general, a committee with institutional recognition

16. Alexander, "They Decide Who Lives," 106.

comprised of some public members and some professionals, as with a hospital ethics committee, provides a mechanism for professional accountability and public deliberations, and shelters the profession from acting in solitude.

4. In Alexander's depiction, the Seattle committee did not receive moral or ethical guidance from the medical society. Hence, even though a committee possesses some form of procedural authorization, its decisions cannot not escape a specter of arbitrariness. Absent a clear set of ethical principles deliberation by a committee of human beings tasked with making decisions regarding the life and death of other human beings seems to bear all the marks of the mystery and inscrutability of the divine will, an appeal beyond which there is no recourse.

5. Insofar as human beings are finite, fallible, and fragile, their decision-making in circumstances of life-and-death is most likely to fall short of standards of both justice and compassion.

6. The shadow of arbitrariness is reinforced by a human process that does not include any structure for public accountability. Playing God means, apparently, never having to say, "We're sorry."

The question of how to ration dialysis machines became so controversial that, within a decade, the US Congress elected to provide dialysis for virtually everyone afflicted with chronic kidney failure. Like the profession, society likewise seeks to evade the anguish of "playing God" by providing the scarce resource to everyone, thereby reinforcing a social mythology that no expense should be spared to save a human life. In general, then, when ethical decisions are perceived to enter some realm of the sacred or religious, they become too difficult to enact or carry out. The lesson for bioethics is not simply about the impact of the technological imperative to use whatever technological means are available, but a second imperative emerges: avoid a religious framing of the ethical question whenever possible.

A second illustration of the technological catalyst for bioethics that bears on the religious presence in bioethical inquiry concerns deliberations over the redefinition of death. This question was of particular salience in the wake of the 1968 proposal of the Ad Hoc Committee of Harvard Medical School to revise the definition of death in terms of "irreversible coma," or what came to be known as a brain death standard.[17] Writing some thirty years afterwards, sociologists Messikomer, Fox, and Swazey use this policy debate of the late 1960s and early 1970s to support a thesis that a shaping influence of religion in the conceptual framework of bioethics is "modest at best."[18]

In their narrative, Messikomer and colleagues contend that the conceptual framework that oriented bioethics from its very beginnings—rationalist, secular, and universalistic—has tended to "'screen out' [religious] questions, or to 'ethicize' them,"

17. Harvard Medical School, "Definition of Irreversible Coma," 337–40.
18. Messikomer et al., "Presence and Influence," 491.

culminating in a restricted influence of religious discourse.[19] They note that "religious voices" (Paul Ramsey, Hans Jonas) were integral participants in broader bioethical reflection on the ethical and ontological questions presented by proposals for redefining death. Ramsey and Jonas raised concerns about conceptually conflating questions that needed to remain distinct for the purposes of maintaining professional and policy integrity, let alone the embodied integrity of patients at the end of life. In particular, the questions of when medical treatment is no longer beneficial or is unduly burdensome and thus can be legitimately withdrawn (an assessment which presumes the patient is alive) needed to be separated from the question of the procedures and criteria for determining that a person has died. Furthermore, these religious voices claimed these procedures and criteria for determining death should not be modified or revised solely for the purpose of increasing the retrieval of transplantable organs.

Though Ramsey and Jonas vocalized their concerns in what Messikomer, Fox, and Swazey designate as "prophetic language," their interpretation contends that the profound assumptions of these religious voices about the human condition of finitude, ethical responsibility, and a "positive transcendent meaning of death" were reduced in professional publications to "perfunctory statements."[20] They attribute the silencing of a prophetic witness to an insistent demand in institutional as well as policy cultures for moral consensus: "this drive for consensus played a significant role in the excision of religious language, concepts, insights, challenges, and angst" on policy problems such as the definition of death.[21] As was the case with Toulmin's analysis, Messikomer and colleagues find that the aims of bioethical inquiry to obtain consensus, to problem-solve, relegates religion to a negligible role especially in policy cultures.

I will return to this sociological interpretation subsequently. For now, it bears observing that what conceptually problematizes the enterprise of ascertaining the influence of religious views in bioethics is, in part, conflict about the concept of "religion." While Paul Ramsey would certainly be a theological or religious voice under any definition, this is not necessarily the case with a figure like Hans Jonas. Questions of mortality and meaning were central to Jonas's speculative philosophy, but to consider this a religious or prophetic voice begs the question. Asking reflective questions of human origins, nature, destiny, and meaning does not require being embedded in a religious community or tradition. This differentiation is a core issue in what I refer to as the declension myth of bioethics.

The Declension Myth

The declension narrative of bioethics presents an interpretation that there is no one decisive moment, event, institution, or founding birth of bioethics, but rather an

---

19. Messikomer et al., "Presence and Influence," 493.

20. Messikomer et al., "Presence and Influence," 497.

21. Messikomer et al., "Presence and Influence," 498.

intertwining cluster of prominent figures, influential cases, and ongoing progress in the medical sciences to which bioethics is one response. The locus of bioethics deliberations is not policy, institutional, or medical professional cultures, but rather primarily among professional academics, including scholars in theology and religious studies. However, over the course of the 1970s and 1980s, this religious presence declines in both visibility and as part of substantive bioethics discourse. On some accounts, this diminished religious dimension to bioethics is part of a larger story of the gradual secularization of American culture and institutions, including medicine, politics, law, and religion. The declension narrative also reflects the emergence of a new moral vocabulary in medicine: The rights of human research subjects and the rights of patients to truthfulness and informed consent emerge as part of broader social movement advocating basic civil rights for minorities and women against social, professional, religious, institutional, and familial patterns of authority. "Rights" discourse is drawn from liberal political philosophy and mediates moral interactions in circumstances of oppression and adversarial relationships. It thereby tends to relegate some models of religious ethical discourse focused on duty and community to the peripheral social margins of religious communities.

In his analysis of what he refers to as a "renaissance of medical ethics," LeRoy Walters identifies forty-nine scholars "who either had strong religious interests or were theologically trained [who] played a principal role in the flowering of the field."[22] Yet, as one of these pioneers, philosopher Daniel Callahan, observed, a process of secularization rather quickly emerged: "once the field [of bioethics] became of public interest, commanding the attention of courts, legislatures, the media, and professional societies, there was great pressure . . . to frame the issues, and to speak, in a common secular mode."[23] In a retrospective analysis of the development of bioethics, Callahan claimed that a secularizing process was essential for professional credibility: for bioethics to move from headline-grabbing legal cases and become recognized as a legitimate academic field of inquiry among academic disciplines, and eventually in medical schools and institutions, "the first thing that those in bioethics had to do . . . was to push religion aside" and demonstrate "that they were quite willing to talk in a full secular way."[24]

As with the analysis of Messikomer, Fox, and Swazey, the contextual dimension is important: the public culture of bioethics, reflected in common public discourse, publically recognized cases, and in public policy necessitates abandoning a religious voice for a secular voice. Callahan furthermore identified some fairly widespread concerns about a religious presence in the professional culture of bioethics, and to some extent in the policy culture and civic discourse as well. While bioethics positioned itself as a source of moral insight and clarity leading to the resolution of moral

---

22. Walters, "Renaissance of Medical Ethics," 12. Only one scholar identified by Walters is female.

23. Callahan, "Secularization of Bioethics," 3.

24. Callahan, "Why America Accepted Bioethics," 8–9.

problems in medicine, religion was perceived as "a source of deep and unresolvable moral conflict."[25] Even in a social context of increasing attentiveness to moral, cultural, and religious pluralism, religious views on ethics and ethical methods often appeared to rely on modes of argumentation that did not seem to recognize a way beyond moral conflict in a pluralistic society. This mode of discussion has its place in professional academic contexts or ethics research institutes, in which it is an accepted part of the culture that the conflict of ideas is the catalyst for dialogue. However, it appears extremely ill-suited for policy settings, wherein religious views could be incorporated into what Callahan considered "single-minded political pressure."[26]

Secondly, Callahan observed an intimidating pressure within bioethics to conform to the canons of secular, public discourse and criteria for publically accessible reasoning, a claim similar to the rational, secular, and universalistic conceptual framework of bioethics proposed by Messikomer and colleagues. Callahan lamented a crisis in discourse in which religious believers "felt the price of acceptance [in bioethics] was to talk the common language,"[27] a language largely shaped by rationalism, individualism, rights, the law, and philosophical constructions of principles. Not accustomed to such asocial and ahistorical abstractions, Callahan observed that many religious scholars "think that [a religious] voice can be expressed with integrity only within the confines of particular religious communities."[28] This crisis of discourse leaves the spheres of professional and policy bioethics as almost entirely a religion-free zone.

Callahan had his own disagreements with religious tradition; he had made an irreparable break with Catholicism in the wake of Paul VI's 1968 encyclical on birth control, *Humanae Vitae*, and initiated the first research center for medical and bioethics, which eventually became known as the Hastings Center. Nonetheless, Callahan was not at all sanguine about the secularizing intimidation and the abandonment of religion in bioethics, because it presented a prospect of ethical default to the law (or a hospital attorney) as a source of morality. Bioethics argumentation neglected the accumulated wisdom and knowledge embedded in the moral memory of religious traditions. Furthermore, in Callahan's understanding, a purely secularized bioethics ignores the concreteness of actual communities (including religious communities) and is agnostic about the goals and meaning of medicine. Lacking communities of moral wisdom and a professional ethic, secular bioethics helps underwrite a medical ethos of moral minimalism and marketplace pluralism (patients become "consumers"), as mediated by "the discourse of wary strangers (especially that of rights) as the preferred mode of daily relations."[29] Without religion, bioethics loses a resource for moral memory and prophetic vision and voice.

25. Callahan, "Secularization of Bioethics," 3.
26. Callahan, "Secularization of Bioethics," 3.
27. Callahan, "Secularization of Bioethics," 4.
28. Callahan, "Secularization of Bioethics," 4.
29. Callahan, "Secularization of Bioethics," 4.

On this declension narrative, bioethics might then provide a fairly compelling illustration of patterns of secularization in several realms of bioethical culture. However, Messikomer and colleagues contend that the declension narrative is a "quasi-mythic" account that they seek to dispel as inaccurate and over-simplified.[30] Instead, they situate the religious problem for bioethics within a social context of controversy within religious traditions, such as the post-Vatican II Catholic context that led Callahan and others to anticipate a change in ecclesiastical teaching on birth control. The tumult in various religious traditions initiated what Messikomer and colleagues designate as a "process of militant secularization on the American scene."[31] With ethics within religious traditions as a matter of contested terrain, religion could not be looked to as an authoritative moral source for the emerging bioethics discussions.

Bioethics develops during an era of reverberating social protest and rebellion against diverse forms of authoritarian dominance and oppression, including medical paternalism, for which the political potent discourse of "rights" was well-suited. Bioethics oriented itself to the moral discourse of rights not because of a special philosophical affinity for liberal political philosophy as such, but because bioethics was sociologically situated in an era of movements for civil rights that converged conceptually with patient rights. Secular forms of intellectual thought were prevalent in bioethics; what is portrayed by Callahan as an intimidating orthopraxis was to Messikomer and colleagues primarily a matter of "conformity" to the core philosophical and conceptual framework: "even at the short-lived height of the presence of religious thought in bioethics," theologians and religious ethicists "were already conforming to what quickly became its predominant, rational secular mode of thought."[32] Bioethicists influenced by religious perspectives become "intellectual commuters" between religious and secular subcultures, "alternately complying to the norms of each."[33]

The narrative of declension into a secular-only bioethics is hence disclosed as a mythic invention; religion, at least in the manner interpreted by Messikomer, Fox, and Swazey, really has never had a substantive presence or influence in bioethics. There is no declension as such because bioethics has always been oriented towards a secular and nonreligious ethic. The minimalist influence of religion is in turn a function of the limited scope of the conceptual framework of bioethics, which reflects and reinforces social agnosticism regarding questions of human nature, identity, destiny, and meaning. These are questions that can be taken up in particular intermediate communities, including families and religious communities, but they have no real import for the public discourse of bioethics, whether carried out in institutional settings, the professional academic culture, or the policy culture. Indeed, the policy culture of bioethics displays a discernible pattern in which "bioethics has characteristically 'ethicized' and

---

30. Messikomer et al., "Presence and Influence," 488–489.

31. Messikomer et al., "Presence and Influence," 491.

32. Messikomer et al., "Presence and Influence," 490.

33. Messikomer et al., "Presence and Influence," 490.

secularized, rationalized, and marginalized religion, and thereby restricted its influence on the mode of reflection and discourse, and the purview of the field."[34]

A Conceptual Critique

The research and technological catalysts and the declension narrative present important differences about the influence and presence of religious views in the emergence of bioethics. These differences are ultimately attributable to (1) who assumes the narrative role, (2) the understanding of bioethics, (3) the culture of bioethics that is taken to be representative of the whole of bioethics, and (4) the concept of religion. For example, the discourse of the declension story tends to be articulated by some medical historians and some moral philosophers shaped by a religious intellectual legacy as well as by theological ethicists. In this narrative, bioethics is understood to be an interdisciplinary or multidisciplinary critical inquiry in which substantive questions of human ultimacy and meaning, of human ends and medical purposes, are disclosed within the practical ethical issues confronted in bioethics. This narrative also takes bioethics to be primarily shaped by ethics research institutes and some professional cultures, within which deeper questions, such as those pertaining to the meaning of mortality, can be more readily explored. Religion brings to this discourse not only traditions of wisdom regarding the substantive questions, including wisdom about the questions to be asked, but also living moral communities that historically seek to embody this wisdom in practical decision-making.

The story of bioethics as primarily a crisis-response to the legacy of research abuses in American (and Nazi) medicine tends to be articulated by historians of medicine and bioethics, as well as by scholars who are focused especially on the policy process. There are some readily identifiable historical markers in this story—the Nuremberg Code, the Beecher publication, the public Tuskegee disclosure—as well as clear policy developments, such as the establishment of the National Commission and the issuing of *The Belmont Report*. In this narrative, bioethics is primarily about the construction of ethical norms and principles and their application in concrete circumstances of moral choice, inclusive but not exhaustive of biomedical research. Nevertheless, the issues and bioethics agenda embedded in the research culture of bioethics tend to stand in for other bioethics cultures. As articulated by Evans, this particular culture is the jurisdiction claimed for the expertise of the bioethics profession.[35] On the crisis-response interpretation, religion is primarily a matter of worldview, whose bearing on questions of practical moral deliberation is remote and whose distinctiveness from philosophical principles or ideological constructions of the world is rather elusive.

The narrative of bioethics as primarily a creation of new questions and dilemmas generated by advances in medical technology has a diverse array of authors, including

34. Messikomer et al., "Presence and Influence," 506.
35. Evans, *History and Future of Bioethics*, xxx.

physicians, journalists, and social scientists. The technological catalyst narrative tends to see bioethics primarily fashioned through vexing clinical dilemmas requiring concrete decision guides about the immediacy of a specific person's life-or-death needs, rather than speculative discourse about the ultimate good of the human person. The clinical or institutional settings of ethical deliberation can generate policy and legal deliberation in which nonreligious modes of justification, such as secular or professional appeals, are a necessity. The necessity of moral-political consensus in a pluralistic society orients bioethics to a quest for a common morality. This emphasis precludes incorporation of particular moralities embedded within religious communities as well as in professional associations, except insofar as they may reinforce the concepts and principles of the common morality.

Although Messikomer and colleagues do not accept the technological catalyst narrative, they do interpret the "modest" influence of religion in bioethics through two examples embedded in the narrative, redefining death and human cloning. Their interpretation of "religion" is critical for their claim that religion as such has never had a significant influence in bioethics. Religion, as they articulate it, is dis-affiliated or disorganized, having little to do with belief, practice, or participation in a faith community. What determines the realm of the religious is rather comprised almost entirely of matters of meaning, ultimacy, and the human condition, rather than praxis. It is in this respect that Ramsey and Jonas are considered religious voices—they are interested in similar questions, although they speak to these issues from very different points of reference and experience.

The question of the scope of bioethical inquiry and its relation to religion is especially central to the declension myth. In his retrospective essay, Callahan maintains that in the early decades of bioethics, a general consensus prevailed that "bioethics should . . . pay most attention to the oldest of human questions, the meaning of human life and human destiny, the dignity . . . of human beings, and the ancient temptation of hubris because of the new powers put in the hands of science."[36] As Callahan correctly states, these are "human" questions, not exclusively religious questions, but they have been addressed theologically and enacted practically by faith traditions and religious communities, and they provide the background for the moral wisdom of the traditions. If these questions mark the issues for bioethics, bioethics necessarily must be a multidisciplinary enterprise of critical inquiry that requires inclusion of religious voices.

Strikingly, Callahan's account of the orienting questions of bioethics overlaps noticeably with the interpretive content Messikomer and colleagues ascribe to religion in their critique of the declension narrative: "[religion] is oriented to basic and transcendent aspects of the human condition, and enduring questions of meaning, to questions of human origins, identity, and destiny; the "whys" of pain and suffering, injustice and evil; the mysteries of life and death; and the wonders and enigmas of hope

36. Callahan, "Bioethics and Culture Wars," 424.

and endurance, compassion and caring, forgiveness and love."[37] These are certainly questions, issues, and virtues of many religious traditions and communities, but they are not the totality of religious experience. Where, after all, is ethics and community in this interpretation? Nor does a person need be affiliated with a faith community to be oriented to the transcendent and contemplate questions of meaning.[38] Thus, while Callahan and Messikomer and colleagues seem to have some overlapping consensus about the concept of religion, their disagreement is about the nature of bioethics and its orienting questions. The definition of religion adapted by Messikomer, Fox, and Swazey allows them to present a particular critical edge to their interpretation, for they can more readily claim that what bioethics, construed as secular, rational, and universalistic, is about is something very different than what religion is oriented towards. Callahan contends that questions of meaning, dignity, and destiny were intrinsic to early bioethical deliberations, and necessarily incorporated concerns of religious traditions and communities. By contrast, Messikomer and colleagues interpret bioethics as oriented to a different set of issues about the expansion of individual choice and scientific progress; in their critique of the declension narrative, the philosophical and secular parameters of the bioethics field screen out religious discourse and questions and effectively domesticate religion.

The partitioning of the philosophical, procedural, and political from the substantive and ultimate is not something, however, that speaks to the intellectual credit and integrity of bioethics. This holds important ramifications for the development of bioethics once its story moves beyond the mythic past and into more contemporary history and living memory. In their critique of bioethical inquiry in general, Messikomer and colleagues maintain that it will become "progressively harder to convince" subsequent generations of bioethicists that "religious thought and traditions could provide valuable ideas, perspectives, and forms of moral analysis that were pertinent and enriching to the bioethical enterprise."[39] This challenge became even more evident as the culture wars began to seep into bioethics.

Compromise, Authority, and Influence

As disclosed in the first chapter, my initial experience of what was really a foretaste of the culture wars was very unpleasant and embittering. My point in this discussion is not to narrate a history of the bioethical culture wars; others have presented very thoughtful interpretations.[40] Instead, I want to identify some of the ways that the evolving politicization of bioethics and the bifurcation of the field from what has been designated as "mainstream" into "liberal" and "conservative" bioethics has made

37. Messikomer et al., "Presence and Influence," 485–86.

38. Childress, "Religion, Theology, and Bioethics," 43–69.

39. Messikomer et al., "Presence and Influence," 490.

40. Fox and Swazey, *Observing Bioethics*, 285–325.

it much more difficult for religious voices to have a meaningful presence in both the professional and public bioethics cultures and provide the compelling case for enriching contribution invited by Messikomer and colleagues.

I begin by drawing out some of the implications of the epitaph pronounced in 2005 by philosopher Jonathan Moreno on what he referred to as "the Great Bioethics Compromise" in the wake of the initial years of the President's Council on Bioethics in the Bush Administration. Moreno maintained, retrospectively to be sure, that the initial two decades of bioethics were carried out under the influence of a *pax bioethica*. However, in what reads as a different kind of declension narrative, indeed, a narrative of the "fall" of bioethics from academic grace, Moreno claimed that subsequent to the dissolution of the compromise, "the field has fully lost its innocence" and that "the survival of bioethics as we have known it" was threatened.[41] Moreno's declension story is suggestive of a historically evolving, if inchoate, compromise among participants in bioethics deliberations that I maintain is comprised of several elements.

1. Bioethics assumed *moral responsibility for oversight of the social implications of scientific innovation.* This represented a compromise position between an ethos of modernist progressivism, with its implicit value judgment that anything new is morally good, and an ethos of prohibition, with its own implicit value judgments, rooted in a moral mythology that expanding technological powers over human nature and destiny inevitably threaten human boundaries and identity. Scholars in religious studies understand this compromise as a middle ground between the views of two pioneering religious bioethicists: Joseph Fletcher's enthusiastic endorsement of medical technologies as a means of expanding autonomy, including autonomy from religious authoritarianism, and Paul Ramsey's more skeptical and prophetic witness against some technologies as evidence of a fabricated humanity.

2. Bioethics assumed responsibility for *developing policy regulations to ensure that scientific and biomedical advances would promote human welfare and a broader common good.* This represented a compromise position between a *laissez-faire* market-oriented permissivism—in which such developments were protected matters of proprietary interest for corporate or institutional benefit, but not public welfare—and a moralistic restriction of new developments on the grounds that such advances would necessarily become sources for oppression, abuse, and violations of certain intrinsic limits on human beings.

3. The field of bioethics *set aside or bracketed certain issues pertaining to the moral status of developing human life,* such as the moral standing of unborn human life, the ethics of abortion, and research on human embryos. This represented an implicit agreement to find common ground and purpose on those issues susceptible to rational moral reflection, such as informed consent to medical treatment,

41. Moreno, "Great Bioethics Compromise," 14–15.

and ethical prescriptions, principles, and prohibitions in biomedical research, and an avoidance of those issues that inescapably push back to incommensurate metaphysical interpretations. This is the method that Toulmin portrays as enabling the National Commission to make as much substantive progress as it did with controversial questions in the ethics of human research; it is also just this bracketing of ultimate concerns that commentators such as Messikomer and colleagues believe worked to exclude or "ethicize" religious considerations in bioethics.

4. Bioethical deliberations in the *pax bioethica* presumed *the necessity of moral civility and respect for different positions in a morally pluralistic culture*, especially in contexts of institutional and public policy-making. The discourse of civility exhibits a compromise between (culture) "war" rhetoric (such as "moral crusades" and "camps" of competing bioethics) and a posture of moral quietism or particularism. The concept of a compromise necessarily presumes certain virtues as critical responsibilities of bioethicists in their roles as citizens, and occasional leaders, in a broader pluralistic society. These virtues include a shared quest for areas of agreement, philosophical charity towards views with which a person disagrees, intellectual humility regarding the fallibility of personal positions, a communal commitment to good faith deliberations, and recognition of the deep complexity of the issues.

5. Bioethics assumed expertise regarding s*elf-appointed responsibilities to engage in responsible, integrity-bearing moral analysis* of the social and practical ramifications of technological development. This process of moral assessment, sometimes retrospective but often prospective as new technologies are introduced, was articulated through ethics commissions, policy task forces, ethics committees, and research review boards. This reflected a compromise between a position held by many in the research and medical professions that scientists, researchers, and physicians were best situated to assess these matters based on their professionalized expertise and a position that medical technologies were broaching questions of ultimate human ends that had been the customary province of theologians and religious communities.[42]

6. *Religion has a restricted role in the public square of bioethics.* This is a disputable part of the "Great Bioethics Compromise": Moreno's narrative never once refers to religion as a factor promoting, inhibiting, or dissolving the compromise. Callahan barely touches on religion in his lamentation on the culture wars in contemporary bioethics, preferring the use of the term "ideology." Similarly, philosopher Ruth Macklin's critique of the conservative bioethics movement takes pains to differentiate religious argumentation and appeals within the context of a tradition and moral community from the reliance on metaphor, emotion,

---

42. Evans, *History and Future of Bioethics*, 3–32.

intuition, and misrepresentation she claims characterizes politically-oriented conservative bioethics.[43]

However, it was but a small jump for other scholars to see the politicization of bioethics, especially as reflected in debates over abortion and reproductive choice, as a proxy for religious values[44] and thereby situate the question of the status of religion in bioethics as the linchpin of the bioethics compromise. On this view, the compromise regarding religion in turn facilitated the other forms of compromise I've delineated. For example, philosopher Vincent Barry drew out a historical analogy and claimed that "the founders of bioethics reached their own 'Jeffersonian compromise' in order to appeal to as wide an audience as possible."[45] This "Jeffersonian compromise" represented an extension of the peace that the Enlightenment philosophical tradition came to with regards to religious difference: Religious liberty and conscience was to be guaranteed to all persons in their private communities, but "the idiom of any particular religion or philosophy was not only inappropriate for shaping policy in a secular, pluralistic society, but potentially divisive."[46] This compromise became the exemplar for the posture of bioethics towards religion in general and towards religious differences specifically.

There are certainly representatives of this kind of rigid separationist position in bioethics, but I don't find Barry's attribution of this grand compromise about religion to the founders of bioethics (including Callahan) to be very persuasive. To his credit, Barry does name the religious aspect to the bioethics culture wars controversy that is overlooked or neglected by the philosophical bioethicists. As I shall illustrate below, the bioethical problematic of religion has subsequently become the central feature for some scholars of what bioethics needs to reject to maintain its independence, integrity, and political neutrality.

I find that, though in certain respects anachronistic, there is moral wisdom articulated in the perspective offered by Alexis de Tocqueville in his nineteenth-century account of how democratic institutions and a republican form of government had been sustained in the United States. De Tocqueville was simply mistaken regarding his assessment of religious uniformity and an orthodox Christian morality; the pluralism of religion and pluralistic religious moralities were clearly in evidence in his era. However, these empirical oversights do not discredit his more philosophical claims. In particular, de Tocqueville maintained that the integrity and sustainability of the political institutions as well as the integrity and sustainability of religiosity was better assured to the extent that religious communities forsook aspirations for political power. De Tocqueville makes a critical distinction between *authority* in civic society

43. Macklin, "New Conservatives in Bioethics," 34–43.

44. Charo, "Endarkenment," 104.

45. Barry, *Bioethics*, 67.

46. Barry, *Bioethics*, 67.

and *influence,* both direct and indirect, in the society. He elaborates on this distinction by contending that an ironic but sustaining feature of the new democratic experience is that religious considerations have greater influence in society the more they avoid alliances with political authority and power.

On his account, the indirect influence of religion is manifest not in addressing laws or political interest groups, but rather in its regulation of the "mores" of citizens, which de Tocqueville defined as "the whole moral and intellectual state of a people."[47] Indeed, in what seems a prescient comment for an age focused on choices at the beginnings and endings of human life, de Tocqueville said that "just when [religion] is not speaking of freedom at all that it best teaches the Americans the art of being free."[48] That "art" is cultivated by citizens as they differentiate between legal requirements and moral responsibilities, between rights to choose and right choices. The indirect religious cultivation of freedom risks diminishment when supplanted by politicization or a quest for the acquisition of political power: "any alliance with any political power whatsoever is bound to be burdensome for religion. It does not need their support in order to live, and in serving them it may die."[49] The argument of de Tocqueville about the influence and integrity of religion resonates directly with the philosophical claims of George Washington in his "Farewell Address,"[50] Thomas Jefferson in the "Virginia Statute for Religious Freedom,"[51] and of James Madison in his "Memorial and Remonstrance Against Religious Assessments."[52] Those foundational documents of the political culture sought to secure the foundations of rights to religious liberty, and in so doing protect both the state from religious authoritarianism and religion from the tyrannical tendencies of political power.

These hard-fought distinctions and compromises have seemed to dissolve or collapse in the cultural wars that have worked towards the politicization of bioethics. This current era has undoubtedly given credence to the concern of Messikomer and colleagues that subsequent generations of bioethicists would be very skeptical that religion could generate insights and contributions "pertinent and enriching to the bioethical enterprise."[53] That challenge is readily evident in the critique of religion presented recently by Timothy Murphy in his defense of an "irreligious bioethics."

47. de Tocqueville, *Democracy in America,* 287.

48. de Tocqueville, *Democracy in America,* 290.

49. de Tocqueville, *Democracy in America,* 298–99.

50. Washington, "Farewell Address," 468–70.

51. Ragosta, *Religious Freedom,* 74–100.

52. Madison, "Memorial and Remonstrance," 309–14.

53. Messikomer et al., "Presence and Influence," 490.

Religion in an Irreligious Bioethics

In analyzing and answering the critique of religious influence in bioethics by Murphy, I want to use the set of conceptual issues identified above that accounts for divergence in the crisis-response, technological catalyst, and declension stories of bioethics: how bioethics is constructed, what culture of bioethics is drawn upon as representative of the field as a whole, the construction of religion, and the relation between religion and bioethics. Murphy provides a fairly immediate conceptualization of what he means by the domains of bioethics: "the concepts of health and disease; the practices, standards, and institutions of health care; and the motives for, and processes of, and the social effects of biomedical innovations."[54] It's not quite clear from this construction what bioethics brings to these domains, although Murphy subsequently clarifies that bioethics engages in "normative" work or "evaluation" in these realms in contrast to what he labels "theological work." It is in respect to this normative work that religion becomes a problem. Bioethical inquiry benefits from interpretive or non-normative descriptive accounts of religion, such as presented by anthropologists or sociologists. However, when it comes to normative evaluation, religion can "interfere" with bioethics and, in a telling metaphor of the political culture of bioethics, Murphy asserts that a "rapprochement" with religion is to be avoided: "bioethics should avoid any rapprochement with religion that interferes with the ability to do its normative work."[55] It is also very noticeable that the policy culture of bioethics, the contested terrain of the culture wars, isn't included initially in Murphy's domains of bioethics.

Murphy clarifies what he has in mind as an "irreligious" bioethics, which does not mean quite the same thing as a secular bioethics. Murphy contends that secular bioethics provides a protective buffer for religions from hard and challenging questions about truth-claims. A secular bioethics might well have made its Jeffersonian compromise with religion, as expressed in a posture of neutrality towards private religiosity and withholding judgment on a religious practice like intercessory prayer; by contrast, irreligion implies not only absence of religious belief or principles, but also an epistemic entitlement and moral requirement to "express disregard, indifference, and hostility to religion." Rather than the compromise of tolerance of secular bioethics with religion, "irreligion treats all religions with a hermeneutic of suspicion."[56] That is, irreligion sees through the illusions of false consciousness of religious adherents and finds hidden agendas of power, oppressive patterns of social structure, and materialism. Murphy's hermeneutic entails that the integrity of religious moral analysis is inherently ethically compromised. The posture of entitlement and obligation of suspicion advocated by Murphy is rather different than that expressed by the early generation bioethicists who, notwithstanding their own secular identity or absence of

---

54. Murphy, "In Defense," 3.
55. Murphy, "In Defense," 3.
56. Murphy, "In Defense," 5.

faith commitments, are described by sociological interviewers as neither "indifferent to religion [nor] inclined to trivialize it."[57]

Murphy is less clear what he has in mind by "religion," although he initially seems to accept the broader construct of religion in which the focus of religion is on matters of meaning and questions of ultimacy. There is a linguistic sloppiness in Murphy's language about religion that carries over into his interpretation of the relationship of religion to bioethics. Initially, Murphy's claim about the interference of religion implies that there is something inherently bioethically problematic with religion per se quite apart from specific bioethical issues presented by different religious traditions. However, as Murphy begins to explicate the interfering nature of religion, his target becomes clearer. Bioethical disregard towards religion pertains more directly to *religions* as *organized or institutionalized* communities that reflect governance through creeds, practices, institutions, and authorities. Religious community assumes a form of heteronomy that contrasts sharply with the ethical principle of autonomy. Murphy's account of religion is then very compatible with the contemporary social ethos in which an increasing number of Americans, and especially among millennials, do not identify with an organized religious tradition.[58]

Within the scope of institutionalized religion, Murphy's critique is at times focused on religious claims with *theological content*, such as belief in deities, revelation, prayer, and miracles (the latter of which pertains most directly to the faith traditions organized through the precepts and practices of the Abrahamic religions—Judaism, Christianity, Islam—and perhaps Hinduism as well). This range of interfering religiosity means that Murphy's critique would not necessarily be relevant to traditions that have been part of bioethical inquiry such as Buddhism, or East Asian traditions of China or Japan, or indigenous religions, such as Native American. Significantly, Murphy identifies an irreligious bioethics with a "philosophy of immanence"[59] to contrast with theologies that posit a transcendent realm. The immanence-transcendence distinction is the core issue in Murphy's otherwise undiscriminating critique of religiosity: "the most valuable approach to religion is to repudiate in all its manifestations the idea that there is a transcendent reality to which the immanent world is beholden."[60] His appeal to immanence seems to function primarily as a philosophy of negation, that is, a "repudiation of any alleged transcendent reality . . . as somehow relevant to the decisions to be made in biomedicine,"[61] and is never given a substantive explication. Murphy's construction of the agenda of bioethics as a project of normative evaluation, and his advocacy of an irreligious bioethics, appears to involve five principal

57. Messikomer et al., "Presence and Influence," 487.
58. Pew Research Center, "Changing Religious Landscape," 3–32.
59. Murphy, "In Defense," 6.
60. Murphy, "In Defense," 8.
61. Murphy, "In Defense," 6.

forms of repudiation of religions primarily understood through features of organized community and convictions of a supernatural realm.

Borrowing. One form of repudiation is what can be called *ethical borrowing*, or in the more evocative phrasing of Murphy, "cannibalizing" good ideas by bioethics from any source.[62] Murphy acknowledges the possibility that religious content could contribute to the goals and methods of bioethics, but ultimately the value of the religious claims would have to be assessed by "moral and logical grounds" independent of the originating theological or religious context.[63] No doubt such borrowing has occurred historically, such as the way that the biblical concept of persons as in the image of God (*imago Dei*) informed concepts of respect for persons, their dignity, and their autonomy, or how an ethic of religious compassion and love was incorporated into a principle of beneficence. Murphy acknowledges that many religious claims converge with secular moral reasoning, which implies the prospect for an overlapping consensus between religious values and secular bioethics, if not the values of irreligious bioethics. This nonetheless comprises a form of repudiation of religion insofar as the theological or communal grounds are not necessary for acceptance of the bioethical value: there is no logical dependence of bioethical morality upon religion.

Moral Immunity. A second form of repudiation is expressed in Murphy's strongly-worded objections to what he portrays as a bioethics-religion relationship constructed around the "deference" or "subservience" of bioethics to religious thought; religious views are given a "privileged status" in bioethics discourse.[64] It is worth closely scrutinizing Murphy's account not only of *how* bioethics is purportedly deferential to religion, but also of *who* makes claims for special privileged status for religion. Murphy initially directs his arguments against *pro-religious commentators*. The critical problem for Murphy about pro-religious discussants (the only commentators so cited by Murphy are the sociologist Fox and the historian Swazey) is their absence of sufficient self-critical reflection.

The specific context that evokes this critique from Murphy is the question of normative moral evaluation of female genital cutting. More generally, Murphy contends that advocates of religion have invariably failed to "call on bioethics to identify and resist false religious beliefs, to resist any religious practices as objectionable because of their effects, or to decouple health care practices from questionable theology."[65] But this seems either over-simplified or simply mistaken. Several religious beliefs or practices have been held to a moral accounting by ethicists within religious traditions, not only regarding genital cutting, but also faith healing and religious-based refusals of

---

62. Murphy, "In Defense," 4.
63. Murphy, "In Defense," 4.
64. Murphy, "In Defense," 3, 4.
65. Murphy, "In Defense," 4.

vaccination.[66] Understanding the rationale for certain practices that seem contrary to health must precede moral judgment, but certainly doesn't preclude moral judgment.

Murphy acknowledges that a significant "amount of work done on bioethics issues from religious perspectives."[67] These perspectives are constructed not by insufficiently critical pro-religious commentators, but are developed by what Murphy refers to as *religious analysts*. Presumably this category could encompass professional scholars in bioethics from numerous disciplines rather than confessional communities, but a form of religious-based hubris is embedded in such analysis that seems to restrict the category of religious analyst to a person of faith convictions: "all religions seem convinced of their ability to address any and all issues in bioethics."[68] I find Murphy's observation perplexing if not mistaken, but his critique points indirectly to a substantive difference he fails to recognize, namely, that as medicine vacillates between being a career and an occupation, and bioethicists are reticent about credentialing and other trappings of a profession, religion is often a way of life that would encompass many aspects of health, disease, and medicine as vocation, that have implications for the array of specific ethical issues addressed by bioethics.

A third religious constituency Murphy represents as addressing bioethics issues is intimated by a further shift in his language from analysts to *religious believers and apologists*. This identity is perhaps more prevalent throughout the entirety of the essay. It is religious believers who are depicted as vulnerable to ideological excesses, who place certain interpretations or beliefs as "off-limits to questioning,"[69] and who are ideologically constrained. Religious apologists reinforce the claims of religious privilege and superiority, for they "see nonreligious analyses and conclusions as ultimately subservient to theology."[70] Only once does Murphy portray persons situated to religious experience as commentator, analyst, or believer as a *bioethicist*, but this bestowal ultimately reinforces his hermeneutic of suspicion about the intellectual honesty, integrity, and independence of religious argumentation. While considering how religion may mask hidden agendas and ideological bias, Murphy contends that "individual bioethicists working from within faith commitments may find it hard to do work in, for example, public bioethics ventures without paying attention to their synods, congregations, or the religious leaders they share deep confraternity with."[71] The intellectual integrity of such commentators may be sacrificed for fidelity to the authority of their tradition or advocacy of a religious commitment.

This critique seems entirely speculative; Murphy adduces no evidence of compromise of ethical integrity by religion in the bioethics realm. Murphy's concern can

66. Campbell, "What More," 1–25.

67. Murphy, "In Defense," 5.

68. Murphy, "In Defense," 5.

69. Murphy, "In Defense," 6.

70. Murphy, "In Defense," 7.

71. Murphy, "In Defense," 6.

itself be situated within some long-standing biases in American political culture that affirm that some persons cannot be trusted because they do not adhere to the state as the ultimate authority in moral and political life. The kind of hermeneutic of suspicion that Murphy advances is precisely the cultural bias John F. Kennedy faced in his bid to become the first president with a Roman Catholic religious identity, when critics maintained Kennedy's allegiance would ultimately lie with the Vatican, not the Constitution.

It is then pro-religious commentators, religious analysts, religious believers, and an occasional well-intentioned but ultimately compromised individual bioethicist that advance what Murphy reconstructs as a claim that religious convictions and values command special or "privileged" status in bioethics discourse. The connection Murphy intends to make between the cluster of religiously-informed bioethicists and the need for special status should now be clear. The assertion of deference and privilege, which Murphy interprets as a request for the immunity of religious convictions from critical moral scrutiny, is necessary to avoid exposing the inherent biases, ethical compromises, and divided loyalties that come with the mantle of religious devotion. The second form of irreligious bioethical repudiation of religion is then not merely about *ethical content* but also *moral character*.

Privilege and Bioethical Integrity. Strikingly, rejecting a privileged status for religious values, beliefs, or practices is ascribed by Murphy to both religious bioethics and secular philosophical bioethics.[72] As noted previously, Murphy implies that secular bioethics tends to give religion a moral pass when it comes to questions about the value or disvalue of religion relative to health care. Rather than presenting a direct challenge to religious understandings, such as whether a belief in a God or a transcendent reality inhibits good health practices or better health care decisions, or the empirical efficacy of intercessory prayer, secular bioethics gives religious thought immunity from such critique.

The secular reticence to critique, a posture of deference presumably rooted in a principle of tolerance and respect for autonomy, in combination with the inability of religious commentators, analysts, believers, and apologists to bring critical scrutiny to bear upon their own traditions or faith communities, culminates in the moral immunity of religious-based convictions. That seems to be the "privilege" that religious approaches to bioethics either enjoy or explicitly claim. Murphy doesn't provide any illustrations or context for his interpretation of religious privilege, although professional refusals to provide certain legally available medical procedures based on religious or personal conscience would be one example of a claim of immunity from generally applicable laws and professional norms (I address issues of conscience in chapter 11). However, the special cases of protection of religious conscience can't be used to generalize about religion or religious practices in their totality.

72. Murphy, "In Defense," 3–6.

The sentiments of disregard, indifference, and hostility to religion cultivated by an irreligious bioethics are warranted in Murphy's view because the moral immunity of religion represents a threat to the integrity of the normative evaluative responsibilities of bioethics (Murphy is not concerned, as was de Tocqueville, about the integrity of religion). In one of his opening salvos, Murphy contends that "bioethics should keep its distance from religion because it loses something important when it presumes in advance that religious views occupy any kind of privileged status when it comes to theorizing decisions about health, health care, and biomedical innovation."[73] Subsequently, in critiquing the composition of the major professional reference work, *The Encyclopedia of Bioethics*, Murray asks, "why not prioritize attention to domains of analysis according to their significance for decision-making, rather than assume that religion has a privileged status above all other kinds of analysis?"[74] The commitment of bioethics to the integrity of moral choice and decision-making is compromised by the moral immunity of religion and its patterns of interference with normative ethics. Moreover, with the culture wars of bioethics as a backdrop, Murphy contends that the "intellectual independence and political objectivity" of bioethics are risked when forms of ideology interpenetrate moral analysis.[75] This interpenetration is evidenced by the arguments of religious believers who are limited in their ability to "follow evidence and arguments where they lead in public affairs."[76]

The example Murphy provides is rather perplexing because it illustrates an assumption about religion apparently embedded in the intellectual infrastructure of bioethics, not a claim for privilege argued for by religious scholars. My own view is that, contrary to a claim of special advantage, religious scholars in bioethics experience a heavier burden of justification in the professional and policy cultures of bioethics because of the necessity to translate a religiously-rooted value into the secular vocabulary of bioethics and its organizing principles.

Epistemic Consciousness. Murphy's claim is that bioethics "loses something important"[77] when the purported posture of religious privilege prevails, and that "something" is in part comprised of intellectual integrity. At least the irreligious bioethics Murphy advocates appears to lose a further "something" already lost by secular bioethics. This "loss" amounts to an interesting, if rather limited, non-normative, epistemological claim: "the advantage that an irreligious bioethics offers [is] a detached vantage point from which to judge the value of religion."[78] Bioethics does its normative work best when assuming the "irreligious viewpoint . . . to the extent that viewpoint enables questions that would otherwise go unasked, to the extent that it thwarts facile

73. Murphy, "In Defense," 3.
74. Murphy, "In Defense," 6.
75. Murphy, "In Defense," 7.
76. Murphy, "In Defense," 6.
77. Murphy, "In Defense," 3.
78. Murphy, "In Defense," 5.

answers, and to the extent that it discloses the total costs of one religion compared to another and the costs of religion compared to non-religion."[79]

The epistemological advantage is the fourth form of irreligious repudiation of religion. Unlike either secular or religious bioethics, an irreligious bioethics will rely on the embedded hermeneutics of suspicion to pose questions alien to the interpretative frames of various religious traditions, including whether religious values and practices are actually beneficial when it comes to health care, good critical reasoning, and moral choices. Murphy gives no specific examples of facile answers; perhaps he has in mind a common default within as well as outside religious traditions to worries of "playing God," or alternatively, as intimated in his critique of intercessory prayer, ascribing certain matters of life beginnings or of life endings to be "in God's hands." More generally, though, the epistemic issue seems to converge with the concerns that Murphy believes confer religion an immunity from critical moral scrutiny. Religious believers or thinkers do not turn the harsh light of moral criticism on religious practices and values, but rather affirm that religious beliefs and interpretations are "off limits to questioning."[80]

In his account of epistemic viewpoint, Murphy's claims about the facile answers of religion resonates with criticisms by biologist Richard Lewontin in the context of debates over human cloning in the late 1990s. Lewontin maintained that traditions of religious reflection purportedly avoid the experience of wrenching moral anguish because their positions are constructed from divine decree or scriptural interpretation: theological reflection on human cloning attempted to "abolish hard ethical problems" and evade "painful tensions."[81] In contrast to moral philosophy, Lewontin asserted: "What religious revelation does is to provide the certainty that in all situations there is an unambiguously right thing to do, as given by Divine Law, and leaves only the question of how to know God's will."[82] Even though Murphy rejects the possibility of answering the epistemic question, both he and Lewontin greatly misrepresent the nature of religious reflection in moral communities and religious ethics expressed in the policy culture of bioethics. Skepticism is moreover warranted regarding the irreligious epistemology of detachment as such a viewpoint is detached from lived experience.[83]

Justice. Although Murphy identifies irreligious bioethics with a "philosophy of immanence" to contrast with theistic transcendence, he does not specify the normative implications of immanence until the concluding paragraph, in which the fifth form of repudiation of religion occurs, namely, a quietism that manifests as callousness and disregard for injustice in the world.

79. Murphy, "In Defense," 5.

80. Murphy, "In Defense," 7.

81. Lewontin, "Confusion over Cloning," 22.

82. Lewontin, "Confusion over Cloning," 22.

83. Walzer, *Interpretation and Social Criticism*, 6–15.

> A key benefit to bioethics follows from the irreligious assumption that the immanent world is the world itself entirely. This view makes it possible to urge reform and work toward progress in bioethics in ways not entirely available to religions that hold that the most important justice available to human beings comes only after death. . . . An irreligious bioethics . . . enables the field to think more critically and independently than is otherwise possible and to work toward justice in bioethics without the expectation of a safety net of a life beyond this one.[84]

That is a rather astonishing indictment, although it apparently is not idiosyncratic to Murphy. Callahan indicated that philosophers in bioethics tend to see religion, or at least some forms of religiosity, as an "enemy" to civil rights.[85] This of course is a core issue in the culture wars, so it's a bit hard to disentangle Murphy's polemic from the cultural context. There are certainly examples of religious traditions that are quietist on matters of social reform. It is also the case that religious traditions can initiate and perpetuate injustice. As a normative claim, however, Murphy is simply mistaken to contend there is a minimal impulse or motivation for a this-worldly justice and for affirming the equality of persons for traditions that affirm convictions of a transcendent reality. That impulse for justice, the dignity of individual persons, the equality of all persons, is part of the essential ethic of good and righteousness in the biblical religions: "What does the Lord require of you, but to do justice, and to love kindness, and to walk humbly with your God?"[86]

The social context in which bioethics emerged was laden with advocacy of civil rights and social justice that was in part inspired by religious commitments and communities. The primary figures in the emergence of bioethics were, as noted by Messikomer and colleagues, influenced by profound patterns of rejection of inegalitarian and hierarchical tradition, including religious tradition, which culminated in their "militant secularization." More recently, the widespread—if not quite universal—support among major religious traditions for universal access to basic health care in the United States should provide a compelling refutation that religious traditions possess little impulse for social justice in the ethics of health care. Religious communities engage in enacting this commitment through establishing community structures for caring for the vulnerable in the absence of universal access, including but not limited to organizing health care institutions.

Conclusion

Much more could be said about the different patterns of religious presence in the emergence of bioethics as well as the critiques of that presence as delineated by Murphy

---

84. Murphy, "In Defense," 9.

85. Callahan, "Bioethics and Culture Wars," 427.

86. Mic 6:8.

and others. My analysis displays that the problematic relationship between religion, religious bioethics, and the field of bioethics reflects different historical interpretations, different understandings of both bioethics and religion, and certainly disputes over the value of religion in human social life and in matters of public policy. My intent in the subsequent chapters is to bear witness to the contributions and critiques that a pluralist religious perspective can offer to the many cultures of bioethics and to the human quest for meaning.

3

Bearing the Image

Persons as Imago Dei

Bioethics addresses issues at the defining boundaries of human nature and identity that are fraught with controversy, including the origins, thresholds, and endings of personhood. Moral conclusions about such issues as embryonic stem cell research, withdrawing treatment from patients in persistent vegetative state, or determinations of death (and hence, permissible organ transplantation), presume interpretations about the characteristics required for inclusion in the moral community, about the responsibilities of moral agents, and the moral protections granted to persons in the moral community but who are not considered moral agents.

My object in this chapter is to present an interpretation of the human person as framed by the divine designation that persons are made in and are bearers of the image of God, a concept the religious traditions have referred to as the *imago Dei*. This designation of ontological and moral standing is articulated in the biblical creation narrative in Genesis: "So God created humankind in his image, in the image of God he created them; male and female he created them."[1] This confers an existentially and morally distinctive status upon human beings. Its moral implications are briefly intimated shortly thereafter in the Noahide covenant, which prohibits the shedding of blood, usually interpreted as a prohibition against murder, insofar as it desecrates the divine image borne by human beings.[2] My interpretation of this foundational religious symbol builds on the relational and ethical content embedded in these (and other) passages from sacred texts, but is not confined to them. My account seeks both

1. Gen 1:27.
2. Gen 9:6.

to identify certain characteristics embedded in the *imago Dei* that inhere in the human person and to advance discussion of the moral meanings of those qualities.

The traditions of theological analysis have emphasized human capacities for rationality, self-conscious reflection, and freedom as constitutive of the *imago Dei*. A focus on these capacities is understandable as they seem in many respects to identify characteristics necessary to differentiate human beings from nonhuman life, serving as one boundary that the concept of *imago Dei* is supposed to mark. The difficulty is making this rationalistic interpretation all-encompassing of the human person. These limitations can be discerned by considering the other boundary the *imago Dei* is to mark, namely the distinction between human beings and God. This boundary is presumed in the oft-articulated prohibition in public discourse on "playing God." The proposal that God is imaged in the world as defined by rationality, consciousness, self-reflection, and autonomy represents an entirely restricted view of God, that is, a god of the philosophers who is detached and removed from, rather than embodied or imaged in, human beings. This god would not have any intrinsic relationship with those earth creatures that lack rational, self-reflective capacities, and thus would find it difficult to acknowledge the awe-inspiring nature of creation as "good." We experience the divine nature as relational; God does not create and depart in some deistic fashion, but is in ongoing relationship with human beings, other earth creatures, and through the ongoing creative ordering of nature. In this respect, persons bear the *imago Dei* through our relationships. Furthermore, we inescapably experience these relations as embodied persons; whatever else the *imago Dei* may mean, it is intertwined with our embodied selves.

Nature no less reflects the handiwork of the creator, and insofar as the creation narratives depict humans as also created from the soil or dust, humans are part of nature. Human beings bear marks of the divine and the natural: We both reflect and bear witness to origins in divine being and in created naturalness. It is a mistake to separate these two features of the person in a rigid dualistic fashion. A central moral and existential human challenge is to maintain an integration of self as bearing both an image of the divine and marks of the natural throughout life. This is a critical consideration in circumstances of medical care in which persons, families, and professionals inescapably encounter inherent limitations of our bodily being.

In the subsequent discussion, I develop and expand on these experiential realities to present elements of a moral anthropology, an understanding of human nature, which informs many of the ethical perspectives presented in this book. In particular, I engage in an exposition of a coherent cluster of eight interrelated characteristics—creativity, narrative, embodiment, relationality, giftedness, covenant, stewardship, and agency—that mark human beings as bearers of the *imago Dei*; I also articulate an array of moral responsibilities embedded in this witness-bearing symbol of human identity. My exposition cultivates an ethic of covenantal responsibility structured around features of gift-responsiveness-responsibility-transformation.

Creativity

Insofar as the bestowal of the identity of *imago Dei* to human beings is embedded in a story of *creation*, it follows that the image of the divine is manifested in part through human capacities for creativity. Insofar as the symbol is embedded in a *story* of creation, it also follows that the *imago Dei* is expressed through narrative. I first turn my attention to the inherent human characteristic of creativity and its ethical implications.

Creativity as a central feature of our humanity emerges in important teachings of many religious traditions. The principle of *tikkun olam* in Jewish tradition, which refers to human responsibility for repairing the world and partnering with the divine in completing creation, presumes human creativity and is a significant theme in Jewish bioethical scholarship. A different way of formulating the point has been expressed by Christian thinkers in bioethics who have advanced the idea that human (and Christian) participation in the development of various innovative medical practices and technologies is illustrative of human responsibilities to be cocreators with God in a continuing creative process (*creatio continua*). The substantive manifestations of our creative nature are intimated in one of the three symbols of human identity proposed by Christian theologian H. Richard Niebuhr, the symbol of "man as maker."[3] A fundamental feature of who we are as persons and how we bear witness to the divine is through envisioning and shaping the world as oriented by certain goals and aspirations.

Technology. Our inclination for creativity, which implies an imaginative visualization of the art of the possible, is clearly manifested in various forms. Most significantly for the purposes of medicine, creativity is displayed through tool-making; tools span the range from rudimentary instruments for subsistence living to those that have significantly shaped modern medicine, from the nineteenth-century invention of the stethoscope to the innovative and invasive diagnostic and life-extending technologies that now invoke awe and amazement about the wonders of contemporary medicine. Tools and technologies extend our reach beyond our body and are unquestionably methods of shaping or altering the natural for human purposes. While creativity expressed in the development of technologies is an inestimable human good, it cannot be considered the sole or only human good; moreover, the uses of a technological device can be severed from the original creative vision and intent. The development of technology and assessment of its applications in biomedicine in particular must be framed by fundamental questions about the purposes of the technology and the nature of the organizations that control its implementation. The ethical implications of this manifestation of the *imago Dei* include a general moral presumption in favor of technological advances in medicine, a rebuttable presumption against technologies anticipated to bring about irreversible and irrevocable change, and a concerted effort

3. Niebuhr, *Responsible Self*, 3.

to resist conflation of ethical imperatives with the so-called technological imperative. That technology gives us the means or the *how* of doing something does not resolve the ethical issue of *whether* the action should be performed. I develop subsequently in this chapter the concept of stewardship as one ethical criterion that seeks to preserve or repair a balance between creativity, control, and moral good.

The Art of Medicine. A second meaningful form of human creativity is comprised of aesthetic expressions through painting, sculpture, dance, acting, music, and numerous other forms. While we often refer to the creative genius of a Mozart or Michelangelo, as well as more contemporary artists, aesthetic creativity is a shared human experience. Aesthetic experience and creativity is often a catalyst for critical thinking and reflection, including ethical reflection, on aspects of the human condition. The connection between creativity and critical consciousness is embedded in the term used to describe various collections of creativity, namely, "museum." The aesthetic sensibility moves us to muse, to be creatively critical, in contrast to more recreational diversions found at amusement parks.

The aesthetic expressions of creativity comprise a good with important ethical and bioethical implications. Our aesthetic sensibility often awakens or elicits from us profound sentiments such as those of awe and wonder, which open the human person to profound engagement with meaning. These profound connections to a meaning larger than ourselves are illustrated in Einstein's observation that the human practices of art and science, as well as religious experience, stem from a common root, an experience of the dispositions of awe and wonder in response to the mysterious.[4] Following out this line of reasoning, we should be capable of finding an intrinsic relationship between the science of medicine and the arts of healing. Failure to recognize this connection would imply a lack of imaginative attentiveness, or in Einstein's phrasing, our "eyes are closed,"[5] and we are willfully ignorant of our nature.

The ethical implications of understanding medicine or healing as an art traces back as early as the formative Hippocratic Oath, which includes commitments of fidelity and loyalty to teachers and students of "the art" and a set of ethical commitments towards patients. The modern understanding is perhaps best expressed in an observation of Sir William Osler: "It is much more important to know what sort of a patient has the disease than to know what sort of disease the patient has."[6] Knowing the disease relies on the scientific method for categorization based on symptoms as well as technical expertise to diagnose that the disease has manifest in a particular patient. Knowledge of a patient requires various skills that must be cultivated through a more humanistic form of education, including observation, communication, listening and interpreting the patient's story, touching and the physical examination, as well as

---

4. Einstein, "Strange Is Our Situation," 202–5.
5. Einstein, "Strange Is Our Situation," 204.
6. Kahn, "What Would Osler Do," 443.

virtues acquired through experience, such as caring, empathy, and discernment, and the physician's presence in the relationship.

The intrinsic relationship of the science and the art of medicine is specified in medical practices that integrate knowing the patient in whom a disease manifests. The omission of interpretive skills, virtues, and relational presence in medicine and medical education can imply that what physician Abraham Verghese has aptly titled the "iPatient" has replaced the actual human patient. The iPatient designates a mode of impersonal and distanced epistemology in which the patient is known primarily through empirical data accumulated in their medical record.[7] A consequence of the reliance on the iPatient is a decline in physician skills in touch and the performance of the physical exam, which Verghese contends is a necessary ritual for cultivating trust in the physician-patient relationship. A capable and competent physician will clearly be proficient in the science of medicine, but it is the integration of the art, including the discerning use of technologies, and knowing the patient as a person, that distinguishes the physician as a *healer* (I provide a fuller exposition of the physician's calling as healer in chapters 5 and 6).

Procreative Generativity. A third manifestation of human creative inclinations with ethical ramifications occurs in creating children or procreation, in which creativity issues in generativity. We use the language of "bearing children" to reflect this creative and generative process, its labor and burdens, and its inherent responsibilities and joys; the biblical metaphors of parenting as "being fruitful" and of children as "fruit"[8] are suggestive of both the necessary labor and planning required as well as the joy and delight of having, bearing, and nurturing children. As any parent can attest, parenting is a very imprecise art that can't be mapped out in advance and yet is as meaningful as any human experience can be. Indeed, the meaningfulness of the experience is related to its improvisational and artistic nature rather than its design as a scientific project.

Children are a sign and witness of hope for the future; a common refrain among members of current generations that it is personally (and perhaps ethically) irresponsible "to bring children into a world like ours," that is, a world in which fear, sorrow, suffering, and premature death are pervasive and apocalyptic anxiety abounds. Procreative generativity may be qualified and shaped by the extent of moral responsibilities present persons assume and should be willing to bear on behalf of the being and well-being of future generations. Parenting takes us into an experience of hope for a future that will not include ourselves.

At least until the advent of assisted reproductive technologies such as in vitro fertilization, procreative generativity necessarily required in human beings the expression of our sexuality. We are sexual beings no less than creative beings. The inclination to reproduce seems in the Genesis narrative to be an intrinsic feature for all

7. Verghese, "Culture Shock," 2748–51.

8. Gen 1:28, 9:7 (NRSV).

natural life and processes. By contrast, the narrative relates that human beings receive a covenantal responsibility of procreation, which implies that persons make choices and exercise their agency about sexual expression in a manner different from the rest of creation. The difference lies not in the sexual act, but in its context, the affection and unity of the sexes that occurs, and the meanings the partners bring to their intimacy. Human sexuality, including but not limited to procreative generativity, is to follow a distinction developed in Roman Catholic teaching, a matter of personalism rather than physicalism. Sexual relations in human beings are not limited to purposes of procreation, but express love and care for the sexual partner, and manifest mutual pleasure; sexuality symbolizes rather than comprises the meaning of their union.

Imbued with mystery, awe, and ritual, procreative generativity has in the past century become among the most medicalized realms of human experience.[9] Technologies to assist and to prevent conception are pervasive and ethical controversies abound. In this regard, it is worth recalling that obstetrics, which comes from a Latin root, *obstare*, meaning "to stand by," was not a developed medical specialization for most of human history, emerging primarily in the late nineteenth century. The language of "standing by" is a valuable metaphor, implying at least initially respectful observance of natural processes and the integration of self and nature. However, in contemporary settings of procreation and reproduction, it is rare that medical technologies stand by; rather, they are developed for purposes of intervention into and facilitation of these natural processes. The oral contraceptive was developed to impede the natural course of a woman's ovulation, while in vitro fertilization works to overcome the barriers imposed by natural processes on conception, including hormonal stimulation for hyperovulation to facilitate egg retrieval from a woman. Various technologies are relied on in an obstetrical setting to ensure minimization of risks to the woman's health and increase the prospects for a safe birth of the child. There is little bioethical controversy currently about medical interventions into human reproductive processes for considerations of safety. However, ethical controversies over medicalized procreative generativity and medicalized childbirth, such as is illustrated in high rates of delivery from cesarean section procedures, reflect concerns regarding the extent and scope of medical specializations in company with associated technologies for diagnosis, monitoring, and safety. That is, given the general moral acceptability of in vitro fertilization in bioethics, a question is whether that acceptance also wants permission for further and more specific interventions, such as pre-implantation genetic diagnosis, medical (or nonmedical) sex selection, or gene editing. Is there some point on the continuum of reproductive technologies at which the extensive medical powers to manipulate human reproduction and procreative generativity diminish its profound personal, relational, and social meanings? Can the awe and amazement at the birth of a child be

9. Martin, *Woman in the Body*, 25–70.

diminished because reproduction has become an engineering problem akin to what transpires in Huxley's novel, *Brave New World*?[10]

Moral Imagination, Empathy, and Vision. Two characteristics embedded in the preceding analysis of forms of creativity are worth brief attention because of their profound implications for ethics. Creativity highlights in various ways the faculty of imagination, and this can be expanded one step further to convey the indispensable concept of moral imagination. Moral imagination involves an imaginative exercise by which a moral agent seeks to recognize, understand, and affirm the experiences of another moral agent by seeing the world through their eyes or "walking in their shoes." Moral imagination is likewise embedded in ethical maxims such as the principle of universalizability, which affirms that a moral judgment applies to all similarly situated moral agents.

The critical feature of the exercise of moral imagination for my current purposes is that it is a necessary condition for the cultivation and expression of the virtue of empathy, which is not only a mediating feature of everyday human interaction, but is often idealized as an indispensable characteristic of an effective physician-patient relationship. In complement with sympathy, or "feeling for" another person (a patient), and compassion, a virtue of "suffering with" another person, empathy is characterized by a "feeling with" the other person, and this feeling "with" is possible only through the moral imagination.[11] As important as empathy is in the context of medical practice, empirical research has determined to the dismay of medical educators that the empathic understanding of medical students undergoes a substantial erosion precisely when students start seeing actual patients in the third year of medical school.[12] This displacement of empathy is one reason for the emergence of various health humanities programs that emphasize literature (and other creative arts) as a way to engage the human condition when medical training is experienced as depersonalizing patients.

A second ethical feature embedded in our inherent creative capacities is what can be termed "vision" or "seeing" a broader array of possibilities. The metaphors of vision and sight are central in the responsive quality of ethical interactions; a lack of awe and wonder in response to the intricate aesthetic, scientific, and religious dimensions of the world reflects a kind of blindness or moral myopia. William F. May has portrayed ethics generally, and applied medical ethics specifically, as a kind of "corrective vision" in which envisioning context, symbols, images, and stories is a necessary precondition for engaging in normative problem-solving.[13]

Persons bearing the image of God not only participate in the created world, but utilize inherent creative capacities through technologies, aesthetic expression, and procreative generativity and nurturing. The imaginative capacity required by creativity

10. Huxley, *Brave New World*.

11. Miller, *Friends and Other Strangers*, 109–16.

12. Hojat, "Devil Is in the Third Year," 1182–91.

13. May, *Physician's Covenant*, 1.

necessarily opens into exercise of the moral imagination and the virtues of empathy and expanded vision. Even in bearing witness through creativity, various values can conflict, but such conflicts in fact represent the importance we ascribe to this feature of our life. The *imago Dei* is more than creativity, but it is not less.

Narrative

The *imago Dei* is an identity and status bestowed in a story or narrative told about creation, a story retold by moral communities for generations and centuries. This narrative is meaningful because it witnesses to who persons are and calls moral communities to remember possibilities of who we can be through the symbol of the *imago Dei*. The clear intimation is that the creative aspect of the human self is also expressed through storytelling and narratives as well as through witnessing and listening to these narratives. Creativity and narrative are especially important ways of engaging and training our moral vision and perception and enhancing empathic relationships. The imaginative capacity requisite for the cultivation of empathy is necessarily exercised as we engage in finding ourselves in a narrative, such as through identifying with a protagonist.

In an existential sense, in the beginning was the story. The narrative mode of discourse in which the *imago Dei* is situated is manifested through community formation and identity, in cultivating analogical discovery and interpretation by the community, and in processes of remembering and what I refer to as "re-storying" as a feature of restoring relationships and communities. These features are moral possibilities and existential necessities of narrative because a narrative does not represent a detached philosophical view from nowhere, but is rather embedded and experienced as a situated story from and about somewhere.

Narrative Community. The practice of storytelling necessarily situates persons in a community; for every storyteller, there must be a listener, a story-receiver, an audience. In the creation narrative, the community is not present in the story, but the community is the reason for the story. The story of divine creativity forms a community that receives an account of its identity, integrity, and responsibility through the narrative. A defining feature of the community, honoring the Sabbath, is given a covenantal meaning as a symbol of creation and provides insight into how the community can live in fidelity to a formative story. The Christian Gospels likewise bear witness to the commitment and character of a community in response to a re-storying narrative of transforming love.

Analogical Discovery. Narrative is explicative and expository rather than argumentative discourse, and thereby invokes analogical reasoning. Narrative invites analogy, metaphor, and symbol—that is, we find identity and even meaning by understanding our own circumstances in likeness to a formative story that provides a base point of orientation. We always find ourselves through the mirror of other stories.

For example, writing in his own memoir, *When Breath Becomes Air*, physician Paul Kalanithi interpreted his diminishing professional empathy through Tolstoy's story, *The Death of Ivan Ilyich*: "I feared I was on my way to becoming Tolstoy's stereotype of a doctor, preoccupied with empty formalism, focused on the rote treatment of disease, and utterly missing the larger human significance."[14] This concept of the story as a moral mirror in turn requires and presupposes skills cultivated through the narrative community of listening, observing, and interpretation. The processes of analogical reasoning and interpretation are why, for some scholars, the fundamental nature of ethics is that of an interpretative inquiry.[15]

Narrative is the medium of a relationship in which there is potential for a shared quest to make sense of human experience, to uncover or discover a common journey for meaning. As Kathryn Montgomery articulates the point, narrative opens to "accounts of the way the world works and how we and our fellow human beings act in every conceivable circumstance."[16] This role of narrative assumes enhanced significance in a social context in which biomedical and other technologies have radically called into question ways by which "the world works" and have instead generated innovative interpretations. Narrative can then provide analogical resources for interpretative understanding in the face of unprecedented technological possibilities. Furthermore, narrative is "concerned with the construction and interpretation of meaning."[17] Montgomery suggests that the pronounced public and professional interest in bioethics "reveals a narrative hunger for meaning in the face of human mortality and the technology that shapes it."[18]

Remembering and Re-storying. The formative and constitutive stories of personal and communal identity are recollected and retold. Memory and remembrance of the past are carried forward by storytelling into a future of possibility. Narrative provides a way of experiencing eternity in time by uniting past and future into a reality of the present "now." The communal act of remembering a foundational narrative calls a community to its profound and ultimate dependency and thereby awareness of its existential contingency. Remembering necessarily invokes virtues of gratitude, appreciativeness, and humility.

It is a feature of human communities and human bodies to become alienated and experience brokenness, including a rupture from constitutive narratives. In such circumstances, remembering is insufficient to the moral task of restoring wholeness, of healing the community and the embodied person. A different narrative may emerge in the context of an experience of woundedness or brokenness that expresses restorative possibilities of identity, integrity, and meaning. A narrative of deliverance

14. Kalanithi, *When Breath Becomes Air*, 85.

15. Walzer, *Interpretation and Social Criticism*, 1–30.

16. Montgomery, "Narrative," 2138.

17. Montgomery, "Narrative," 2139.

18. Montgomery, "Narrative," 2141.

from oppression may augment and supplant a narrative of creation, or a narrative of redemptive reconciliation can emerge from a witness of covenantal solidarity. The construction and articulation of a narrative that is responsive to the experience of broken communities and broken bodies is what I refer to as the re-storying nature of restoring wholeness and healing.

Re-storying narratives have profound ethical implications for bioethics. The narrative possibilities in the context of the rupture and brokenness of illness are probingly articulated by sociologist Arthur Frank. Frank contends the re-storying that emerges in the experience of illness may take three primary forms, those of restitution, chaos, and quest.[19] These forms of re-storying narrative are especially significant for making sense of and bearing witness to suffering.

Narrative discourse is thereby a profound way of bearing witness of the *imago Dei*. Narrative both presupposes and is a catalyst for community formation and identity. It invites the exercise of moral imagination and analogical forms of reasoning that display the necessity of metaphor, symbol, and symbolic rationality in the experience of moral life. Narrative opens to engagement with the deep questions of the human condition and the human quest for meaning that are inescapable in confronting bioethical issues. Significantly, the essential virtue of empathy cultivated by narrative is experienced by telling stories in and through the body.

Embodiment

The narrative bestowal of the identity of *imago Dei* occurs when the human body is formed and receives the breath or spirit that marks the creation of a living person. Subsequently, in the laws that mark the beginnings of the Noahide covenant, the prohibition of (unjustifiable) killing is connected to the image of God that each person bears.[20] Both the creation and the renewal narratives bear witness to the religious and moral significance of embodiment, a status that holds significant implications for bioethics.

The human body has long been problematic for philosophic and theological traditions. For Socrates and Plato, the body was a prison that inhibited the soul from achieving realization with the ultimate forms or reality. Descartes understood the body to be inert matter, an organism that functioned as a machine, and the source of various illusions that prevented persons from acquiring true knowledge about the self and the world. The traditions of meditation and yoga in various south India traditions, including Hinduism and Buddhism, historically rooted these practices in a soteriology of release or escape from physical corporeality. In our own era, the Cartesian philosophical perplexity of the mind-body distinction continues to organize academic debates, with the mind understood as a consciousness that emerges from the physical

19. Frank, *Wounded Storyteller*, 75–136.
20. Gen 2:7; 9:6.

organ of the brain in the course of encountering and processing experience in the world. An interpretative metaphor for the body in the modern context of individual rights and market economies is that of property, through which the individual affirms claims of ownership that warrant respecting their privacy and their control over their bodily integrity against claims by others. The social context of contemporary biomedicine interprets the human body through reductionistic mechanical and engineering metaphors of "fixing," "fabrication," and "design." Embodiment is bioethically problematic insofar as bioethics has privileged a disembodied self or will that makes autonomous decisions even as the experience of disease and illness requires medicine to directly attend to bodily pathology, integrity, and restoring wholeness.

Each of these accounts of embodiment as prison, machine, or property has a certain experiential plausibility, as exemplified in our finitude and fallibility and in the separateness of self from body inherent in the experience of illness, but they mistake partial experience for the totality of our embodied life. Whatever else may be true about our apprehension of our own embodiment, my claim is that the body is a bearer and witness of the *imago Dei*. The body is revelatory both of the divine and of the human person. Our embodiment is intrinsic to our identity and integrity as persons, not contingent or accidental, in the manner presupposed in the prison, machine, or property accounts.

Religious Narratives of the Body. It is not simply philosophical, cultural, or medical traditions that have encountered the body as an obstacle. The moral status and meaning of the body has certainly been contested historically by Christian thinkers, who themselves are heavily influenced by modes of bodily discipline shaped by Pauline injunctions. The ethos of the disciplined body introduced its own form of self-body dualism into Christian theological and ethical teaching that connected conceptually with Socratic and Platonic understandings and provided a theological background for the Cartesian mechanistic interpretation of the body.

However, underlying the injunctions and warnings about the body and embodied action in Christian thought are profound claims and symbols about the significance of embodiment; that is, the proscriptions presuppose and are given intelligibility only through an assumption of the intrinsic integration of body and self. The incarnation of God in Jesus, who is portrayed in Christian Scripture as *imago Dei*,[21] is absolutely critical to the Christian story of salvation. Furthermore, the biblical narrative depicts Jesus, following his death and resurrection, manifesting himself in physical bodily form to his disciples, consuming food such as bread and fish. These narratives form the basis for the theologies of incarnation and resurrection that are subsequently incorporated into Christian doctrinal creeds.

The rituals and symbols of the tradition likewise manifest the significant soteriological and moral status of embodiment. Virtually all communities in the Christian traditions require adherents to at some point bear witness of their convictions and

21. Heb 1:3.

commitment by participating in the rituals of baptism and the Eucharist or sacramental supper. Not only do both rituals involve embodied activity, as symbols they underscore that participation in Christian life is embodied. The baptismal ritual symbolizes cleansing and purification from sin as well as the eschatological hope of a bodily resurrection, while the sacramental ritual involves remembrance of the embodied nature of Jesus as Christ and his offering and gift of body and blood so that human beings can be reconciled and restored to the divine presence. Moreover, participation in Christian life means a joining of the person to the church, which is symbolized as the *corpus Christi*, the ongoing embodied manifestation of the presence of Christ in the world. The rituals, symbols, and theological teachings of Christian embodiment do not make room for an anti-materialistic dualism or spiritualism.

The embodied witness of the *imago Dei* means a person's body is ultimately neither prison, machine, property, nor commodity, but is rather a *temple, tabernacle*, or *sanctuary*. The human body is vested with sacredness that evokes awe and amazement at its intricacies and organic totality. Bioethics has been mistaken to focus all moral inquiry on the disembodied will as autonomous decision-maker, for there is a wholeness of the self that is experienced only as an embodied person. We simply have no experience of our self as disembodied.

My interpretation of the religious and ethical implications of embodiment is influenced by teachings specific to my own faith tradition: the "soul" of a person is not a separate metaphysical entity, but is rather constituted by an integration of body and spirit.[22] Persons are embodied souls or ensouled bodies, and the deprivation of embodied experience represents its own form of imprisonment and bondage.[23] Bearing the body as a witness of the divine generates ethical responsibilities rooted in qualities of sacrality, gift, relationship, and teaching regarding the intricacies and mysteries of the body.

Embodied Wonder. Reflective experience of the body should elicit dispositions of awe, wonder, and reverence. Yet there are multivalent meanings to the experience of awe and wonder that are especially pertinent for ethical reflection in medicine. We can wonder about our body in the sense of recognizing it as a unique medium for self-revelation, trust in the body's own restorative and healing capacities, and marvel over the distinctive achievements in aesthetics or athletics and ways of being in the world we experience only through our embodied life. However, we also express wonderment about our body when we experience illness; we may well "wonder what is going on" with us.

These two senses of wonder, the "awesome" and "awful" aspects of embodied life, are deftly intimated by Frank in his observation that "the arts of being ill and of practicing medicine should converge in mutual wonder at the body."[24] The illness ex-

---

22. *Doctrine and Covenants* 88:15.

23. *Doctrine and Covenants* 138:50.

24. Frank, *At the Will of the Body*, 62.

perience leads the patient to engage in wondering as confusion, uncertainty, and fear, though it is not separated from wondering as trust and hope for healing. The physician who practices the art of medicine must share the wonder of the body, including both wonder as trust and as marvel at mystery, even if some aspects of puzzlement emerge. The initial shared sense of wonder will set restraints and moral limits on treating the person's somatic symptoms as merely a scientific puzzle. Einstein's critique of persons who have lost the sense of wonder at mystery is effectively echoed in Frank's critique of physicians who practice in the absence of wonder: "A physician who does not have this sense of wonder seeks only to cure diseases" rather than be an agent of healing to the person.[25]

The philosophical and bioethical priority of the disembodied self acquires some intelligibility through differentiating the sources and senses of wonder and points to a profound existential experience of our body. In much of our everyday experience as persons in good health, we are barely aware of our bodily life; embodiment recedes into the background of consciousness. The object of my conscious awareness at the present moment is the reflective mental activity of developing ideas and communicating thoughts that can be translated into images and words on a computer screen. That this activity requires the bodily medium of my fingers (as well as other physical functions) is seldom in my thought process. It is often difficult in everyday life to make our bodies the focal point of consciousness. This reality of embodiment underscores the pedagogical purpose of religious symbolism and ritual to provide embodied reminders of identity.

Bodily Consciousness and Medicine. Given this embodied situatedness, philosopher Drew Leder has insightfully suggested the philosophical and ethical importance of differentiating between the "disappearing" and the "dys-appearing" body.[26] Our common experience is that the body "disappears" as our conscious, reflective activity is directed beyond the body (such as to images on a computer screen). The contrasting phrase of the "*dys*-appearing" body, which resonates with Frank's senses of "wonder" over the body, refers to circumstances in which our consciousness is rammed inward into our bodily life, and we cannot but experience awareness of our embodied selfhood, and perhaps only such awareness, as in pain. The body appears to us when we experience dysfunction in some regard. In the simple activity of typing right now, for example, I am very much aware of a splint on one finger from a recent physical injury that impairs my ability to go from mental reflection to embodied action to words projected on a computer screen. Heightened bodily appearance and awareness in consciousness is also experienced in confronting the limits of extreme exertion in physical activities, or through practices requiring unusual or difficult bodily postures, such as in meditation or yoga. In experiencing the "dys-appearing" body, reflective activity is directed towards the immanence of our embodiment rather than to a sense

25. Frank, *At the Will of the Body*, 62.
26. Leder, *Absent Body*, 69–99.

of self-transcendence by extension of embodiment through instrumental or expressive actions.

Most commonly, however, the body "dys-appears" in the context of sickness and illness; a "bout" with influenza leaves a lasting memory of our bodily selves. We recover from these episodes of embodied consciousness through the body's natural healing processes and, if necessary, the aid of some medicine. The implications of embodied awareness for medicine and for ethical reflection on medicine should be clear. The disappearing body is the emblem of good physical health and defies a need of medical treatment, so much so that we will seek alternative explanations for symptoms or aberrations in bodily life that may prove disruptive to our projects and preoccupations. It is the dys-appearing body that most often compels persons to visit their physician. A disembodied bioethics, an intellectual meeting of bright minds or thoughtful deliberations about decision-making, cannot do justice to medicine and its encounter with human embodiment.

Sensitivity, judgment, and discretion by the medical profession is important in such circumstances, lest a person's entire health and bodily organism be medicalized, as historically has occurred with women's reproductive life, including menstruation and pregnancy. Part of Frank's critique of contemporary (or post-modern) medicine is directed at ideologies and practices of medicalization that issue precisely from the diminishment of wonder about and over the human body. As an aspect of the property metaphor of the body delineated here, Frank briefly narrates "the story of medicine taking the body as its territory" in ways that manifest symbols and practices of "colonization."[27]

The responsibility of medicine practiced in a manner disposed by wonder is nonetheless directed towards care of the physical bodily organism as part of caring for the person; healing that reconnects and reintegrates the person with their body, that restores a fullness of wonder, or ameliorates symptoms or conditions when healing is beyond the realm of medical expertise, is the end aspiration. This is an especially compelling responsibility when the dys-appearance of the body is common and recurrent, such as repeated insulin treatments for persons with diabetes, the inescapability of bodily limits for persons who experience chronic disability, or the embodied experience of terminal illness.

The sustaining power of cultivating wonder for both patients and physicians can occur in part through stories that disclose that the body bears within itself biological resources for healing. A person's body may sustain a paper cut or a broken bone; it may become afflicted with the common cold or the perennial new strain of influenza. In these and like circumstances, healing and restoring of health come from within the body, its immune system, and its capacities for cellular and bone regeneration. Human healers, whether shamanistic or professional, must first learn from the wisdom the body bears and its own organismic regenerativity in order to be successful

27. Frank, *At the Will of the Body*, 50–58.

in their own vocation. Sentiments of awe and wonder are important in cultivating moral restraints on what is done to the body in medicine, permit medical space for attentiveness to the intrinsic healing properties of the body, and can provide a basis for critique of ongoing professional or cultural objectification and instrumentalization of the body. The practice of medicine as a healing profession in large measure begins, as expressed by physician-writer Sherwin Nuland, only as physicians are "awestruck at the amazement within us."[28]

Embodied Narrative. The body can thus become a site of a remarkable interaction and tension between the sacred, the cultural, and the medical, permeated with competing interpretations and stories. The narrative nature of embodied life, including the embodied experience of medicine, is underscored in a metaphor advanced by Verghese of the body as "text." The first imperative for physicians, dictated by principles of both beneficence and respect, is to engage in "reading" the body.[29] The body is a teller of stories, and it is a professionally deficient physician who only reviews charts and test results, and treats the iPatient. As with any embodied narrative, the physician as healer acknowledges the restorative powers inherent to the body, and must rely on interpretive skills, discerning observations, empathic understanding, and embodied connection through laying on of hands in a physical examination.

The embodied initiating rituals and symbols in religious experience have parallels with indispensable features of medical practice. As one illustration, Verghese invokes the language of ritual to portray the significance of the physical exam in cultivating trust between patient and physician, without which the relationship is diminished of meaning and reduced to a transactional interaction. The embodied ritual of touch in the exam may have no direct or instrumental medical significance, but illustrates symbols with profound relational meaning. The physical exam expresses a "crossing of thresholds" and presents the prospect of transforming identities of patient and physician from strangers to a partnership in healing.[30] Verghese and other medical educators contend that this ritual of embodied wisdom is becoming a lost art in a profession oriented more by time, tests, and technological proficiency.[31]

The foregoing account of the medical and bioethical implications of how embodiment bears the *imago Dei* should not be interpreted as advocacy of a thoroughgoing materialist theology or religious ethic. The body *is* the medium of revelation of the self to others and to the world, but a person is more than their bodily experience or organism. However, as displayed in the attitudes and symbols of religious traditions, various practices of medicine, and in cultural rituals, there is moral and religious significance to the body and embodiment beyond imprisonment, mechanistic, property, commodity, or colonialist interpretations of the body that are pronounced in bioethics

28. Nuland, *Wisdom of the Body*, xix.

29. Verghese, "How Tech Can Turn Doctors," para. 1.

30. Verghese, "Treat the Patient," para. 19.

31. Sanders, *Every Patient Tells a Story*, 109–28.

discourse. The body bears the marks or image both of the handiwork of the divine and of experience in the world.

The symbol of the body as temple or sanctuary implies both respectful wonder regarding the body and boundaries to instrumentalization and medicalization of the body. This invites a narrative interpretation of the body as a text that requires of physicians skills pertinent more to the art of medicine to read and interpret the stories of affliction told in and through the body. This account of embodiment as an inherent characteristic of the *imago Dei* also bears witness against some contemporary paradigms of bioethics. There is a meaningful moral difference between the ethical principle of respect for persons and the principle of respect for autonomous choice. The body is rendered morally extraneous and invisible in the ethics of autonomous choice.[32] It is a striking irony that the moral self presupposed by the bioethical principle of respect for autonomy is most often portrayed as human will, a decision-maker, a disembodied being. The moral traditions of religious embodiment can help us draw back from advocating a self we do not know and have no experience of, and witness to an imperative in bioethics to discover the moral wisdom of the body.

Relationship

The creation narrative ascribes the status of *imago Dei* to human beings not only as individual selves, but as relational beings. From a symbolic unity of being, two persons emerge who are in essential relationship as sharers in the divine image. We are not complete beings without relationship.[33] We are fully moral selves as we are in relationship, or as social creatures in the Aristotelian interpretation.

The narrative likewise conveys an understanding that two persons through their relationship manifest the *imago Dei* without diminution despite differentiation. The symbol of the *imago Dei* thereby provides a profound basis for the principle of equality of persons. I do not wish to idealize this concept: hierarchy and power quickly emerge in most relationships, and the cultivation of equality remains an elusive moral aspiration. Nonetheless, our core identity as image bearers of the divine witnesses to a basic equality in relationship and to an essential commonality with all persons whom we otherwise encounter as other-than-self or as strangers-from-self.

Relationship is identity-creating, identity-sustaining, and identity-transforming. In a very central manner, we acquire, maintain, and cultivate a sense of who we are within formative settings of family, friends, schools, churches, workplaces, and professional and civic groups, or other settings that are designated as intermediate communities. Relationships are identity-conferring through various roles and correlative responsibilities we assume in those roles. I am in relationships as child, sibling, spouse, father, educator, friend, coach, congregant, civic participant, and not least of

32. Meilaender, *Body, Soul, and Bioethics*, 37–88.
33. Buber, *I and Thou*, 3–34.

all, patient; moral commitments inclusive of, but not limited to, equality of respect is embedded in each of these roles. Relationships are necessarily identity-transforming as well: I am quite sure I learn more life lessons and acquire a deeper understanding of my responsibilities from my children, my students, and my basketball players than they learn from me. I am a parent who is nurtured and tutored, a teacher who is taught, and a coach who needs to be coachable.

In my own religious tradition, relational identity and responsibility is also expressed through lineage with respect to both predecessors and progeny. The moral commitments of gratitude and remembrance with respect to predecessors are intimated by Danish philosopher Soren Kierkegaard, who in his critique of the preferential loves of friendship and erotic love, observed that the purest form of love is manifest in remembering the dead, as those who have preceded us cannot reciprocate gratitude, generosity, and care for legacy.[34] There are moreover few better exemplifications of extensive moral commitments than those assumed by parents in their relationships with children. Parents express affirming or accepting care and love, sustaining nurture and transforming care, and fidelity through time, and in health and sickness, towards their children.

These two examples of relationships of lineage necessarily invite important distinctions in relationship-initiation and meaning with important implications for contemporary bioethics. Our relationships with our predecessors generate unchosen or involuntary responsibilities whereas relationships with our posterity characteristically reflect invited, chosen, or voluntary responsibilities towards persons we hope will outlive us. In the tradition of liberal political philosophy that has been enormously influential in bioethics, it has often been difficult to justify any kind of concept of involuntary or unchosen responsibility. The paradigm relationship within this tradition is that between the authority of the state and the individual sovereign self. In very pronounced respects, familial relationships with their admixture of involuntary and voluntary responsibilities are a kind of moral anomaly. Bioethics has continually worked within a tension created by relationship models that derive from political metaphors and contexts, such as contract, and those that derive from domestic or familial metaphors.

The choice of relationships through which exemplary moral connection and commitment is mediated is important. Formative narratives and religious imperatives regarding love of neighbor as well as experience of moral life leads me to contend that a starting point for a thick ethic of relational responsibility resides in relationships of intimacy and shared bonds that reflect an aspiration for both equality and unity amidst diversity. This suggests an initial moral affinity of relationship with what philosopher Stephen Toulmin has referred to as an ethic of intimates.[35] This underlies my emphasis on a covenantal account of ethics delineated shortly. It must be

34. Kierkegaard, *Works of Love*, 317–29.
35. Toulmin, "Tyranny of Principles," 34–39.

acknowledged, however, that the historical context for the emergence of bioethics is an era of repudiation of authoritarianism (political, gender/familial, religious, medical) and assertion of the primacy of respect for the civic rights of individuals. Those origins have influenced the trend in bioethics to present the civic or political relationship of strangers as morally paradigmatic, accompanied with an explicit rejection of the domestic relational model of paternalism that may seem embedded in an ethics of intimates, and similarly, to confer moral priority on voluntary forms of relationship. It is important to examine the implications of these different relational sources for moral responsibilities further.

A common moral thread in the construction of voluntarily chosen relationships is respect for self-determination. This emphasis meshes well with a conception of rights-mediating individualism and the ethics of personal autonomy. It is often unclear, however, if respect for autonomous choice implies a correlative responsibility of personal accountability for one's actions. The question of accountability is important, for the primacy of moral voluntarism is claimed to reside in its rejection of heteronomy in which accountability is imposed on others in order to explain and even excuse personal failings. Moral voluntarism often then seems to support a conception of personal rights shorn free of relational responsibilities and accountability.

This does not mean moral voluntarism necessarily has no space for non-voluntary relationships, but rather confers on them secondary significance. This is an experiential paradox insofar as commonly, the most formative and ethically significant relationships we experience are non-voluntary relationships encountered in family settings. This includes commitments of care by children for their parents, as displayed in the narrative with which I began the book.

It is instructive that in many aspects of living out a religious witness, a person may be called into a relationship not necessarily of one's own choosing. Jesus informed many of his early followers: "You did not choose me but I chose you."[36] It is important to acknowledge the importance of voluntary moral relationships without at the same time maintaining that such relationships encompass the totality of the moral life. Moral space for responsiveness to various callings not of our own choosing seems especially significant in the context of medicine and health care since assuming a patient role and relationship is seldom voluntarily chosen.

Unquestionably, one of the signal achievements of the Enlightenment in western culture was the articulation of a philosophical (and theological) justification for liberation of the individual from tyrannical oppression and servitude to authoritarian governance. On the social contract narrative articulated by figures such as Hobbes and Locke, a moral agent possesses certain rights in virtue of his or her humanity that precede the formation of civil society and government and furthermore holds these rights in equal measure with all others. Rights language, which is considered the most prevalent form of global moral discourse and of international law, thus originates as

36. John 15:16.

a revolutionary discourse presuming adversarial relationships with strangers that manifest profound differences in power. The organization or agent possessing political, economic, scientific, or ecclesiastical power is presumed to be a threat to infringe or deprive another of their basic interests to liberty, welfare, or equal respect: the language of rights thereby provides protections in a context of distrust and of rampant self-interest. It is a powerful political and moral narrative, and as a moral discourse, the inherent rights of persons aim to affirm a grounding for the moral equality of persons, even in the midst of disparities in power. The commitment to equal respect can then give rise to practices of cooperation that mitigate self-interest and cultivate procedural, if not personal, trust.

In general, then, rights language is most at home in a relational context of distrustful and self-interested strangers rather than a context of mutually nurturing intimates. In the context of a responsible relationship of intimates, it would be very odd, if not entirely inappropriate, to assert one's human rights against the other person. Rights language does not emerge in the everyday give-and-take of domestic life, for example, because of the assumptions of cooperation and shared goals constitutive of the family. Rights language may prevail when a couple is going through divorce proceedings and there are deep disputes over possessions or over child custody; it is indicative of a deep, perhaps irreparable, rupture in trust and the prospect for adversarial conflict and heightened distrust. Rights provide protections in the context of relational ruptures.

The discourse of rights derived from the social contract narrative provided moral justification in the formative years of bioethics for the critique of professional paternalism and authority and the advocacy of various rights of vulnerable patients or research subjects to information, truthful disclosures, consent to or refusal of treatment, and protections of privacy and confidentiality. The inadequacy of the medical traditions of paternalistic beneficence is held by bioethics scholars to reside precisely in the omission of rights of the person.[37] The ongoing and expanded use of rights discourse in bioethics discloses a presumed underlying structure of inequality in the relationship of physician and patient, and the disempowerment of patients relative to health care institutions and the health care system. This relational presupposition has supported the emergence of the economic discourse of "consumerism" in contemporary medicine and health care, with its ethos of *caveat emptor* to express caution and distrust about an interaction embedded in self-interest and power. Insofar as rights language continually mediates the relationship of physician and patient, it symbolizes the fragility of relational trust, the mutually shared interests of the parties, and the necessity of cooperative practice.

My claim is that the relational presuppositions of the *imago Dei* are delineated through mutuality, reciprocity, partnerships, and trust, rather than the adversarial character of rights language. The creation narrative offers a perspective for moral

37. Veatch, *Hippocratic, Religious, and Secular*, 10–29.

relationship and responsibility that is very distinct from the narrative of social contract: a moral anthropology rooted in the *imago Dei* will not presume the asocial egoism from which relationships are only entered into for collective protection against the powerful.

The implications and complications for bioethics of identity-bestowing, sustaining, and transforming relationships will be developed in subsequent chapters addressing the meaning of healing in medical relationships. For current purposes, however, I want to expand further on the relational nature of the human person as witness of the *imago Dei* by proposing three forms of identity-bearing relationships and responsibilities: *gift* relationships, *covenantal* relationships, and *stewardship* relationships. My contention is that these forms of relationship share some common features with other forms of relationship, including relationships mediated by rights, but also go beyond alternative accounts in expectation and responsibility. I interpret relationships mediated by the moral discourse of rights to be a necessary moral minimum or floor for interactions between strangers, while relationships embedded in gift, covenant, or stewardly trust bear witness to a morality of ideals within communities.

Giftedness and Gift Relationship

Embedded in the creation narrative is a portrayal of the divine as self-giving in care and love. In the creation chronology, following the bestowal upon male and female life and form reflecting the divine image, and prior to the presentation of any commands or instructions, human beings are blessed. The form of relationship exemplified in the creation narrative is established through care and grace; human life as part of and as distinct from the natural world is characterized by a profound receptivity and responsiveness to an existential experience of what I refer to as "giftedness." The bestowal of blessing means that persons are first and foremost beneficiaries and recipients who are entrusted with their bodies, lives, and relationships, as well as responsibilities for the natural world. As no human being is self-created, human agency and claims of entitlement are necessarily secondary to the givenness and giftedness of our existence and experience. The symbol of the *imago Dei* witnesses to this gifted character of our relational identity.

The giftedness of our relational experience embeds us within an ethos of gift-response-responsibility. Although we may not recognize a gift or blessing when we receive one, in everyday experience we are seldom indifferent to them. At our best, the receipt of a gift elicits dispositions of responsive gratitude and appreciation towards another situated as a giver. The dispositional responsiveness to gifts generates a responsibility of caring for what we have received, including our life, our embodied self, our relationships, and other ways that blessings manifest as gifts (e.g., the gift of children, or the gift of health).

Situating human beings as both initially and ultimately beneficiaries of gifts and blessings (creation narrative) rather than as egoistic rights-holders (social contract narrative) displays profound ethical implications. The ethos of giftedness invites us first to consider what we share in common with other persons. Insofar as the experience of giftedness is shared with all persons, the *imago Dei* expresses that we are profoundly shaped by our interdependency with others and our solidarity with their neediness and vulnerability. Gifts have a powerful way of symbolically and ethically binding members of the human community to each other. Gifts evoke a "coming together" that can counter the atomistic individualism of the modern world.

Secondly, an awareness and experience of radical dependency opens the scope of gift-based responsibility to encompass commitment to an expanding moral community in human relationships. An analogical discourse presented in the LDS scriptural text, *The Book of Mormon*, is illustrative of the relationship of the moral commitments embedded in shared vulnerability. The narrative context for the analogy is a prophetically prescient concern about communal responsibility to care for the needy, vulnerable, and marginalized, as exemplified in the image of a "beggar." The prophetic teacher (Benjamin) expounds: "Are we not all beggars? Do we not all depend upon the same Being, even God, for all the substance which we have, for both food and raiment . . . Now, if God, who has created you, on whom you are dependent for your lives and for all that you have and are, doth grant unto you whatsoever you ask that is right, . . . then, how you ought to impart of the substance that you have one to another."[38]

The ethical analogy rests on two capacities inherent in the *imago Dei*. First, the radical dependency of all members of the community on powers beyond their control for gifts of life, sustenance, and nurture must rise through accumulated cultural experience to a level of awareness and recognition. Secondly, persons possess epistemic capacities to identify with and to empathize with vulnerable persons because vulnerability and dependency are shared and common features of the human condition. This empathetic imagination incorporates a supposition of human equality of need. The vulnerability of some persons, the needy, the stranger, the beggar, exerts itself in various subsistence needs all persons have, including food, clothing, shelter, and care in time of illness, as well as for nurturance and education. This radical dependency for our being, life, body, and health on powers we do not control entails that we are also necessarily interdependent with each other. Our responsiveness to various gifts of grace is manifested in commitments of solidarity, empathy, and fellow-feeling or compassion as expressed in caring for other equally vulnerable persons in a manner in which we have received. The witness borne by the *imago Dei* gives rise to responsibilities of care and gratitude: caring manifests gracious responsiveness to the blessing of care and grace bestowed on us. The circumstances of giftedness and interdependency,

---

38. Mosiah 4:19–21.

which are initially generated in an involuntary relationship, become a source for relationships of responsibility and meaning.

The foregoing interpretation of the human condition as fundamentally one of giftedness is arguable and contested. My interpretation of the essential giftedness of the human condition not only bears witness of equality, radical dependency, and human interdependency, but it also bears witness against contemporary constructions of our existential strangeness as subject to forces beyond our control that are indifferent to human welfare or indeed are arbitrary, abusive, and cruel, rather than creative, nurturing, and reconciling.

Alternatively, the interpretation of giftedness may seem rather alien to the ethos of the modern self that manifests as an independent moral agent who possesses in virtue of their humanity certain rights against others, but seems to have had moral responsibilities for others shorn off except those to which the agent has voluntarily consented. The prevailing cultural standard of minimally decent morality, reflected principally through rights discourse, is constituted by the negative responsibility to not inflict harm on others and by respect for their equal freedom. Moral philosophy categorizes actions to positively benefit others in the ways embedded in the relational ethos of gift-response-responsibility as an imperfect or discretionary responsibility, or as bound to social role (including professions) or as supererogatory. Responsiveness to the ill, the beggar, the homeless, the starving, and the refugee thus becomes a matter of optional philanthropy rather than a gift-initiated call to caring. Ultimately, the moral content of the modern self is situated in affirmation of respect for self-determination and formalized in the principle of respect for autonomy, and its responsibilities are self-generated by voluntarily acceptance. The resonance of such intellectualized positions in contemporary life must be conceded.

What is shared by the existentialist and the individualist paradigm is the question of power, of both subjection to arbitrary power, including natural and political and biomedical power, and of aspirations to control and mastery by the empowered self. Such a philosophical presupposition structures the interpretation of social institutions and intermediate communities—familial, educational, religious, professional—in particular authoritarian ways; it is no surprise that the emergence of the empowered patient in bioethics coincides with an interpretive structuring of medicine, the medical profession, and the medical model as the mediator of specific powers and knowledge in ways that are authoritarian, domineering, patronizing, oppressive, and paternalistic. My contention is that both the existentialist and individualistic interpretations of the human condition lead to the same kind of social and professional outcome, expressed in Camus's profound parable *The Plague* as "fighting against creation"[39] for control over ontic realties beyond our control, including beginnings and endings of our own biological being.

---

39. Camus, *Plague*, 127.

Without presuming to have resolved this metaphysical dispute, my claim is that in many aspects of everyday life, we act as if we live in a world where giftedness, manifested through creative, nurturing, and reconciling forms of interaction, is more compelling and meaningful than a world structured by indifference, arbitrariness, and egoism. Existentially, each person initially is situated as a profound recipient from others for their life and identity prior to being able to make assertions of the hostility of the world to humanity and/or the necessity of the individual self to affirm their will-to-power. We may want to start, at any rate, with a presumption of giftedness, even if that subsequently is revised and reconstructed by other experiential realities. With this presumption in mind, I present two examples that display the ethical structure of gift-response-responsibility, selected because of their profound influence in self-understanding and the shaping of a life.

The fragile and contingent giftedness of our experience complements the creative features of the *imago Dei* through the identity-conferring, relationship-constituting, and transforming experience of parenting. Each child is a gift that bears to its parents its own unique way of being. A parent's responsiveness to their child's being and vulnerability is shaped by a dynamic of unconditional love and transformational love. A parent displays near speechless wonder and awe at birth, and grateful appreciation and care for the very being and existence of the child, regardless of circumstance or distinctive identifying features. A parent's responsiveness to the gift of their child is inextricably interwoven with the parent's assumption of responsibility for the child. For, while the child's self is often identified with that of the parent, it is also ultimately beyond the parent's control. Parental nurturing, through teachings, education, and the life experiences a parent seeks to make available to his or her child, reflect a form of love to advance the well-being of the child beyond the needs of mere subsistence. Transformational love is represented in the aspiration of every parent of every generation to "give my child more opportunities" or "a better life" than the parent experienced. The possibilities inherent in gift-based responsiveness of creative and transformational love are to be distinguished from a transactional parent-child relationship in which, for example, the parent becomes a kind of domestic ATM to fund projects and purchases of the child's choosing.

A second exemplification of the ethos of gift-response-responsibility that, like parenting, I have come to appreciate from different experiential perspectives, is the profound giftedness of learning and of teaching. My academic mentors were not academics beholden to the confines of some ivory tower; they were teachers, and their concern for both the learning and the well-being of their students went well beyond the quasi-contractual expectations of a course syllabus or of academic position descriptions. Having subsequently entered the teaching profession, I seek to become for my students what my mentors were for me. I cannot reciprocate their actions, but I can expand their influence through generations by offering some transformative educational experiences for my own students.

The context for these two illustrations of a gift-bearing relationship is important to note: everyday interactions that influence the core character of our lives, rather than the interactions of strangers, which characterizes the relationship of a business to consumers, or the state to its citizenry. An important question for subsequent inquiry is whether, on a continuum from an ethics of intimates to an ethics of strangers, the physician-patient relationship is better situated within a gift-based relationship or a stranger-based relationship organized around economic or civic assumptions. That is, to what extent does this core relationship in medical ethics embody the character of giftedness and the ethos of gift-responsiveness-responsibility, and to what extent is the relationship structured by an ethos of rights-based individualism with its assumptions of adversarial power and mistrust? These questions can be approached in certain respects through the witness of the *imago Dei* to a second form of moral relationship, that of covenant.

Covenant

The moral reality of giftedness to being and experience and the incorporation of an ethical dynamic of gift-response-responsibility gives rise to a specific form of relationship described in the religious traditions as covenantal. The symbol of the *imago Dei* situates persons with a context of giving and receiving identity-affirming and identity-transforming covenants. A covenantal relationship, such as embedded in a marriage, is transformative rather than transactional in nature.[40] The transactional relationship, as intimated in the ATM example, interprets relationship as a means to the exchange of goods extraneous to the self. In the context of a covenantal commitment, a person's identity and self are intrinsically bound up in and found through the relationship, and consequently, their way of being in the world with others is altered. Consistent with the reciprocal gift-character of the relationship, a covenant binds the covenantal parties to each other.

Although bioethics discourse occasionally conflates covenant with agreements in a contractual relation, a covenant implies a very different moral structure and logic. A covenant is always conveyed in a relationship-initiating gift, such as in the pronounced goodness of creation and gifts as blessings bestowed on human beings, as well as the giving of self in a loving or marital context. An invitation to a covenantal relationship symbolizes giving rather than merit, grace and mercy rather than negotiation, and delineation of terms for agreement. The moral structure of covenant thereby reinforces the ethos of gift-response-responsibility and expands the ethic to incorporate an identity-transforming dimension. The moral structure of a covenantal ethic is organized according to the following features: *giftedness, responsiveness, binding promise, relational fidelity, transformed identity, embodied trust,* and *renewal.*

40. May, *Physician's Covenant*, 124–36.

Although numerous covenantal relationships are attested to in religious narratives, the central illustration of the meaning and structure of covenant is presented through the archetypical Exodus narrative: Hebrew slaves are delivered from bondage in Egypt, and following a perilous journey in desert wilderness, enter into a covenantal relationship with Yahweh in the holy mountain of Sinai, and thereby assume a responsibility of fidelity that will transform their identity into the people of Israel chosen as an example to other nations. The narrative illustrates that covenantal relations and identity-transformation are experiential processes: Yahweh's gift of deliverance of the slaves from oppression is accompanied by a reminder of their giftedness prior to the covenantal commitment. The preface to the covenant of the Decalogue reiterates to the former slaves their history and calls them to memory of their deliverance: "I am the Lord your God, who brought you out of the land of Egypt, out of the house of slavery."[41] Having been delivered from involuntary bondage, the covenant represents a voluntary form of binding of Israel to God.

This narrative history prior to the covenant and this call to remembrance of the gift of deliverance differentiates a covenantal ethic from a contractual ethic, and also differentiates a gift-responsiveness ethic from a command-obedience ethic. Giftedness is enacted through the deliverance of the slaves from oppression; responsiveness is manifested by the willingness of the people to bind themselves as a moral community with a covenantal commitment to their deliverer; responsibility involves an acceptance of, and binding to, a way of life shaped by moral obligations as well as a promise of presence and a witness to live in fidelity to the covenant over time; and the covenant, as expressed in the Decalogue, symbolizes transformative liberation from enslavement as individuals to freedom as a community called to bear witness in the world.

The covenant at Sinai has moral content, containing restrictions, responsibilities, and promises. As biblical scholar Walter Harrelson observes, the intent internal to the covenant is to provide moral parameters for the common life of a free people and community: The Decalogue "refines the character and ethos of Israel's life with God, and it does so in ways that liberate and also confine the life of the community."[42] The responsibilities inherent in the covenantal commitment highlight the binding nature of a covenant, but as responsibility is preceded and framed by the gift-source of covenantal relations, a covenant does not imply a relation of oppression and disempowerment.

The covenant is ratified by the new moral community through a mutual promise of ongoing fidelity that is to be continually remembered and renewed through practice and ritual. The prior gift of deliverance from oppressive power is carried forward and shapes the present covenantal partnership and the promise of a common future. The relationship is identity-transforming for both parties; persons whose basic identity has been shaped by tribal membership and oppression are invited to become a

41. Exod 20:2.
42. Harrelson, "Decalogue," 146–47.

unified and free people, while a God associated with particular persons (Abraham, Isaac, Jacob) becomes a God of a choice and treasured people.

The external and visible nature of a covenantal relationship is often witnessed to through an embodied enactment of a ritual that includes an embedded promise or vow. In diverse religious settings, believers participate in rituals such as baptisms, sacraments, or mitzvah celebrations that acknowledge the identity-creating gift, embrace the binding relationship, and embody their commitments. In the covenants that mediate human relationships, marriage partners exchange vows and emblems of commitment such as rings, parents offer both accepting and transformative nurturing and care to children, and friends make oaths of loyalty to each other. Even young children understand that engaging in a "pinky swear" or becoming "blood" siblings invests a relationship with a deeper commitment than a signed agreement that represents the transactional nature of contractual relations.

The coming together that occurs in establishing a covenantal relation is not simply a one-time occurrence that forever lasts. The renewal of a covenant presupposes a remembering of the formative promises and responsibilities, a retelling and a re-storying of the relationship, and a restoring of fidelity, presence, and the solidarity of being bound together in partnership for a common purpose. A covenant situates a person or community not only in place, but also within history, within time, entering an open future even while looking backward. The narrative embeddedness of a covenant means a covenantal ethic can unite past, present, and future. The processes of remembering, re-storying, and renewing provide sustainability, resilience, and resolution to live up to covenantal aspirations. The covenantal relation does not become a relic, but always permeates the present and thereby shapes the future. Just as promises are not made to be broken, so also a covenantal relation is not created to be forgotten.

The profound transformation of identity embedded in a covenantal relationship is underscored by the biblical symbol for human neglect or violation of the covenant as infidelity. The covenant is an expression of relationship premised on trust, giftedness, gratitude, fidelity, and mutual care; a broken covenant symbolizes not simply rejection of ethical responsibilities, but also of the binding character of transformed identities and ethos embedded in the covenant. A covenantal ethic is in part comprised of "giving back" in the context of a gift-initiated relationship; by contrast, betrayal involves "going back" on responsiveness and commitment and cannot be a matter of moral indifference.

A central issue in explicating the covenantal meaning of the *imago Dei* is the scope of gift-based covenantal relationships. In a thoughtful analysis, Bouma and colleagues contend that moral covenants in human relationships share three primary features with religious covenants. Human covenants are rooted in events, gifts, or actions that make persons vulnerable to others; covenants form and provide the bond of moral community; and covenants persist over time in an open-ended and unspecifiable manner.[43] These features distinguish the moral relationship of a covenant from transactional, contract-based relationships as typified in a commercial exchange of services. The covenantal commitment is not a relationship for book-keeping about transactions and exchanges, or for delineating the decent minimum of relational interaction. Such an account implies the resonance of a covenantal relational structure in marriage, family, and perhaps in some friendships, as well as in the relationship of some focused communities, including religious communities.

In marriage, family, and some friendships, the covenantal bond is initiated and solidified through the reciprocal responsiveness of gratefulness and promise that call each person to go beyond personal interests through fidelity and loyalty to the covenantal partner. This implies patient commitment and the virtue of long-suffering as witness to the continuation of the relationship over time and circumstance. These virtues are embedded in practices that cultivate renewal of the ethos of gift and display a gracious, caring response to the needs of the other person.

The open-ended feature of covenantal commitment to the ongoing nature of the relationship enables the relationship to persist even through what Aristotle describes as the shared "salt" of difficult times.[44] The metaphor of salt notes that salt is difficult to consume directly, but its presence also preserves, enlivens, brings out differences previously hidden, and offers the promise of transforming. In contrast to contractual and transactional exchanges, the absence of specific performance clauses in covenantal relationships implies that the moral focus of covenant is on dispositions of character and virtues including caring, fidelity, forgiveness, gratitude, mutuality, reciprocity, solidarity, and trust. It follows that the open-ended character of covenantal commitment does not entail that anything goes, but rather is framed with the ethos of gift-responsiveness-responsibility-transformation that is open to continual renewal.

Beyond the ethics of intimates, the question is whether the scope and ethical structure of covenant can be extended to other human relationships. Some recent literature on medical professionalism portrays the relationship between medicine and society through the language of covenant. A 2005 report issued by the Royal College of Physicians, for example, observes: "[Medicine's success] has been and remains founded upon a covenant between the medical profession and society . . . The terms of that covenant will change as the relationship between doctors and society changes."[45] However, covenantal language appears very infrequently in the report relative to the relationship between members of the medical community or between physician and patient.

An instructive appeal to covenantal language is also provided in the APA Code of Ethics for Pharmacists, the first precept of which refers to respect for the "covenantal relationship between the patient and the pharmacist." An explanatory

43. Bouma et al., *Christian Faith*, 84–85.

44. Aristotle, *Nicomachean Ethics*, 220.

45. Royal College, *Doctors in Society*, 1.

statement embeds the covenant within a gift ethos, that is, the covenantal framework is appropriate since a "pharmacist has moral obligations in response to the gift of trust received from society."[46] I have found that the meaning of covenantal language is often lost on professional pharmacy students. However, the important question is not so much whether the specific language of covenant is used in statements articulating the professional commitments of medicine, pharmacy, or of other healing professions as much as whether the ethical structure of gift-responsiveness-responsibility-transformation can be discerned in professional relationships or in relationships between professionals and their patients.

For now, I will leave the questions about the scope and applicability of a covenantal ethos for medical professionalism and bioethics open with the intent to engage these issues more fully in my analysis of calling, healing, and covenant in medicine (chapters 5 and 6). My principal claim at this stage is that a distinctive form of human relationship is embedded in the *imago Dei.* Covenant provides a different model of being-in-relationship that directs moral attention to transformative relationships as distinct from transactional exchanges mediated by rights-claims. The covenant responsibility embedded in the gift ethos serves as a potent moral ideal and aspiration and bears witness of alternative moral structures in relationships.

Stewardship

A third form of relational identity embedded in the *imago Dei* is an entrustment of stewardship. The stewardship metaphor provides direction about how to enact gift-bearing covenantal responsibilities. The context in the creation narrative within which a principle of entrusted stewardship is most commonly derived is through the mandate or covenantal responsibility bestowed on humans to assume dominion over nature. I invoke the language of stewardship rather than dominion as informed by discourse in my own tradition which stresses a pervasive tendency in human beings to engage routinely in "unrighteous dominion."[47] Moreover, "dominion over" rather than "stewardship of" implies a fundamental separation of humanity from creation that diminishes the embedded gift ethos and its accompanying responsibilities of care and trust. The problematic implications of the language of dominion are reinforced by critiques of the Christian tradition since the beginning of the era of environmental consciousness that the dominion mandate of the creation narrative has been enacted through anthropocentric domination and exploitation.[48] My claim here is not that nomenclature absolves responsibility, but rather that stewardship responsibilities cannot be uncoupled from their embeddedness in an ethos of giftedness and of covenantal relationship.

46. American Pharmacists Association, "Code of Ethics," principle 1.

47. *Doctrine and Covenants* 121:39.

48. White, "Historical Roots," 1203–7.

Though the moral status of human beings is expressed through the symbol of the *imago Dei*, we are nonetheless creatures of the earth, an identity that is reinforced through the shared etymological roots of "human" and "earth" in the term *humus*. The divine gift that bestows the blessing of covenantal responsibility enjoins commitments of both caring for and cultivating the earth and the natural world. More generally, insofar as the *imago Dei* is expressed through stewardship of various gifts we have received, whether these are ecological or pertain to our personal life, our embodiment, or the lives and welfare of others-in-relation, such as children, a balance of caring for and cultivating of such gifts is required. As delineated in the discussion of parenting above, this balance can be conceptualized as a dynamic between accepting and transforming responsiveness; accepting responsibilities in the absence of transformative intent may reflect ungracious apathy, while transforming in the absence of caring acceptance may obscure the original giftedness and manifest egoistic expressions of power. My intention in the following is to provide seven distinguishable features that serve as moral criteria by which a responsible stewardship ethic can be assessed.

Entrustment. The entrustment of stewardship is part of the covenantal blessing bestowed upon human beings. Stewardship is a gift-bearing responsibility within which is embedded gracious responsiveness and conduct. Stewardship thus witnesses to matters of grace and gift rather than right or merit. Stewardship presupposes a recognition that ultimately "the earth is the Lord's,"[49] a reality that imposes restraints of accountability. The divine call and trust of caring for and cultivating creation or other gifts is constituted at its core by mutual trust—that is, by the mediating moral conditions of covenant fidelity. Human persons embodying the *imago Dei* must be attentive to the qualities of character that must be embodied and enacted to be worthy of an ongoing commitment of trust.

Authorization. The covenantal relationship delegates to persons authorization for responsible use of what they have received through the nexus of giftedness. Moral responsibility is thereby situated within a context of accountability and answerability rather than anthropocentric authoritarianism, unrestrained dominion, or isolated individualism. The "binding" nature of covenantal commitment both liberates and constrains. Persons as stewards can exercise moral agency, but they do not have authorization to act in ways that betray the giftedness of the relationship. The concept of stewardship authorization means responsibility and accountability for ensuring that decision-making processes and outcomes reflect fidelity to the prescribed intentions of caring and cultivating the gift, blessing, or trust.

Agency. Persons are moral agents who have responsibility for acting with creativity and initiative in a manner that accords with their status as *imago Dei* rather than waiting for directions about specific performance as implied by a contractual exchange. This stewardship reliance on creative agency symbolizes the open-ended and unspecifiable moral commitments embedded in the covenantal ethos. The exercise of

49. Ps 24:1.

moral agency requires the use of imagination, discernment, interpretation, deliberation, and informed judgment to enact responsibilities. Stewardship responsibilities thereby become a tutorial for moral character.

Beneficence. As embedded in the ethos of gift-responsiveness-responsibility-transformation, the substantive moral direction for personal agency in the context of a stewardship entrustment consists in seeking to bring benefits to other persons. The stewardship call to balance the responsibilities of caring and cultivating entails subordinating personal self-interest or the self-serving interests of a larger community to the good of the commons. Biblical teaching interprets the beneficence of stewardship as a matter of service to other persons: "Like good stewards of the manifold grace of God serve one another with whatever gift each of you has received."[50] This construction of stewardship implies neither self-renunciation nor self-indulgent egoism, but rather a balanced moderation such that many benefit without detriment to the welfare of others.

Sufficiency. The core evil in the biblical traditions that manifests infidelity to the covenantal relationship and betrays entrustment is neglect of the poor, the vulnerable, the needy, or the stranger. The point is not simply that those with excess are indifferent to the basic needs of others, but more fundamentally, they do not even notice those who experience deprivation and bypass the vulnerable, the stranger, or the wounded. The exemplification of this pattern of culpable obliviousness in the Gospels is conveyed in the narrative of the Good Samaritan parable (I devote chapter 4 to an exposition of the bioethical relevance of this parable).[51] The moral threshold for responsible stewardship is that of sufficiency: a minimal level of goods sufficient for the basic needs of living is necessary for each person. There is no room in the ethics of covenantal stewardship for prioritizing advancement of the "1 percent" economic elite.

There is furthermore no conceptual room in the ethics of responsible stewardship for the concept of a "prosperity gospel" or "prosperity theology."[52] The basic features of the prosperity gospel movement all run contrary to the ethical concepts I have emphasized, including contract rather than covenant, entitlement rather than giftedness, empowerment rather than embodiment, and dominion rather than stewardship. I have claimed moreover that an essential feature of the gift-bearing covenant is an assessment of our radical dependency; our fundamental nature as "beggars" who receive manifold blessings from the divine analogically entails a moral commitment of hospitality to the stranger within the moral community.

Prosperity as an end-in-itself is an illustration of unjust stewardship and unrighteous dominion. The purpose of prosperity is to cultivate dispositions of empathy,

---

50. 1 Pet 4:10.

51. Luke 10:25–37.

52. Bowler, *Blessed*, 3–40.

solidarity, and charity. The moral presupposition of covenantal sufficiency is our capacity to identify with the other, the stranger, the beggar, or the vulnerable.

Creative Expansiveness. The entrustment of responsibility requires exercise of agency as directed by divinely-bestowed creativity to cultivate the gift, blessing, and trust and so expand or magnify its extent and impact for a greater number of persons. Cultivation or transformational responsiveness need not violate caring or accepting responsiveness. So long as the sufficiency criterion is satisfied, persons may use their agency and their creative capacities to enhance or expand the gifts they have received. This includes cultivating and expanding the gifts of knowledge regarding nature and the human body to provide caring and treatment for ill persons. It appears to be part of human nature that some persons will express gracious responsiveness for all good gifts by expanding the goods with which they have been entrusted, while others will assert entitlements to the detriment of their trust and the deprivation of others.

Accountability. The person called to responsible stewardship is ultimately accountable for oversight and exercise of their trust as guided by these seven ethical concepts of a stewardship ethic. Moral agents who bear witness to the image of the divine in the world must give an accounting of moral choices undertaken and present an assessment of the extent to which they have engaged in a fair, expansive, and beneficent stewardship, or instead have practiced in a manner illustrative of an unrighteous dominion.

The relational commitments and trust of stewardship stresses not only actions and processes, but also exemplary characteristics or virtues. These include trust, fidelity and loyalty, joyful acceptance of gifts, gratitude, empathy, moderation, benevolence, justness, creativity, and accountability. These characteristics bear witness against the qualities implicit in a consumer or transactional paradigm of relationships, which tends to permeate contemporary health care and even professional-patient relationships. In the name of instrumentalized efficiencies, the transaction or exchange model implies diminished trusting relationships, maximized self-interest, and absence of accountability. In a complex global economy, and a complicated and convoluted health care system, not all actions or outcomes can manifest responsible stewardship, but the virtue characteristics can be cultivated and sustained.

Moral Agency

Our capacity for moral choice is not only an aspect of the *imago Dei*, but a necessary condition for the manifestation of each characteristic of the *imago Dei*. I have situated the discussion of moral agency last not because it is the least important of these eight foundational concepts, but rather to emphasize that any argumentation on the moral self that neglects agency is incomplete and inadequate.

I frequently use the language of moral agency to signal some of the differences between the secular principle of respect for autonomous choices and the religious principle embedded in the theological concept of the *imago Dei*; moral agency is more closely aligned with a principle of respect for persons, including their embodied life, than the narrower principle of respect for choices of an autonomous self. Furthermore, moral agency is necessarily coupled with accountability, just as rights to choose are correlated with responsibilities for choices and outcome. Moral agents are answerable to various audiences of moral accountability, including conscience, community, professional peers, and the divine. Our finitude and fallibility make it difficult to predict and control the courses and outcomes of actions that we initiate. If we make mistakes in judgment, or err in decisions, it is morally preferable to err on the side of decisions that are reversible and revocable. Moral agency is then differentiated from autonomy in the sense that a context-oriented form of the precautionary principle is embedded within agency.

A second difference is that human beings do not come into personal accountability as moral *tabula rasa*. There is little question that our values are inscripted through parental upbringing, peer influence in schools, religious education, and other forms of socialization. However, beyond socialization processes of values, each person possesses a minimal knowledge of right and wrong that presents foundational moral standards of accountability for actions. In Christian and even forms of secular philosophical thought, this minimal moral content has often been articulated through the concept of conscience. Moral agency implies then that some minimal standards of morality are intrinsic to our personhood; such standards do not require discovery through revelation, nor construction through social interaction, nor invention in radical, existentialist freedom, though these methods all have a place in social morality.

This is not to deny that the content of rightness and wrongness can vary from culture to culture, from time period to time period, or that the overlay of the accretions of culture can become predominant in personal decision-making. Anne Fadiman's masterpiece of medical anthropology, *The Spirit Catches You and You Fall Down*, marvelously illustrates contrasting worldviews about health and disease in the Hmong community from those of American medicine.[53] While both shamanistic traditions in Hmong culture and the practices of American medicine are oriented by a commitment to healing, what comprises healing is culturally conditioned. In the specific account narrated by Fadiman, conflicting worldviews influenced different courses of action desired by a Hmong family about the care of a young female child for her epileptic seizures that were contrary to those prescribed by the physicians.

The situatedness of ethical commitments within background (and sometimes, foreground) worldviews makes the articulation of ethical reflection a very challenging enterprise, and it is the primary reason for placing this chapter preceding any ethical analysis of concrete bioethical issues. Nonetheless, the intrinsic standards of moral accountability resist a collapse of morality into ethical relativism, subjectivism, or a post-modernist ethic of "speak your own truth." This means it can be appropriate to

53. Fadiman, *Spirit Catches You*, 20–118.

say to someone who rationalizes or excuses a morally reprehensible action as compatible with cultural practices that they could not not have known the action was wrong. It is also the case that our conceptions of wrongness are often more refined than conceptions of the right or good; we are more capable, or at least more vocal, about determinations of unfairness than of fairness, or about specifying what comprises indignity in dying than we are about the meaning of a dignified death.

Agency and Moral Conflict. The criteria and standards of moral agency and accountability are especially demanding when we encounter circumstances of moral conflict or dilemma, that is, when a choice needs to be made between various goods or between lesser evils than in circumstances when we confront a choice between a manifest right and wrong. These latter circumstances often pose considerations of moral psychology, of weakness of will, of human finiteness and fallibility. The moral question in this analysis concerns having the dispositions or inclinations to *do what one knows* to be good.

The moral questions encountered in bioethics seldom are of this kind of conflict, but are more frequently infused with our finitude and uncertainty about *knowing the good* when basic values may be in conflict with each other.[54] It is a basic good of moral experience as well as medical practice to act in ways that promote the welfare, interests, and embodied experience of other persons. It is also a basic good to relieve the pain or suffering of wounded or sick persons. In the account of the *imago Dei* I have presented, these goods are implied by the commitments to gift, covenantal, and stewardship relations. Yet, it is not uncommon in contemporary medicine for the commitment to protect and prolong life to conflict with the commitment to relieve pain and suffering. This conflict resides at the core of ethical and professional disputes regarding legalization of physician-assistance in hastening a patient's death (discussed more fully in chapter 9). An ethical dilemma requires choosing one responsibility or value as primary, even if it infringes or compromises the validity of another good or value. These kinds of conflicts are embedded in the moral landscape of contemporary bioethics.

The accountability implied by moral agency thereby emerges predominantly in the context of ethical conflict of good with good (or wrong with wrong) and is manifested through bearing witness to a process of integrity in answering. The moral logic of answering is structured by several interrelated considerations arranged here in a sequential, albeit existentially arbitrary, fashion.

Moral Rationale. A first criterion for accountability is the good or value that is protected or promoted by the action under deliberation. This good should be related to an aspect of the *imago Dei* as delineated in this chapter—that is, the value should reflect on the fundamental welfare (physical, emotional, relational, spiritual) of a person or community. This consideration enables an initial differentiation between ethically acceptable and ethically unacceptable courses of action insofar as the infringement or

54. Lemmon, "Moral Dilemmas," 139–58.

compromise of one value should not occur in the absence of promoting or protecting a value of equal or greater value.

Moral Deliberation. Moral agency incorporates the creative and imaginative aspect of the *imago Dei* to require an imaginative rehearsal of alternative courses of action and a reflective method to assure a selected action can protect or promote the value. From an array of ethically acceptable actions, the moral agent engaged in deliberation can discern ethically preferable actions.

Moral Necessity. A further element of answering with moral integrity involves assessment of whether there are any alternatives that could express the value or realize the good without any infringement on the conflicting value. This requires both imagination and fact-finding to ensure that compromise of one value is really necessary. It is often claimed, for example, that many ethical issues in end-of-life care are ultimately attributable to obstacles or problems in communication. There is no need for moral infringement if a different communication pattern will remedy the conflict. The proposed course of action should be both ethically preferable and morally necessary.

Effectiveness. A basic pragmatic test of ethical integrity must consider the extent to which the contemplated action will be effective in protecting or promoting the particular good or value. This demonstrates the importance, though not sufficiency, of instrumentalist rationality in ethical reasoning. In philosophical parlance, an act that "can" be performed does not mean it "ought" to be performed, but an act that "cannot" be carried out precludes the action from being considered as a plausible alternative in moral deliberation. Answering in moral agency thereby adds to both moral necessity and ethical preferability a condition of practical feasibility.

Moral Residue. If the expression or realization of one value necessarily requires infringement of another value, the action should be designed to minimize the impact on the infringed value rather than erode its significance. The value chosen against cannot be dismissed as irrelevant or extraneous; it retains influence for the dispositions and intentionality of the moral agent. The experience of moral residue places restraints on ethically warranted infringements so that they do not become habitual violations to the extent that the good disappears from the moral landscape. Some process of restoring the meaning and relevance of the value chosen against is symbolically necessary.[55]

Publicity. The course of action chosen as well as the agent's process of deliberative integrity should be capable of being explicated and defended before and acceptable to a range of moral audiences, inclusive of but not exhausted by professional peers and a broader community of ethical witnesses.

With this account of the integrity of answering embedded in the feature of moral agency of the *imago Dei* in mind, let me turn in conclusion to an overview of some of the implications of this interpretation for the ethics of respect for autonomy in bioethics. It is important to recognize that few aspects of bioethics have had more

---

55. Walzer, "Political Action," 160–80.

practical import than advocacy of the self-determination of decisionally-capable patients to make choices regarding their own health care, their own bodies, their own determinations of how and when to die. The bioethics literature has appropriately focused on respect for patient self-determination given the historical legacy of physician dominance and patient passivity and disempowerment ascribed by identification with the sick role of the patient.

In the wake of advocacy of the moral authority of patients, however, bioethics has struggled to articulate a morally reasonable balance between empowerment and accountability, particularly within the relational context of health care professional and patient. When moral cues turn from the family (paternalism) to the market (contractarianism), the model of patient as consumer emerges as an extension of an active, participatory role assumed by patients with autonomy but substantially diminished accountability.

A robust conception of moral agency does not mean patients are duty-free in the way the principle of respect for autonomy presupposes. Moral agency affirms that persons are empowered with freedom for action, and seeks to strike an appropriate balance of freedom with accountability. This balance of agency and accountability is differentiated from an authoritarianism that makes persons passive objects that are acted upon, and also from a libertarianism that avoids accountability.

A first implication of moral agency is that patients are agents with responsibilities to engage in actions most conducive to good health. While I certainly advocate for universal access to basic health care as a matter of social justice and covenantal stewardship, such a claim to a positive moral right is correlated with positive responsibilities for personal health and caring for the gift of one's physical body. Empirical knowledge that lifestyle behaviors and the social determinants of health are much more significant for good health than the receipt of quality medical care[56] means patients who have received health care education have primary responsibility for enacting healthy lifestyle behaviors, and for relying on the health care system to first provide preventive health care and secondarily sick care.

Secondly, within the context of a clinical relationship, patients assume a positive responsibility for truthful disclosure; patients are accountable for a truthful witness of their story. "Everyone lies" was the cynical view of the primary physician-diagnostician in the popular television drama *House M.D.* I am unclear that there is empirical evidence to back up this claim; it made for good entertainment, but may be detached from the moral realities of the relationship. The emphasis on patient privacy and the documented experience of interrupting physicians may mean that patients do not so much lie as withhold very personal information. Physicians who are patient and are healers do not interrupt the patient's narratives within twelve seconds,[57] nor seek through interruptions to divert the patient from the moral witness of storytelling. For

56. Schroeder, "We Can Do Better," 121–28.
57. Rhoades, "Speaking and Interruptions," 528–32.

a patient whose body is exposed and whose person is vulnerable before the physician, a veiled rather than a naked personality is understandable. This in turn entails that it is the physician who needs the virtue of patience such that the trust necessary for complete disclosure of the patient's story can be cultivated.

A third implication of this account of moral agency is that when the patient, or a patient's family, rejects the recommendations of the physician, they should have a morally coherent reason. Moral accountability requires answering others when they inquire as to the nature of a refusal. Often, refusals appeal to the values the patient espouses, or has lived by their entire life, which would be compromised or negated by a medical intervention. However, it is sometimes difficult to sort out such values, particularly in the context of surrogate decision-making. I live in a region of the nation that has among the highest rates of parental refusals of vaccinations for their children, with one city having approximately one-quarter of their school children not having had pre-school vaccinations. While I accept that in many circumstances, such decisions do reflect family values and lifestyles, the absence of a legal requirement for the parents to give voice to the rationale for their objections is morally and culturally problematic. Consequently, the public and professional default has been that the parents' reasons or values are religious in nature, even though state law permits exemptions based on philosophical and ethical reasons. Significantly, a recent study implies that none of the parental reasons for refusing vaccination for children are religious-based.[58]

Fourth, moral agency protects freedom of conscience from being disregarded or silenced by authoritarian imposition. This is applicable not only to patients, or parents of minors in the vaccination context, but also is relevant to physicians and health professionals. An appeal to conscience is a form of moral agency that pertains to the preservation of personal integrity.[59] Morally controversial circumstances, most often pertaining to reproductive choices or to end-of-life decisions, arise when a physician, whose professional commitments are bounded by responsibilities of presence and non-abandonment, refuses a patient request for a particular procedure on the grounds that participation would violate the physician's personal integrity and moral self. The commitment to non-abandonment, however, does not disappear; the condition of moral residue entails that the physician who refuses to participate in the procedure has a professional and moral responsibility to provide information about the procedure and offer to transfer the patient to another physician or health care facility when requested. (I develop a more extended discussion of conflicts of conscience in chapter 11.)

Moral agency is equally important in the context of citizens who may be confronted with oppressive or unjust laws or institutional systems. The principle of self-determination provides social space for the autonomy of religions as well as professions.

58. Hough-Telford, "Vaccine Delays," 2127.
59. Wicclair, *Conscientious Objection*, 1–8.

Such communities function to protect the freedoms and agency of persons and their constituent communities from the oppression or tyranny of other religious communities, from professional authoritarianism or from the power of the state. My forebearers, for example, walked a thousand miles across the Great Plains and into a deserted desert wilderness of a different country (Mexico) so that they could exercise moral agency with respect to religious liberty. The opportunities for responsible exercise of agency are greater in a liberal, democratic, and pluralistic society, but likewise so are the prospects for irresponsible agency.

Conclusion: *Imago Dei* and "Playing God"

The central claim of moral anthropology in this chapter is that human beings are bearers of the image of God or *imago Dei*. The content of this phrase is informed in part by interpretations about the divine nature and about our world, and in part through interpretations of the formative creation narrative within which the phrase is initially articulated. I have sought to provide substantive expositions of ethically relevant concepts embedded in the phrase, including those of creativity, narrative, embodiment, and relationship, as enacted through gift, covenantal, and stewardship relations, and moral agency. This exposition has supported my claim that the *imago Dei* is inclusive of, but must mean more than, our capacities for conscious self-reflection. Subsequent chapters display the bioethical implications of this interpretation of the *imago Dei*. I want to conclude this chapter by briefly distinguishing the concept of *imago Dei* from the oft-criticized concept of "playing God."

The metaphor of "playing God" is one of several conversation stoppers in bioethics. It has been critiqued by scholars as well as by national bioethics commissions.[60] In general terms, the phrase is invoked as a reaction to and against medical developments and technologies that have placed immense powers of creation and extension of life and god-like powers to design miraculous machines into the hands of researchers and the medical profession. Decisions about use of these powers and technologies are pervaded by human finitude, fallibility, and fragility, and consequently may be interpreted as both arbitrary and over-reaching of important limits.

As such, the concept of "playing God" bespeaks a different concern than I present in this interpretation of the *imago Dei*. The advent of new technologies, as one expression of human creativity, has shaped bioethics from its very inception. The claim that, as a further expression of human creativity, medicine must be construed as an art in complementarity with the science of medicine, informs understandings about the purposes and goals of medicine. The development of these technologies not only fits within a prevailing narrative of linear scientific progress and mastery of mortality, but also may require reinterpretations and re-storying of other narratives. The human

---

60. Childress, *Practical Reasoning*, 14–16.

body is inescapably the object of both the science of medicine and the art of healing, and the bioethical question is, in part, how it may be possible for patients, for members of the healing professions, and for citizens to maintain the dispositions of awe and wonder invoked by the body as *imago Dei* while engaging in invasive procedures of bodily integrity even for the purposes of healing.

The ethos of gift-response-responsibility-transformation has salience for several important bioethical questions, including the relationship between physicians and patients, the distinction between therapeutic and enhancement interventions, gifts of body tissue for research, transplantation, and education, and fairness in the allocation of medical resources, as well as whether medical care is best understood as a good of the public commons or a private commodity organized primarily by a market structured around consumer preference.[61] The concept of moral agency embedded in the *imago Dei* is similarly at the core of numerous questions, such as the moral responsibility of physicians for listening to the stories by which patients truthfully bear witness of their illness experience, and the contested issue of patient requests to die with dignity through a prescription from their physician of a lethal medication. All these manifest ways that human beings bear witness to the prevalence of meaning in their encounters with medicine and bioethics.

61. Goldhill, "American Health Care," 38–55.

4

Bearing the Story

The Good Samaritan in Bioethics

In late May 2017, a white supremacist directed verbal insults and assaults at two young women, one of whom was wearing a *hijab* or head covering, while they were riding a mass transit train in Portland, Oregon. Three men intervened and requested that the man cease his hateful speech and leave the train at its next stop. Instead, Jeremy Joseph Christian used a knife to stab each of the men, inflicting fatal wounds in two of them, and injuring the other person critically, before departing the train and eventually being captured by police.

In the midst of mourning and public outcries for civility, the three persons who sought to protect the young women—Ricky John Best, Taliesin Myrddin Namkai-Meche, and Micah David-Cole Fletcher—were valorized as heroes and "good Samaritans." Oregon's governor encouraged citizens to "take the example of the good Samaritans who sacrificed their lives for the safety of others" and come together in unity rather than support cultural divisiveness.[1]

Living in relative proximity to these events, I found myself surprised at how frequently the discourse of "Samaritan" was invoked in both news media and by public officials to refer to the actions of the three men. They were more than just good citizens, more than heroes even; their interventions were taken to embody self-sacrificial concern for others that had a profound moral and religious character. Although the Samaritan allusion escaped most of my students, the civic resonance of the "good Samaritan" language would not have made much sense in the absence of a moral culture comprised of a few shared narratives. Ultimately, the designation of a person as a "Samaritan" traces back to a biblical parable related by Jesus. The Good Samaritan

1. Marco et al., "Portland Train Stabbings," para. 35.

parable retains meaning not only within religious communities, but also within professions, especially the medical profession, as well as in the broader society.

The parable has come down to us in an account given by a physician, Luke. Jesus initially is responding to a question about the greatest commandment in the *Torah*. His reply to love God and love one's neighbor is problematized by a legalistic questioner who inquires, "who is my neighbor?" Jesus answers not from Scripture but with a story:

> A man was going down from Jerusalem to Jericho, and fell into the hands of robbers, who stripped him, beat him, and went away, leaving him half dead. Now by chance a priest was going down that road; and when he saw him, he passed by on the other side. So likewise a Levite, when he came to the place and saw him, passed by on the other side. But a Samaritan while traveling came near him; and when he saw him, he was moved with pity. He went to him and bandaged his wounds, having poured oil and wine on them. Then he put him on his own animal, brought him to an inn, and took care of him. The next day he took out two denarii, gave them to the innkeeper, and said, "Take care of him; and when I come back, I will repay you whatever more you spend."

Using this re-storying as context for understanding the teachings of *Torah*, Jesus then continues the conversation, asking the questioner, "Which of these three, do you think, was a neighbor to the man who fell into the hands of the robbers?" He said, "The one who showed him mercy." Jesus said to him, "Go and do likewise."[2]

Few stories in the moral legacy of western culture are as evocative of moral imagination and responsibility. The parable is the definitive expression and exemplification of Christian love for the neighbor and the stranger. As evidenced by the numerous health care institutions and programs denominated by the term "Samaritan," the parable has also had a profound influence on the historical and institutional ethos of medicine. The medical appropriation of the biblical narrative as a symbol for and witness to the caring and compassionate nature of medicine extends to members of the healing professions. Ethicist Larry Churchill observed, "The one figure of virtue which most forcefully and clearly has captured the imagination of physicians is the Good Samaritan."[3]

There has been a dynamic of discourse about the role of the parable in bioethics discussions, with some scholars finding it to provide an influential moral frame, while others contend that it is of limited moral relevance, even morally uninteresting, for contemporary bioethics. Its manifest focus on a dyadic interpersonal relationship between a giver of care and a recipient in need seems to provide little moral direction when moral horizons expand to encompass the social. The parable emphasizes love,

2. Luke 10:25–37.
3. Churchill, *Rationing Health Care*, 3.

mercy, empathy, compassion, and expressions of beneficence, all valuable virtues in interpersonal interactions, but arguably has limited applicability to competing claims of rights or principles of justice.

In this discussion, I wish to examine the different approaches and uses of the Samaritan parable in bioethics (and in the medical humanities more broadly) as illustrative of the moral potency of narrative. My interpretation analyzes five possible methods for incorporation of the parable in contemporary bioethical discourse, highlighting features of (1) moral perception and corrective ethical vision; (2) professional identity; (3) moral aspiration; (4) limited moral maxims in circumstances of scarcity; and (5) a form of prophetic witness and solidarity. The feature of prophetic witness, which I take to be central to the purpose of the parable, seems to have been missed entirely in bioethical discussions.

Moral Perception

One reason the Good Samaritan parable has a continuing relevance to contemporary medicine and secular bioethics is suggested by medical ethicist and historian Albert Jonsen: Along with other formative stories in religious and classical texts, the parable helps shapes our moral vision and perception. Jonsen contends, "A parable, like a myth, stimulates our imagination to see in ancient words a modern problem."[4] Jonsen's metaphor of "seeing" conveys critical meaning. As much as bioethics is recognized for providing various tools and methods to resolve moral problems in medicine and health care policy, the first moral task concerns recognizing the problems and issues, both as problems and as moral problems, as distinct from scientific or economic or political problems.

Narratives, stories, parables, and myths provide moral framing to envision what questions need to be raised. The moral power of any parable, metaphor, story, or mythic symbol resides in significant measure in its impact on moral perception and imagination, and in its evocative capacity for empathic presence. The story as moral parable aims to reform or transform our way of seeing the moral world: stories, symbols, and images provide what William F. May describes as "corrective vision."[5] Such narratively-structured corrections open the prospect of moral community in which strangers, outcasts, and enemies may become moral neighbors. Seeing and doing, identifying and enacting, recognizing and resolving, are inextricably connected.

The Good Samaritan parable directly enjoins moral envisioning through the concluding phrase of Jesus, "Do likewise." That is, the parable invites its dramatic audience as well as its expanded audience of religious believers, professional communities, and the broader culture to extend the moral imagination and consider circumstances of moral action similar to the situation confronted by the Samaritan. The

4. Jonsen, *New Medicine*, 40.

5. May, *Physician's Covenant*, 1.

moral admonition invites finding oneself in the story and then exercising imagination and discernment in subsequent situations that are analogous to those presented in the parable. In the parlance of moral philosophy, the parable assumes a responsibility of its moral audience to find similar circumstances where moral wisdom requires similar action.

Living out the injunction in a similar or analogous fashion means it is first important to interpret what the Samaritan was portrayed as "doing." As shown before, Jesus relates the parable in response to a query from a person reported in the narrative as seeking both clarification about the centrality of the status of the *Torah's* commandment of neighbor-love and self-justification regarding his own moral and religious status. Jesus affirms the first claim, but radically challenges the second by presenting the Samaritan as the moral exemplar of love; the radical challenge stems from the identification of the moral exemplar with an ethnic group, the Samaritans, vilified within Jewish culture of antiquity as morally inferior and spiritually compromised. The spiritual elites, represented by the characters in the story, may know about the moral law, but the moral stranger knows the person in need and lives the *Torah*.

As the story unfolds, the first moral consideration is the assault on the traveler that leaves him lying by the side of the road half-dead. This means the story initially invites the audience to identify not with the rescuing character of the Samaritan, but rather with the plight of the wounded person. The wounded embodiment of the traveler discloses our shared human vulnerability to bodily harm and suffering. Each of the three moral agents in the parable sees the wounded traveler, but while the religious figures display evasion or avoidance, only the Samaritan is moved to act. Part of the doing exemplified by the Samaritan, then, that others are called to emulate involves seeing the wounded and vulnerable person and subsequently identifying with their experience. An aspiring Samaritan is first attentive, a witness to human loss and vulnerability, and then experiences that loss as in some way his or her own deprivation. This imaginative process cultivates in the moral agent the moral capacity to identify with the needy and afflicted in order to enact compassion and share in the suffering of the other person.

The moral capacity for identification with the other person is the context for the emergence of a core feature of moral and professional experience, the virtue of empathy. Empathy is not the response of "I'm sorry for the loss you've experienced," which has a closer affinity to sympathy; it is also different than the response of "I'll share in your loss and suffering with you," which is the path of compassionate presence. Rather, empathy represents an imaginative identification with the other person, as expressed in "I understand your vulnerability, and I can see myself in your experience of loss."[6] Empathy bridges an epistemic divide without which compassion and healing become very difficult to achieve or will otherwise devolve into paternalistic pretensions ("I know how you feel"). The religious leaders portrayed in the story were witnesses to

---

6. Miller, *Friends and Other Strangers*, 109–16.

loss, but their moral failure did not simply reside in a failure to enact compassion: it encompasses as well the failure to exercise the virtue of empathy with the vulnerable.

The parable thereby presents a challenge to the moral imagination of its audience: doing as the Samaritan requires abandoning self-justifying tendencies, seeking to envision a moral world more expansive than personal and necessarily limited horizons, and cultivating empathy in the settings of shared human vulnerability. Seeing this moral world from the perspective of other persons and other cultures, moral agents recognize that fundamental moral virtues and norms are embedded in both integrity of character and witnessing actions of persons we consider strangers. The point here is not just that the Samaritan came to the rescuing assistance of a wounded stranger, but rather that persons who bear witness to following the moral path of the Samaritan must enter into the strangeness of the moral world envisioned by the Samaritan.

Furthermore, the parable presents a radical challenge to our moral imagination with respect to the scope of neighbor-love and compassion. The questioner asks Jesus "who is my neighbor?" but at the conclusion of the parable, Jesus re-stories the issue entirely by posing to the self-justifying lawyer the question of which of the three figures portrayed in the parable "was neighbor" to the wounded and dying traveler. The lawyer's question presents an intellectual and juridical classification that is necessarily restrictive. The question presumes certain persons in my moral world are neighbors for whom I assume some responsibility for their welfare and other persons who are strangers or enemies for whom I have negligible responsibility. The reframing question of Jesus breaks down the confining intellectual and legal schema and illustrates that moral agents are to live as neighbors to anyone in need.

"Neighbor" is thereby not determined by proximity or by ethnicity but as a moral construct situated by responsiveness to need. Love, empathy, and compassion are enacted rather than intellectualized. The neighbor is not so much found in the external world but cultivated and discovered in the self through witnessing and responsiveness to any person. The concluding admonition of the parable to "go and do likewise" thereby expands the scope of moral responsibility from the particular situation to broader, general realms of action. Put another way, part of the ethical imperative consists in refraining from judgment about who is in and who is excluded from the moral community. That question has already been decided because each person, prior to ethnic or tribal identity or religious affiliation, bears the *imago Dei*. The ethical question is instead about ways to enact gift-bearing responsibility.

The horizons of moral imagination are similarly expanded by the word "likewise." The phrasing implies that though moral agents may not encounter the circumstances that directly replicate those of the Samaritan and the wounded traveler, there are pervasive opportunities to rise to the challenge of attentive witnessing, availability, and responsiveness to others in need. The vulnerable, the wounded, the stranger, the persons experiencing ordeals, are *always* a feature of our moral landscape and are invariably encountered in the context of caring for the ill in the healing professions.

The parable's subversive conclusion presents an implicit responsibility for initiating circumstances where a person can be a neighbor to the stranger in need rather than only reacting to crisis after harm or violence has been inflicted. Becoming a neighbor to others as known and witnessed through empathy and compassion can mirror the sharing of giftedness that engenders a covenantal moral relationship.

The selection of a paradigmatic narrative, story, or symbol is laden with internal ethical and epistemic limitations. When certain aspects of our moral vision are corrected, other elements in our moral world may become blurred or obscured. Even though Churchill attests to the professional significance of the Samaritan parable, he also acknowledges its capacity to confine, restrict, and stop: "the power of the story has become truly an arresting power, paralyzing our imagination, to stretch beyond those whom we encounter as identified individuals in distress."[7] In particular, Churchill is concerned that the parable as conventionally understood and applied isolates moral attention on persons whom we directly encounter, and to dyadic relationships, and consequently can neglect background issues of social structure and justice. It might well be asked why the journey of the traveler to Jericho wasn't safe in the first place. These difficulties inherent to correcting, expanding, and confining the moral imagination are illuminated in considering the ways the symbol of the Samaritan has been appropriated in professional as well as institutional identities.

Witnessing Professional Identity

Jonsen contends the parable of the Good Samaritan historically was invoked by various writers within the Christian tradition to "exemplify the duties of the Christian physician."[8] The parable shaped Christian conceptions of hospitality and responsibilities of caring for the sick, wounded, and vulnerable. It was interpreted by Christian writers as presenting two especially ethically expansive provisions: (1) Caring is inclusive, not exclusive, and extends to persons outside the immediate religious community, thereby building on and expanding the religious traditions of care and hospitality to the stranger; (2) caring is shaped by an altruistic commitment of responsibility even in circumstances of cost to self, such as time, resources, interests, or financial considerations.

This inclusive and altruistic legacy of the parable continues to be influential in theological and religious views of the health professions. Fisher and Gormally observe that "the Good Samaritan parable has long inspired the Christian vocation of healthcare: the response to a transcendent call to care lovingly for the sick person, to treat all those in need of such care, and to do one's best to save, heal, and care."[9] The responsibility of doing as the Samaritan has been emphasized particularly within recent

7. Churchill, *Rationing Health Care*, 7.

8. Jonsen, *New Medicine*, 39.

9. Catholic Bishops, "Catholic Social Teaching," 138.

Roman Catholic teaching on the professions. The *Ethical and Religious Directives for Catholic Health Care Services* portrays the commitments of Catholic religious communities to sponsor or provide health care services as a "modeling [of] efforts on the gospel parable of the Good Samaritan" through which these communities exemplify "authentic neighborliness to those in need."[10]

As important as the parable is for cultivating religious vocation and professional identity within Christian religious traditions, Jonsen contends that the story contains broader implications for professional ethics and integrity. The moral features of inclusive and altruistic caring embedded in the parable give rise to and shape what he designates as a principle of contemporary medical ethics: the "Samaritanian principle" of compassion, which complements the principle of physician competence that emerges from the Hippocratic ethical tradition. In Jonsen's account, the parable offers a bridge between virtue and duty ethics: The Samaritan portrays both "the picture of the compassionate physician" and the responsibility for rendering compassionate service to vulnerable persons in need.[11]

This interpretation is echoed by other scholars. Despite his reservations about the social applicability of the parable, Churchill contends that "'Samaritanism' has . . . become shorthand in our culture to express those essential dimensions of physician morality which are the *sine qua non* of the profession."[12] The story provides "the most powerful, sustaining image which medicine holds up to itself,"[13] a vital correction of vision to professional self-images of parent or of technician.

These claims of seeing professional identity through the narrative are directed through identification with the Samaritan as rescuer to a person in need rather than the broader sense of human vulnerability evoked through identification with the wounded traveler. My claim here is that the cultivation of empathy and the expression of compassion require professional identification with both the Samaritan and the traveler. If professional identity is directed only by the sustaining image of the Samaritan, then moral perception may not see some persons who are wounded and in need of healing, or not be oriented by an active "going out" to care for the most vulnerable, such as the homeless, uninsured, or abused. Compassion with diminished empathy for the wounded might instead be expressed by waiting for persons who have the physical and financial resources to "come in" to visit a physician.[14]

Professional Witness. A striking illustration of how the Samaritanian principle of Jonsen could be appropriated as a partial image for professional identity found expression in the writings of physician Walsh McDermott. McDermott maintained: "Everything the physician does is some combination of technology and what we might call

10. United States Conference of Catholic Bishops, *Ethical and Religious Directives*, 7.

11. Jonsen, *New Medicine*, 40.

12. Churchill, *Rationing Health Care*, 33.

13. Churchill, *Rationing Health Care*, 36.

14. Kullberg, *Ragged Edge of Medicine*, 1–23.

'samaritanism.'"[15] Although McDermott sought to differentiate what he referred to as "samaritanism," or the human support of the physician, from acts performed out of love, it is evident he saw samaritanism as intertwined with the virtues of compassion and caring and the principle of beneficence. In an evocatively titled article, "Technology's Consort," McDermott portrayed samaritanism as intimately connected with the physician's use of technology, in short, as the "consort" of medical technology: samaritanism "forms the guidance system that eases the acceptance of technology and hence allows it to be applied."[16] The metaphor of guidance reflects the complementary nature of the twin principles presented in Jonsen's analysis: samaritanism guides professional competence in the use of technologies.

In his philosophy of medicine, McDermott viewed technology as rooted in medical science and directed towards preventing or altering the disease process; samaritanism represented acts that reassured and provided support to a patient afflicted with disease or illness. The samaritanism of the physician pertains to the art of healing that must necessarily inform and guide the professional's scientific and technological competence, the care for the person that must couple skilled assessment of the disease. The "Samaritan tradition" is a necessary complement to the various sciences that bestow on medicine professional and social authority. "These two functions—the technological and the samaritan—are separable in theory but not in practice."[17] So indispensable was the Samaritan ethic to medicine's professional and social identity that McDermott expressed concern that within an era of modern scientific rationalism, medicine must constantly affirm and reintegrate the image of the Samaritan physician within its science-based technology. Otherwise, medicine would "continue to lose ground as an important healing social force."[18]

McDermott's caveat about diminishing healing in modern medicine as embedded in the "Samaritan tradition" is of particular salience in considering the meaning and symbolism of the Samaritan ethic as witnessed by health care institutions. Historically, hospitals emerged from moral communities who related stories of hospitality to strangers and sought to enact this commitment in an organized manner. These formative narratives provided a moral memory for the numerous hospital systems and medical centers that have adopted the symbol of the "Good Samaritan" in their institutional identity. In some instances, this identity is a vestige of a one-time affiliation with a religious tradition that understood its mission of witness and its traditions of hospitality to be manifested through the delivery of health care services to the ill and sick. However, even when these substantive professional and religious affinities have withered, a symbolic witness remains: secular hospitals and medical centers that retain the language of Samaritan in their institutional identities intend for the quality

15. McDermott, "Evaluating the Physician," 136.

16. McDermott and Rogers, "Technology's Consort," 353.

17. McDermott, "Evaluating the Physician," 136.

18. McDermott and Rogers, "Technology's Consort," 353.

of excellence in health care they provide to be understood not through technological competence, medical innovations, or economic incentives, but fundamentally as a manifestation of caring and compassion and a commitment to healing presence.

Institutional Witness. The appropriation of the story of the Good Samaritan by health care institutions in fact presents some striking paradoxes. Quite apart from the moral legacy of the story, it is not difficult to see why it is compelling to transform the Samaritan into an institutional symbol of compassionate provision for health and medical care. Health care institutions in the contemporary setting are critiqued for (mis)managing the delivery of health care to patients in several respects. As journalist Walter Cronkite expressed the point: "The American health care system is neither healthy, nor caring, nor a system."[19] The health care system is more appropriately designated a "sick care" system, with the vast proportion of resources devoted to treatments for persons who are acutely sick, and a much smaller proportion of resources committed to programs for prevention and keeping persons healthy in the first place. Institutionalized care is not caring; it is controlled by regulations and procedural oversight developed with the good of the institution and the interests of its patient community as a collective body in mind rather than with the particular needs and concerns of a specific vulnerable patient. Consequently, institutionalized settings diminish personalized care while giving emphatic priority to instrumental rationality, efficiencies, and quantitative outcome measurements; patients who utilize an institutional or hospital setting for needed treatment often receive standardized surveys post-visit with scaled metrics for assessment of patient satisfaction. The patient's narrative is rendered invisible.

One reason professional and bioethical discourse emphasizes the rights of patients to control the decision-making process regarding their treatment is that following admission to a hospital, the patient loses control over most everything else. The hospital's schedule for effective and efficient usage of its staff dictates when the patient must awake, eat, take medications, undergo tests or procedures, is seen by their physician, and receives visitors, not to mention the manner of dress. The totalizing environment of the modern hospital leaves little room for patient choices; autonomy over treatment decisions seems to be the last vestige of the person's claim to dignity and respect. Furthermore, historical traditions of hospitality to the stranger seem neglected by patterns of access to hospital services that stratify the populations served and stratify the care provided. Modern hospitals certainly face questions of resource allocation that the Samaritan tradition of McDermott didn't address, but the institutionalized provision of care is directed by embedded values of an industrial and market-place model of health care delivery.

The inherent moral inertia of institutions and the external constraints imposed by law, government, and marketplace efficiencies and priorities converge to push the health care institution and hospital away from a caring context. Patients requiring

19. The Clinton Foundation, "Health Care is Local," para. 1.

hospitalization can expect to receive technical expertise, but not necessarily human-istic caring. It is within this context that the appropriation of the Good Samaritan as institutional symbol becomes especially intelligible. It is one public way that an institution can gesture to both prospective patients and to its professional staff that what lies at the foundation of what is perceived as a depersonalizing and bureaucratic profit-maximizing enterprise is a commitment to care for other vulnerable persons in their need and extremity. The Samaritan as symbol witnesses to care, compassion, and healing as the basis for medical care, even as certain methods of institutional-ized delivery rooted in business models and practices undermine those commitments and instead give credibility to Cronkite's observations of an unhealthy, uncaring, nonsystem.

The institutional appropriation of the Samaritan as a symbol for care reflects symbolic rationality that works to soften and constrain the impersonal if efficient models of technical bureaucratic expertise and its paradigm of instrumental rational-ity. As stated by the Catholic Bishops' Joint Bioethics Committee, "health systems, like the Good Samaritan's acts of rescue and care, can be symbolic demonstrations of crucial values, such as generosity, respect for the dignity and equality of persons, for the inviolability of human life and the good of health, special concern for the vulner-able and powerless, [and] solidarity with and compassion for those who suffer."[20] In this regard, the Good Samaritan parable can be a source not only of moral direction, but also moral memory and moral critique of hospital and institutionalized settings of treatment.

The public effectiveness of this institutional witness to caring is, in large measure, contingent on the public accessibility and knowledge of the framing narrative. In an era in which persons who state "none" in response to religious affiliation surveys are the fastest growing segment of the population,[21] broad cultural apprehension of the Samaritan parable as part of a background civic religion can no longer be assumed. That is in part why the appeal to "Samaritan" language to portray those who sought to intervene in the harassment episode I described at the beginning of the chapter is so striking. Indicative of a declining religious literacy in the culture at large,[22] most of my students have no awareness of the narrative, the values historically embedded in the term, or their biblical origins. For them, "Good Samaritan" is a corporate name and entity; their exposure to the moral concept is largely filtered through legal or policy discourse about "good Samaritan laws" rather than a narratively-constituted ethical identity.

The articulation by one US hospital of its rationale for appropriating the Samari-tan symbol and language is instructive. As indicated on a webpage describing its mis-sion, the institution seeks to cultivate an ethos of Samaritanism among both recipients

---

20. Catholic Bishops, "Catholic Social Teaching," 138.

21. Pew Research, "Changing Religious Landscape," 3–32.

22. Prothero, *Religious Literacy*, 21–38.

and providers of care. The institutional statement makes explicit reference to professional and institutional cultivation of the Samaritan ethos. Although the hospital has recently undergone acquisition by a larger corporation, the institution continues to keep "Good Samaritan" as part of its title, and retains a compressed and succinct statement of its current vision: "We are Good Samaritans, guided by Catholic tradition and trusted to deliver ideal healthcare experiences."[23]

An ethical claim is embedded in this hospital's account of its symbol as well as by the numerous similar organizations that have appropriated the Samaritan ethos and narrative into their institutional discourse. Through their language and symbols, health care institutions tell stories about the kind of care they provide and the kind of practitioners they aspire to cultivate. This symbolism is articulated perhaps best by theological ethicist William F. May in his writings on the covenantal nature of health care institutions. May contends that "institutions, consciously or unconsciously, embody a covenant, a social purpose, a human good, which they avow and serve."[24] May recognizes that callousness and depersonalization are defining characteristics of large-scale organizations, but he argues that a moral commitment of covenant can generate the human activity of organized caring. Caring and healing are the primary ends and purposes for health care institutions, upon which subordinate purposes, such as the business or transactional nature of the organization, ultimately rest.

May contends: "Underneath the contractual edifice of the modern hospital lies a covenanted base of giving and receiving that ought to infuse it."[25] This ethic of giving and receiving, which May contrasts with a commercial model of selling and purchasing services, mediates not only the relationship of physician or nurse to patient, but initially, the relationship of society to profession and institution. The generative gift ethic in medicine is initiated through a broad-scale commitment of public funds to support medical education, hospital construction, and biomedical research, as well as through various philanthropic donations of funds from private persons to support specific goals of particular interest, such as cancer research or palliative care. The moral hinge in May's construction is "ought": though such a covenantal commitment morally ought to be the basis for health care mediated through institutionalized settings, this is no guarantee of its presence. Ought may imply "can be done," but not "will be" enacted. If through patterns of secularization, bureaucratic rationalization, and the instrumentalized rationality of competition, acquisition, and consolidation, this foundational moral commitment is lost, or becomes only a symbol lacking substance, then the institution (or profession) has become a different kind of organization. The language of corporatism and industry will then be infused into the relational interactions of the professions and the transaction of services will supplant the transformation

---

23. Medstar Good Samaritan Hospital, "Mission, Vision, and Values," para. 1
24. May, *Physician's Covenant*, 189–90.
25. May, *Physician's Covenant*, 190.

of service. Ultimately, this raises the question of whether the Samaritan ethos serves more as a moral ideal or aspiration than a moral norm.

Moral Aspiration

The parable of the Good Samaritan provides a memorable exposition of a fundamental requirement of Jewish law and, as illustrated in the examples of professional identity, it has resonance beyond the particular religious communities for whom it originally had meaning. However, the various "Good Samaritan statutes" in contemporary civic law reflect a view that in a secular, pluralistic society, the relevant moral norms required for social cohesion and minimal moral decency are those of non-infliction of harm and respect for the free choice of autonomous persons. In this construction, the moral precepts embodied by the Samaritan cannot be embedded in positive law or establish standards of required legal conduct for which citizens of a society are accountable. That does not imply that the moral teaching of the parable is irrelevant to a good society; the very existence of such statutes implies that it is possible to acknowledge the narrative symbolizes a moral ideal. It can then be claimed that a Samaritan ethic for modern moral life, as well as that of professional vocation, perhaps is best situated within a morality of aspiration rather than a morality of obligation.

An exemplary use of appropriation of the Samaritan narrative as expressive of the symbolic rationality of moral ideals and aspirations is represented in one of the first philosophical contributions to bioethics discourse: Judith Jarvis Thomson's classic essay, "A Defense of Abortion."[26] Thomson relies on an analogous case of rescue of a stranger—that is, the scope of responsibility of a pregnant woman towards her unborn fetus. In the course of her exposition, she draws explicitly on the parable, significantly making an appeal to a common moral memory in commenting that her readers "will remember" how the story goes (though she then proceeds to quote the parable for those with a failing memory). Thomson subsequently distinguishes between a "minimally decent" Samaritan and a "good" or virtuous Samaritan. She claims the two religious leaders in the story who literally bypassed the wounded traveler and crossed to the other side of the road failed to meet even the moral standard of minimal decency. Morality, if it is to have meaning at all, is not exhausted by legal responsibilities of noninterference, but must include some active regard for promoting the positive welfare of others, or some minimal requirement of beneficence. However, the morality of minimal decency also means "we are not required to be Good Samaritans or anyway Very Good Samaritans to one another."[27]

Thomson's analysis of the scope of minimal moral responsibilities is then explored within the context of the circumstances and choices confronting a pregnant woman. The standard of minimally decent samaritanship implies that a pregnant

26. Thomson, "Defense of Abortion," 121–39.
27. Thomson, "Defense of Abortion," 137.

woman should have a choice to determine whether to continue her pregnancy and to assume the implicit commitment of altruistic self-sacrifice, based on the level of risks (physical, emotional, financial, career, relational) posed to herself and her interests. It seems conceptually possible on Thomson's account, even if rare in the real world, for a pregnant woman who determines to terminate her pregnancy to fail to meet the standard of minimal decency: she observes in her concluding section that "it would be indecent in the woman to request an abortion, . . . if she is in her seventh month, and wants the abortion just to avoid the nuisance of postponing a trip abroad."[28]

It is also possible for women to enact good or virtuous samaritanship by continuing the pregnancy while accepting substantial self-sacrifice, not only during gestation, but in assuming responsibilities of parental nurturing. Thomson contends, however, that this alternative suggests the ethics of a Good Samaritan belong to a morality of aspiration or an ethical ideal, for "nobody is morally required to make large sacrifices, of health, of all other interests and concerns, of all other duties and commitments, for nine years, or even nine months, in order to keep another person alive."[29] Good Samaritans will accept some sacrifice of personal interests to advance the well-being of others, but this standard surpasses the minimal sacrifices embedded in what is morally required by the standard of minimal decency. Thomson's account of minimally decent samaritanship contravenes the open-ended duration of ongoing commitment to the welfare of another implied in a gift-based covenantal ethic and relationship.

The different tiers of moral responsibility—good or virtuous, minimally decent, indecency—are invoked by Thomson, not only to show the parameters of moral choice faced by the pregnant woman, but also those encountered by physicians considering whether to act on behalf of the pregnant woman by providing an abortion. At the time of writing of her essay (1970), with abortion illegal in most states and lacking constitutional warrant, Thomson was able to say that in some situations, such as those of a woman impregnated by sexual assault and subsequently bed-bound during pregnancy, physicians would act as Good Samaritans in extricating the woman from the situation by performing an abortion. I do not think that the same point would hold some forty-five years and over fifty million abortions post-*Roe v. Wade*. What is required of physicians is minimally decent professionalism—that is, physicians are obligated to provide sufficient information for informed consent, respect a pregnant woman's choice, provide a safe setting, and perform a technically competent procedure, or provide a referral to another physician in the case of conscientious refusal. Physicians can fail to be minimally decent professionals most commonly by withholding information from pregnant women or by refusing to provide referrals. By introducing into her reconstructed story an element of conflict between different parties that was not present in the original story, Thomson extends the moral scope of the parable to situations beyond those of rendering direct assistance to a

28. Thomson, "Defense of Abortion," 138.
29. Thomson, "Defense of Abortion," 135.

vulnerable person in need. The moral complexity of this extension occurs because the pregnant woman assumes the role of both Samaritan who can rescue and of harmed or wounded person in need of rescue. The duty of empathy towards the vulnerable person is extended to the pregnant woman, but not to the fetus.

Thomson's use of the parable of the Good Samaritan is instructive for differentiating between a morality of obligation and a morality of aspiration or supererogation. Our obligations to not inflict harm on others (any others) are very stringent (though not absolute), while our responsibilities of assistance, beneficence, or rescue to a vulnerable person in need are very limited and restricted in everyday interactions. Outside voluntary acceptance of such obligations in particular relationships (such as parent-child, physician-patient, teacher-student), responsibilities to assist are characteristically specified by the morality of minimal decency. Whether a person has a specific obligation to assist another person will depend on such features as (a) whether the other person is in need of basic subsistence; (b) whether there are more effective ways of meeting these basic needs; (c) whether the individual considering the rescue or assistance is the only person who can meet these needs; (d) whether providing assistance will impose substantial cost, risk, or self-sacrifice on the person who may assist (the condition at which Thomson draws the line of moral decency); and (e) whether the benefits to the person in need are proportionately greater than the burdens assumed by the person rendering assistance. The framework of obligatory beneficence can enable determinations of which role-related actions meet the threshold of minimal decency, which fail to meet that standard, and which exceed the standard and are supererogatory.

In relationships of moral intimacy, such as within families, or friendships, and in some religious traditions and communities, this parsing of obligation and aspiration may make less sense; self-sacrifice for the benefit of one's child, for example, is embedded in societal and personal expectations of parenting. In encounters with moral strangers, a Good Samaritan will go beyond minimal decency, but such a person embodies more of an ideal for moral life rather than an obligation. Thomson's account recognizes that self-sacrificial love may be an aspiration for some persons, but also holds that moral blame cannot be attached to agents who enact different standards of conduct that reflect minimal decency. The significant question embedded in this discussion is what kind of morality—obligation or aspiration—is manifested in the appropriation of the Samaritan symbol as an expression of professionalism in contemporary medicine.

Illuminating Moral Maxim

As suggested by Thomson's appropriation, in one respect, the parable of the Good Samaritan might be considered morally uninteresting from the perspective of contemporary bioethics. The story of the Samaritan's actions do not contain a moral conflict, and the circumstances by which the Samaritan was called to act seem largely beyond his (or the traveler's) control, that is, the pervasiveness of violence in a society, the perennial needs of the vulnerable, and the obliviousness or indifference of cultural or religious elites. The wounded traveler requires assistance because of the violence and physical harms inflicted that have left him half dead; the Samaritan arrives at the scene of the assault "by chance," in the apt wording of the parable, and ministers to the traveler's wounds. While the Samaritan exemplifies the radically subversive demands of the commitment of neighbor-love, the Samaritan seems to not experience any internal or external constraints on performing the healing actions needed by the traveler; the Samaritan experiences neither uncertainty about the good that needs to be done nor weakness of will about doing the good.

While the parable does not then present an occasion of conflict of moral values, the "do likewise" injunction at its conclusion implies that this is more than just an idiosyncratic story, but rather has resonance beyond the immediate situation. As noted previously, the story aids moral perception, helping us see, frame, and envision moral issues (such as those developed by McDermott or Thomson), provides a symbol of moral and professional identity, and generates insight and corrective vision regarding the responsibilities of love and beneficence in similar situations of rescuing a stranger. I suggest here that the moral vision embedded in the parable can function as an illuminating maxim in moral deliberation.

Many contemporary questions in bioethics in which conflicting values emerge, and particularly those that raise broader issues of social justice, resist appropriation into the "likewise" injunction. The Samaritan's goodness is, in part, a matter of moral luck, attributable to the good fortune of encountering a situation of clear human need and moral action without any complicating contexts that may have raised moral conflicts. The exercise of creative moral imagination can develop several different kinds of circumstances in which the "chanced" nature of the encounter may have been substantially different such that the Samaritan might have experienced at minimum a dilemma of moral uncertainty about the requirements of loving one's neighbor and of being a neighbor to the vulnerable stranger.

Self-defense: The Samaritan might have undertaken his journey to Jericho and "by chance" himself been the person assaulted by the robbers. The Good Samaritan had the good fortune of being able to provide needed assistance rather than having to fend off violence. This reframing of the narrative raises the issue of whether the responsibility of love for neighbor and the virtues of compassion, mercy, and hospitality can accommodate use of physical force against another person for the purpose of protecting one's physical security (and possessions).

Risk-filled Rescue: The Samaritan might have come upon the wounded traveler not after the assault, but "by chance" as the assailants were surprising the traveler and the assault was just beginning. In the biblical narrative, the Samaritan had the good fortune of being able to provide needed assistance without placing himself at serious risk of harm. A re-storying that introduces an element of personal risk into the story presents an issue of the scope of love for neighbor when providing care and benefit for another comes at significant cost to one's own interests and well-being. These were the circumstances presumed by those who designated the persons killed in the Portland transit incident as "Good Samaritans." This is also precisely the moral consideration Thomson introduces to differentiate between minimally decent and aspirational or supererogatory conduct.

Stigma or Contagion: The Samaritan might have "by chance" come upon a wounded person who was suffering from some kind of socially stigmatized disease, such as a common contagion like leprosy; indeed, such a stigmatizing condition and associated social ostracization may even have presented the robbers with an exclusivist rationalization for harming. In this context, close contact with a diseased individual, including binding up the wounds, could have caused the Samaritan to violate purity codes or even for the Samaritan to be a vector of contagion. The Samaritan had the good fortune of being able to provide assistance to a person who otherwise was in good physical health and did not present any underlying risk of indirect harm. This form of reframing poses a question similar to that of the previous scenario regarding the applicability of love of neighbor when seeking to benefit may present risks to physical health or moral or religious integrity, though in this circumstance the risk is posed through contact with the wounded traveler rather than from the assailants.

Rescue Refusal: The Samaritan could "by chance" have come upon a conscious wounded traveler who, aware he has been left half-dead, refused the Samaritan's assistance and requested only to die without pain. The Good Samaritan had the good fortune to render assistance to a person who did not (or could not) refuse or resist the proffered help. This re-storying scenario presents an issue about the moral adequacy of love or beneficence when the rescuer's understanding of the welfare of the vulnerable person is different from the person's own understanding of their best interests.

Restricted Access: The Samaritan might "by chance" have encountered on his journey a wounded traveler from a disparaged minority or foreign culture such that there was no wayside inn that would give refuge or sanctuary to the wounded man and continue to provide care for him as he recovered. The Good Samaritan had the good fortune to find accommodations and willing caregivers for the traveler that he rescued. This reframed narrative poses a question about the moral sufficiency of love and beneficence in the context of social and structural discrimination and injustice.

Financial Barriers: The Samaritan might have been able to provide care for the immediate needs of the traveler but "by chance" lacked the financial resources (at least in the time of need) to compensate those who could provide lodging and continuing care as the Samaritan continued on his journey. The Good Samaritan was fortunate that he had the resources to provide for the ongoing recovery of the stranger. This reframing requires consideration of how love of neighbor can be enacted in the context of an institutionalized system that limits access to care according to ability to pay.

Prioritizing Care: The Samaritan "by chance" might have encountered a situation in which several persons had been assaulted, each of whom needed assistance to live. Several persons, including the religious figures, might have been injured at the same place, or persons might have been injured at a further stage in the journey due to multiple attacks by the robbers. The Good Samaritan was fortunate to have been able to provide adequate resources for the wounded traveler to meet the person's immediate needs for care as well as their need for continuing care while recovering at the wayside sanctuary. It is just as plausible, however, to consider the circumstances where not only the traveler but also the religious authorities were beaten and left for dead in the road.[30] This scenario raises questions about enacting the commitment to be a neighbor when there are multiple neighbors in serious need.

The creative moral imagination can formulate various practical and real-life analogies to these narratives where the Samaritan would have experienced some chance misfortunes that impeded his exemplification of care, empathy, compassion, hospitality, and love. Martin Luther King Jr. reframed the parable so as to raise questions about structural violence and the inadequacy of quick, one-time fixes for institutionalized systems of hierarchy and power.[31] Each of these reframed stories presents certain limitations to the direct applicability of the moral commitment to love and benefit another person because of a moral conflict with other competing values such as self-regard, respect, solidarity, and justice. The stories illustrate why the parable, though certainly relevant as a moral ideal or an illuminating maxim for moral deliberation in bioethics, is in need of supplementation by other values and principles. This issue has been developed most substantively by bioethics scholars with respect to the last scenario in which the Samaritan confronts the equally weighty needs of multiple neighbors.

Love and Justice in Scarce Resources

The question of scarce resources is a perennial issue in bioethics; on Jonsen's account of the history of bioethics, rationing resources is a generative issue in the emergence of bioethics as a distinctive field of academic inquiry. Although some writers assert that "the Gospel parable of the Good Samaritan is a useful model for good practice in health care allocation,"[32] I here wish to illustrate the complexities of resource allocation through an analysis of two approaches that frame allocation questions through the moral perplexities that a Good Samaritan would encounter. On both analyses, it is morally challenging for the Good Samaritan to remain good given the conflicting values embedded in resource and rationing settings.

---

30. Churchill, *Rationing Health Care*, 37.

31. King, "I've Been to the Mountaintop," para. 31–34.

32. Catholic Bishops, "Catholic Social Teaching," 138.

Jonsen contends samaritanism is one of the central principles for contemporary medical ethics, and he recognizes the influence of the symbol of the Samaritan for professional identity. Nevertheless, this ethic can extend only so far when the Samaritan, as physician, directly faces a scarce resource quandary in a gate-keeping role. In Jonsen's imaginative reframing of the biblical narrative, the Samaritan provides the immediate care and transport needed by the wounded traveler and continues on his way, only to encounter another person likewise seriously wounded by the robbers. As the Samaritan has previously expended his life-saving resources on the first traveler, he does not have the medicinal or logistical resources to assist the second traveler. He cannot care for both injured persons (at least not without risking having both persons die). The ethics of being the neighbor and enacting compassionate service is thereby portrayed as inadequate for moral guidance when there are more neighbors in need than available resources for care.

In Jonsen's retelling, the Samaritan leaves the second victim—that is, engages in abandonment in order to save the first person. However, the pattern continues; on his journey to find hospitable refuge for the first wounded traveler, the Samaritan repeatedly encounters additional wounded individuals whose needs exceed what he is able to provide in the way of care and assistance. Jonsen takes this circumstance of unending encounters with the ill to be the nature of contemporary health care. Without some kind of providential intervention, the Samaritan faces a moral quandary: "how to distribute his resources among all who can benefit from his attention, now and in the future."[33] As the Samaritan comes to comprehend that while competence and compassion are morally necessary, they are neither individually or collectively sufficient to address the issue of scarce resources, Jonsen frames the moral perplexity at levels of both organizational integrity and personal integrity: "Can the institution of health care be equitable in its essential features of access and quality? Can the compassionate Samaritan be a just Samaritan?"[34]

The conceptual assumption in this rendition is that the norms of love and justice are in inescapable conflict, a claim that may be disputed on many accounts.[35] Justice may be the form that love takes in the social setting when the needs of many neighbors must be considered. Or, alternatively, love may inform a preferential option for the most poor and vulnerable.[36] Although theoretical reformulations of the relationship of love, including compassion, beneficence, and justice as fairness, are certainly possible, and may even be generated by contexts of moral conflict such as rationing resources, Jonsen's insight that an exemplary ethic of samaritanism is ultimately limited in scope and application is certainly valid. As he contends, "Even the Good Samaritan found that his charity had its ethical limits: the strength of his donkey, the

---

33. Jonsen, *New Medicine*, 42–43.

34. Jonsen, *New Medicine*, 48.

35. Outka, *Agape*, 75–92.

36. United States Conference of Catholic Bishops, *Ethical and Religious Directives*, 10.

availability of bandages, and the supply of oil and wine in his flasks."[37] The Samaritan ethic will necessarily be inadequate for the ubiquitous need pervasive in contemporary health care.

Before analyzing Jonsen's argumentation of whether a physician seeking to emulate the Samaritan can display both compassion and justice, I wish to introduce a second account of Samaritan perplexity in the face of limited resources, as developed by theological ethicist Allen Verhey. After quoting the biblical parable, Verhey affirms its ongoing relevance in laws, professional and institutional identities, or the moral formation of religious communities. Yet, Verhey subsequently acknowledges that the parable, as situated in the context of modern medicine, is also "a strange story," for "the Samaritan did not face the issue health care is forced to face today, the issue of scarcity. The limitless compassion of the Samaritan makes his story seem more odd than exemplary: unlimited care seems not a real option."[38]

When the issue of scarcity is acknowledged as a chronic reality in modern medicine, Verhey finds himself posing precisely the same sort of conceptual thought-experiment and moral question raised by Jonsen: "Can we still be Good Samaritans—or Fair Samaritans—in the midst of tragic choices imposed by scarcity?"[39] Some important shifts from Jonsen are made in Verhey's question: the Samaritan's goodness is interpreted less along the lines of love, compassion, and mercy and more as fairness as a form of justice. Furthermore, the "we" in Verhey's inquiry is not limited to physicians, as was the case for Jonsen, but encompasses an array of moral communities, religious and professional, who have found in the Samaritan a symbol or image of caring for the ill and the vulnerable.

Situating the Samaritan ethic within a context of scarcity changes the ethical applicability of its moral guidance, and in fact may change the story itself. However, Verhey suggests that we don't fully apprehend the significance of the moral conflict for a Good Samaritan if we focus only on the scarcity issue. Many disciplines, after all, are devoted to addressing circumstances of scarcity without becoming morally undone. It would be quite possible to develop certain criteria for prioritizing the needs of some rather than others through a cost-effective methodology or similar methods of instrumental rationality. Such approaches nonetheless risk changing individual persons into so-called "statistical lives."

What is existentially wrenching and morally vexing for the Samaritan is witnessing the harm and pain of a person endowed with sanctity (or what I have referred to as the *imago Dei*), as a being nurtured and sustained through the unbounded love of the divine, when it is not possible to meet the person's needs. In the absence of the initial theological perception of endowed sanctity, resolving an issue of scarcity comprises little more than working out an interesting intellectual puzzle. The Samaritan ethic

37. Jonsen, *New Medicine*, 50.
38. Verhey, *Reading the Bible*, 361.
39. Verhey, *Reading the Bible*, 361.

may become a strange, if not inapt, story in modern medicine, not simply because of increasing situations of scarcity, but also due to diminishing commitments to sanctity. The ethic embedded in the Samaritan narrative thereby witnesses to the necessity of a dialectical relationship between sanctity and scarcity rather than policies shaped by prioritizing one concept. This dialectic is sharply posed by Verhey in a brief discussion of microallocation issues: "When the scarcity of commodities forbids a Good Samaritan from helping all who hurt, sanctity forbids a Fair Samaritan from making godlike judgments that one's person's life or health is 'worth' more than another's."[40] In circumstances of limited resources, how then is it possible to be both good and fair?

The common question—how can a Samaritan, whether as embodying moral commitments of a physician, a health care institution, or as a religious community, be good (that is, just or fair) in the context of chronic scarcity—leads Jonsen and Verhey to present proposals that both converge and contrast. Jonsen emphasizes extended and active compassion that is supplemented by the principle of justice. Insofar as the virtue of compassion "is unable to tolerate the obscene spectacle of the sick and wounded lying untended,"[41] the Samaritanism ethic requires a physician or institution to seek out the ill and sick persons that have been abandoned and ensure they receive necessary and beneficial care, rather than waiting until a person in crisis appears in the emergency room. Compassion can take the form of developing procedural rules that give moral preference to some persons based on considerations of medical utility: equal regard; competence in providing effective care; serious need; and prospect of benefit.

Jonsen contends that the impulse of compassion ultimately requires engagement with broader structural or policy level considerations that shape the nature and extent of scarcity. This would mean compassion expressed as prevention rather than as exclusively crisis-intervention. The Samaritan who aspires to compassion and justice must embody courage before decision-making authorities, including not only institutional administrators but also legislators, challenging them to consider that the moral character and identity of the broader society are at stake: "Is this a society that we can be proud of? a society in which the sick and the wounded lie unattended?"[42] Moral integrity and wholeness can be realized insofar as compassion, love, and beneficence are complemented with and directed by principles and processes of justice; the Samaritan ethic can bear a prophetic witness to professionals and policy leaders that the scarce resource issue cannot be resolved one patient at a time, but requires a substantive structural reformation: "The good Samaritan can be a just Samaritan, giving to each his or her due, recognizing that behind each presenting patient awaits another

40. Verhey, *Reading the Bible*, 392.

41. Jonsen, *New Medicine*, 54.

42. Jonsen, *New Medicine*, 54.

patient in need of service."[43] This entails reforming the system so that it authentically promotes health care rather than prioritizes sick care.

Verhey's analysis likewise requires moral engagement of the Samaritan with public policy; he frames what policymakers must hear as not simply a bold approach, but as a "prophetic protest against policies that lead to injustice in access to health care."[44] The content of what comprises justice in the context of scarcity of health care resources is situated by Verhey explicitly within the biblical tradition and its commitment to the vulnerable rather than the stories of the autonomous self of the Enlightenment and philosophical liberalism: "Our test for justice is not a pinched view of individual entitlement, but the care given to the poor and weak."[45] Verhey's account reflects the stewardship principle of the preferential status of the poor.

While Verhey and Jonsen concur that the morality of contemporary Samaritans must encompass not only compassion, but also justice, Verhey frames justice as a virtue that qualifies and directs compassion rather than as an independent moral principle: "The contemporary Samaritan cannot be good with *only* compassion but *just* compassion is indeed required. The virtue of *justice* is essential to those who would be good in the midst of scarcity."[46] This construction retains the primacy of love and compassion for a religious-based bioethics. Furthermore, compassion must be informed by more virtues than justice. These supplemental virtues include truthfulness to remedy the human inclination to deny either or both the sanctity of the person or the scarcity of resources, humility as manifested in recognition of human limits of finitude (and mortality) and fallibility, and gratitude for opportunities to effect change and transformation and to express compassion and care by being with the person suffering when cure is not possible.

Verhey's norm of "just compassion" implies not simply limits on resources, but limits on moral integrity. His language in the policy setting shifts in a morally significant way from that of the "Good" Samaritan to that of the "Fair" Samaritan; he elaborates, however, that "the Good Samaritan longs to be more than fair."[47] The fairness inherent to just compassion requires advocacy of a first priority in resource allocation, that of ensuring that all persons have access to an adequate level or decent minimum of care irrespective of a person's ability to pay. However, the longing of the Samaritan to be and do more persists: "not to provide the best care for any patient is not, therefore, good. It remains tragic."[48]

Verhey's moral distinction between fairness and goodness, between unbounded compassion and just compassion, echoes the views of two other prominent expressions

43. Jonsen, *New Medicine*, 59.

44. Verhey, *Reading the Bible*, 371.

45. Verhey, *Reading the Bible*, 375.

46. Verhey, *Reading the Bible*, 369. Emphasis original.

47. Verhey, *Reading the Bible*, 386.

48. Verhey, *Reading the Bible*, 386.

of a Samaritan ethic. Insofar as fairness requires a standard of access to a decent minimum of care, Verhey makes the same differentiation that informs Thomson's analysis between minimally decent and good Samaritans. This reiterates the importance of distinguishing in realms of both personal moral choice and defensible public policy between what is morally obligatory and required (access to a decent minimum for all) and what is aspirational or ideal (optimal care for all needs). However, as informed theologically, Verhey does something with this difference between the minimally decent and the aspirational that Thomson does not, namely, designating it as "tragic." A falling short of the moral ideal can generate experience of moral anguish and even regret. It may be possible for a minimally decent or fair Samaritan to reach the requisite threshold and find moral contentment in their actions; meanwhile, a good Samaritan will, in Verhey's language, "long to do more" than the moral minimum.

Verhey's construction of the moral conflicts presented by resource scarcity is then compellingly close to the love ethic of theologian Reinhold Niebuhr. The Good Samaritan's aspiration is to provide the best care to everyone, but scarcity makes this impossible. However, providing a decent minimum is "both possible and . . . required by a just compassion."[49] In this fashion, Verhey appropriates Niebuhr's celebrated construction of the love ethic of Jesus as an "impossible possibility."[50] The norm of justice establishes a moral floor below which policies and actions must not fall; in this context, the floor of a minimally decent level of health care for all persons. Love motivates aspirations beyond justice, and beyond any moral ceiling to the provision of care, though ultimately it demands the impossible—that is, the absolutely best quality of care for every person. The goodness of the Samaritan ultimately reflects and symbolizes the "impossible possibility" in health care ethics and resource allocation.

This account means that the ethic exemplified by the love, empathy, and compassion of the Good Samaritan is relevant for health care allocation in two important senses. First, it may be possible for individual physicians to provide the best care to their patients, and the professional vocation should be bound up with that commitment. Even though "a Fair Samaritan will acknowledge that in response to scarcity there are moral limits on what a Good Samaritan may do for a patient,"[51] there are not limits with respect to what a physician *may be* for their patients. Moral character and integrity persist through the expression of compassion, caring, and empathic presence, as well as truthfulness and humility, even if the physician encounters restrictions in enacting all these commitments.

With respect to broader policy and professional implications, the ethic as interpreted in the Samaritan narrative functions in a manner similar to Niebuhr's portrayal of the Christian ethic of love as a discriminating standard of indiscriminate criticism.[52]

49. Verhey, *Reading the Bible*, 386.
50. Niebuhr, *Christian Ethics*, 62–83.
51. Verhey, *Reading the Bible*, 388.
52. Niebuhr, "Christian Church," 301–13.

As a standard of indiscriminate criticism, the Samaritan ethic means that all policies for distributing scarce resources will inevitably fall short of the requirements of love and compassion. This lies behind Verhey's (and ultimately Niebuhr's) view that we cannot call moral choices in the context of scarcity "good," but rather "tragic."

However, it is also possible to use the standard of just compassion to differentiate between or discriminate among alternative kinds of policy arrangements that most closely approximate justice or fairness as informed by compassion. A Fair Samaritan will reject an allocation method based entirely on merit or on ability to pay, but instead require that the most important moral priorities are constituted by securing access to the threshold of a decent minimum of healthcare for all persons, and in expressing preferential concern for individuals who comprise the most vulnerable persons in society. This presents an important corrective to arguments such as those presented by Churchill or by market-driven allocations that suggest that samaritanism must necessarily be abandoned when it comes to institutional, structural, or policy issues in resource allocation.

The Prophetic Critique

My interpretation thus far has largely been oriented on the moral applicability of the parable of the Good Samaritan for dyadic relationships, including those in medical care, as a symbol for professional identity, and as story through which distinctions between the obligatory and the supererogatory can be developed. The ethic of love and care embedded in the parable seems especially compelling in circumstances of personal moral choice about rescue or providing assistance to strangers, but as suggested by several commentators, the parable seems inadequate to the moral challenges presented by institutional inequities and structural or social injustices. With respect to issues that pertain to the institutional and structural, the parable retains the kind of indirect relevance developed through Verhey's conception of tragedy; in other accounts, it seems devoid of moral significance in the social realm of ethics.

We clearly can't ask an ethic embedded in a parable to be a panacea for all social ills, and yet I can't help but wonder whether this construction of the Samaritan narrative as containing personal and professional relevance (but diminished institutional and social significance) encompasses the entirety of the moral meaning of the parable. If Jonsen is correct in claiming that an ethic rooted in samaritanism is "unable to tolerate the obscene spectacle of the sick and wounded lying untended,"[53] then the ethic seems to require and entail more than taking care of the injured and ill while neglecting underlying social causes.

It seems important to situate this particular parable within the context of other teachings of Jesus, and more broadly within the moral witness of the biblical prophetic

53. Jonsen, *New Medicine*, 54.

tradition. That tradition bears witness to the equal worth of all persons and the special care that should be directed to the vulnerable, even as it bears witness against oppression of an economic, social, or political nature, an oppression which becomes especially pernicious and hypocritical when mediated through dominant religious institutions or systems. Jesus's audience would have heard the parable not merely as a heartwarming story about caring for the needy, but more as a prophetic denunciation and critique of an ossified and oppressive social structure facilitated by a tradition of religious practice that had lost sight of what religion was supposed to be about and was characterized more by hypocrisy than by integrity. As distilled through the prophetic call of Micah, the religious way of life should cultivate doing justice, loving mercy and kindness, and walking humbly in the path of God.[54] From that prophetic perspective, neglecting the needy, including the sick, is indeed an "obscene spectacle."

The intimations that the parable of the Good Samaritan is embedded within the traditions of prophetic witness against social oppression and moral (and religious) hypocrisy are fairly evident. There is, first of all, the nature of the pre-story, in which Jesus converses with an inquiring lawyer about the requirements to inherit eternal life. That is a legitimate religious question in certain respects, but the question of personal rewards for living in fidelity to *Torah* is asked only by those of the ruling elites of the society; it is *not* asked by those who are seeking to practice *Torah* in everyday interactions. It may be asked by people in social, religious, or professional power who find their social roles and privileges threatened by the tradition of prophetic witness; it is not asked by persons who have been marginalized by the social status quo.

The pre-story is characterized by an implicit critique of both legalistic morality and the human tendency to self-justification. After responding to Jesus's question about the teachings of *Torah*, the pre-story indicates that the lawyer sought to "justify himself" and fortuitously asked the question that sets up the Samaritan parable, "who is my neighbor?" The question of eternal life has been framed by a legalistic classification of the identity of the neighbor. Jesus is consistently portrayed throughout the Gospel accounts as radically challenging and even subverting the efforts of the ruling political and religious elites to establish a legalistic religious and moral code of conduct that would serve their interests, particularly about Sabbath observance.

The discourse on the identity of the neighbor similarly becomes an occasion for Jesus to critique and subvert conventional interpretations of the moral community. While the lawyer seems to have sought for a legal definition that would draw the boundaries of the commitment to love very narrowly, through the parable Jesus erases the ethnic boundaries and expands the moral community in such a way that anyone in need assumes the identity of neighbor. This reiterates and develops the covenantal responsibility of the people of Israel to witness hospitality for the stranger insofar as Israel had once been strangers in Egypt.

54. Mic 6:8.

This does not yet complete the prophetic witness. Jesus's claim, as related through the parable, is that the neighbor is not found "out there" in the world in terms of proximity, religious commitment, or ethnic affiliation. Rather, the lawyer's question is inverted so that the responsibility falls to the moral agent to become a neighbor to others in need through their actions. The efforts to self-justify, rationalize, or exempt oneself from certain actions because the other person encountered does not meet a socially constructed classification is betrayed by this radical and subversive demand to *be* neighbor to others, and especially to those to whom a moral agent might be inclined to dismiss any claim of moral responsibility whatsoever.

The clearest form of prophetic witnessing in the parable, which would not have been lost on any of the immediate audience, is the identification of neighbor with the Samaritan that displayed mercy, rather than the two figures in religious roles, the priest and the Levite. It may have been the case that such persons had religious duties of purification and non-contamination with blood or a cadaver that circumscribed their sense of responsibility of care for the wounded stranger. However, this is precisely the allegiance to legalistic prescribed duty that leads to indifference to human welfare that draws forth the prophetic critique in the first place. A person cannot fulfill *Torah*, let alone receive eternal life, while being in a mindset of casual obliviousness to needs of vulnerable persons.

The problem that the prophetic witness of the parable is ultimately directed at is moral hypocrisy, publically affirming a set of moral standards and beliefs that a person is not willing to live by. The parable witnesses to how the primary exemplification of love can be embodied in the person of a despised ethnic group, a Samaritan. The irony is rich and compelling: The professional classes, the politically powerful, and the religious elites are instructed to emulate the moral example of a person belonging to an ethnic group that they would customarily go out of their way to avoid just as the priest and Levite in the parable bypass the traveler.

The Samaritan character in the parable symbolically expresses a social critique of moral hypocrisy and of community neglect of the vulnerable. In keeping with Michael Walzer's account of prophecy as a form of social criticism,[55] the parable functions prophetically as the moral memory of a religious community and a reminder of its constituent moral values. The prophetic recovery of the moral tradition witnesses to the community of its need for rediscovery of its moral character. Through the symbol of the Samaritan, a social outcast, Jesus reiterates a core moral teaching of the *Torah* to an audience of the social elite who oppressed rather than welcomed the stranger and marginalized the poor. The prophetic critique presumes a moral tradition and community whose practices contravene constitutive values of both tradition and community.

How might this form and content of the prophetic witness of the parable be meaningful for bioethical inquiry? The form does imply that religious voices can bear

55. Walzer, *Interpretation and Social Criticism*, 57–80.

witness to values that are socially inconvenient and disruptive, perhaps even interrupting conventional discourse and practices in bioethics. More directly, when former President Obama introduced the Affordable Care Act before Congress in 2009, he quoted the words of Senator Ted Kennedy with respect to health care reform: "What we face is above all a moral issue; at stake are not just the details of policy, but fundamental principles of social justice and the character of our country."[56] Obama reflected that the social ethic and character of the country was embedded in overarching basic principles, including those that represented a tradition of freedom and self-reliance and also those that represented traditions of equality and solidarity with the vulnerable, including persons that lack insurance coverage and could access health care otherwise only through an emergency room.

There are a variety of policy alternatives that could reflect the values and character of a nation committed to social justice in the distribution of health care resources and access to medical care. My point here is simply that, in the context of Cronkite's observation of the failure of the current health care structure to provide a coordinated, systemic approach to provide caring that both preserves good health and treats disease and illness, Obama's appeal to the character of the country expresses the prophetic responsibility of witness to the moral memory of the society. Ultimately, the moral integrity of a society is to be assessed according to its treatment of those persons who are on its social margins.

Prophetic Witness as Symbolic Rationality

Bioethics aspires to universalizable moral claims and the avoidance of particularism, which means it trades meaning for moral minimalism as well as moral tradition and community for existentialist freedom. Religious discourse, by contrast, embodies a tradition of ethics, narrative, symbols and prophetic critique that is particularistic and most meaningful in the context of a moral community. The concept of symbolic rationality, a form of moral reasoning in which values are expressed and witnessed to by stories, provides social and moral space for the incorporation of religious traditions of meaning and ethics in bioethics. Through the symbol of the Samaritan and the element of prophetic witness delineated earlier, it is possible to discern elements of an overlapping consensus of secular and religious bioethics, which is why the Samaritan parable continues to possess professional, institutional, and cultural resonance and meaning. Part of the deep moral substance of the consensus is that it is morally wrong, and a symbol of a deep moral deficiency of the social order, that the powerful live well because of their oppression of the vulnerable. Those in power bear accountability for allowing "the hungry, and the needy, and the naked, and the sick, and the afflicted to

---

56. Obama, "Speech on Health Care," paras. 56–57.

pass by, and you [social elites] notice them not."[57] The moral violence of oppression is in part a function of distorted vision, of moral myopia, and in part moral hypocrisy.[58]

The prophetic witness of the parable is thus radically demanding and radically subversive of conventions of power, custom, and tradition. The critique of power is especially relevant for the current system of health and sick care in America. Insofar as political proposals and economic considerations lead persons in power to disenfranchise persons from health care insurance, or to provide access to medical care only through a market-based model, the system bypasses the vulnerable and creates an obscene spectacle of sick persons who are not cared for and are not cared about. The ethic of the Samaritan, rooted in love, mercy, justice, humility, and prophetic passion and preference for the vulnerable, cannot allow a callous neglect of the sick to become politically or professionally normative. This prophetic witness is a moral responsibility of all persons in the diverse cultures of bioethics.

57. Mormon 8:39.
58. Campbell, "Metaphors We Ration By," 254–79.

PART TWO

Witnessing the Burdens
A Bioethics of Healing

5

Healing Here

A Bioethics of Calling and Healing

I was walking the corridors of a children's hospital when, just outside of the pediatric oncology unit, I found myself struck by a prominently displayed poster. The poster portrayed a cartoon figure of a young girl underneath script that read: "Use my name, not my diagnosis." This concern about depersonalized medicine is not at all a new development; Francis Peabody, one of the iconic physicians of the early twentieth century, expressed concern in a classic essay that physicians were becoming so enamored of the science of medicine that the art of medicine, which for Peabody was primarily comprised of a personalized relationship with the patient, was being displaced. Peabody concluded his essay with a memorable maxim: "The secret of the care of the patient is in caring for the patient."[1] Nonetheless, several decades into the bioethics-influenced era of treating patients as moral agents and collaborating partners in health care, the poster disclosed that physicians require visible reminders of their commitment to not only the science of medicine, but the arts of healing initiated by knowing their patient's name.

In a presentation to professional caregivers at a local hospital, theological ethicist William F. May told a story of a history professor at a famous university who would answer his phone, "History, here." The implication of this greeting was that, beyond any specialized discourse, a person who had a conversation with the professor would acquire knowledge of history. May posed a question as to whether patients and others who make inquiries of health care professionals should receive a similar invitation to relationship expressed briefly in the phrase, "Healing, here." Embedded in his inquiry

---

1. Peabody, "Care of the Patient," 882.

is a claim that both the self-presentation and the public perception of what medicine should ultimately be concerned with is healing.

Of course, these two vignettes push in opposite directions. The poster pointedly displays the systemic difficulties of caring for the patient, especially in contexts such as an oncology unit, where success is defined by the cure of disease, or prevention of premature death, rather than relationship with a patient. The analogy made from the story of the history professor, by contrast, points to the possibility and even responsibility that individual caregivers, and the profession as a whole, have for breaking through institutional or regulatory inertia and placing their own defining mark on what they do. The ideal of healing as a defining and unifying feature of the medical profession is underscored by the collaborative effort of American and European physicians in internal medicine to develop a set of principles and responsibilities for medical professionalism in the twenty-first century. This "Physician's Charter" affirmed: "The medical profession everywhere is embedded in diverse cultures and national traditions, but its members share the role of healer."[2] Whatever else medicine is engaged in, its defining characteristic involves healing. The Charter has subsequently been endorsed by over ninety other medical organizations and sub-specialties in the United States.

My aim in this chapter is to explore in what respect medicine is in substance, and not just in nomenclature, a healing profession; indeed, perhaps the quintessential healing profession. What would it mean, in practice and in relationships with patients, for modern physicians to strive to be healers and witnesses of healing to the patients? In what ways can religious or biblical portrayals of healing bear witness to healing commitments in medicine?

My approach to these issues begins with a short analysis of what I believe are foundational concepts for healing in medicine, an understanding of medicine as a "calling" or a "vocation," as distinguished from an occupation, job, or career. The construction of the vocation of medicine can be illuminated by the residual historical influence of religious interpretations of calling and vocation. I then develop convergences and contrasts in religious and medical patterns of healing and healing relationships. My claim is that secular philosophical bioethics, wedded to medical science, neglects healing in its interpretations of the purposes of medicine; consequently, making sense of the claim that the core identity of medical professionals pertains to being healers can be productively shaped by religious-based narrative witnesses of healing.

On Call

In "The Calling," physician Abraham Verghese writes of his concern about current and future generations of physicians who have been raised in a visual, cyber, and

2. ABIM Foundation et al., "Medical Professionalism," 244.

digital age, and may consequently experience "cortical atrophy." He inquires: "Where will their sense of calling come from?"[3] Verghese's experience of a call to medicine occurred not in the form of a dramatic health issue, an epiphany of the body, or through familial mentoring, but involved a quiet form of transformative experience through an engagement with literature. Verghese observes that reading various books of fiction invited learning about "humanity in the rough."[4] The narrative dimensions of moral experience disclose realities of the human condition, extend the empathic and moral imagination, and expand the horizons of the possible. Good literature presents an opportunity for reflection and insights into a person's life, and even "may reveal its [life's] purpose."[5]

Physicians in residency and on into their practice experience what it means to be "on call": they are deemed to have acquired the requisite professional knowledge, skills, and training to assume responsibility regarding medical decisions for patients without depending entirely on the assistance of mentors and colleagues. But, as intimated by Verghese, the medical profession exudes a deeper sense of being "on call"—that is, a "calling" to be a physician, a calling to heal and care that extends beyond attending to responsibilities for treating a patient with a health problem. As Sir William Osler wrote, "The practice of medicine is an art, not a trade; a calling, not a business; a calling in which your heart will be exercised equally with your head."[6] Even as contemporary practices and social pressures push medicine towards a business, trade, or marketplace model that concerned Osler, the concept of calling retains resonance within the profession. Let me illustrate with some narrative-formed accounts of calling.

I frequently ask both physicians and aspiring medical students about why they sought or are seeking to become part of the medical profession. Seldom does the word "career" come up in this conversation. The language of career conveys a form of self-directed, autonomous choice, but the aspirations to medical practice run deeper; this something provides the motivation to endure medical school and the frustrations intrinsic to contemporary medical practice, such as insurance provisions, regulatory and legal oversight, electronic records, and administrative bureaucracy, not to mention demanding patients who have assumed the consumerist approach to medicine. It is an other-directed sensibility often phrased as "my calling to care" for others, or "I just felt called to it."

For some, the catalyst for the calling is a life-transformative medical experience in one's early life, such as a physician's treatment that was instrumental in saving the life of a family member, close friend, or significant other, and that symbolized the moral power of caring. In the *life-saving narrative* of calling, medicine is viewed as a

3. Verghese, "Calling," 844.
4. Verghese, "Calling," 843.
5. Verghese, "Calling," 843.
6. Osler, "Master Word in Medicine," 17.

practice by which one can genuinely "make a difference" in the world and in the lives of particular persons. This experientially-grounded source of calling is necessarily connected with a commitment of responsibility for the welfare of others. Writes one aspiring physician who interpreted his decision to attend medical school as a calling rather than a career choice, "To heal a person, whether it be his body or soul, requires both additional humility and more carefully defined goals . . . Work which affects the lives of other human beings carries with it additional moral and ethical weight."[7]

For other persons, the call to medicine is bestowed not through a dramatic miracle of life-saving, but rather through witnessing the workings of the human body, its wondrous intricacies, the functioning of its various organs, and its fragility and vulnerability as well. Most particularly, a surgical procedure such as the opening of the chest cavity to reveal a human heart can be an overwhelming and ever-remembered experience that can render one speechless, a form of in-breaking of the ineffable. This brings appreciation for the body's own healing capabilities that do not require medical intervention, as well as a form of awe and wonder that approaches a religious or spiritual sensibility. The *narrative of awe* as a source of calling situates medicine as a form of connection with something beyond oneself.

For yet still others, the inspiration of a mentor, particularly a family member in medical practice, makes a difference in life and vocational direction. This is the *exemplary narrative* of calling. I ask my students whether they have a most memorable physician or mentor, and it is striking how many do. The interaction of a primary care physician with their patients, at whatever stage of life, is understandably influential. What commonly distinguishes this memorable physician is their relational commitment, their genuine caring for their patients as manifested in listening to a patient's story fully, conversing in such a manner that a vulnerable person feels comfortable in expressing trust, and the effort made by this professional exemplar to take the time to address a full array of concerns a patient may have, including physical, emotional, or relational, and sometime spiritual, considerations. The most ubiquitous way that the exemplary narrative is characterized is as an interaction that cultivates trust between physician and patient who had heretofore been strangers.

I do not mean to suggest that all physicians experience a call in some transformative manner, be it through literary engagement, witnessing a dramatic reversal of another's (or one's own) health condition, the emulation of a mentor, wonder regarding the human body and its organs, or experiencing genuine care. For many knowledgeable, skilled, and competent physicians, medical practice is a matter of rational choice between various career options. Medicine as a profession continues to be held in high professional and social esteem, it can provide intellectual stimulation through collegial interaction and ongoing learning from professional literature, and gratification and meaning emerges through the care of patients. A calling by contrast, while certainly informed by reason, includes an emotional or trans-rational component that

7. Keller, "Is Medicine a Choice," lines 16–19.

"pulls" one into the profession or vocation. In the transformational experience of a calling, a life passion emerges, a way of being in the world is initiated, and the physician begins a journey to become a healer. And, as shall be developed subsequently, healers transform patients and their identities in ways that careerists do not.

There is some empirical support that distinctive attributes, attitudes, and patterns of treatment occur among physicians who understand their professional role as a calling rather than a career or occupation. A recent national study of 1,504 primary care physicians revealed that those who considered themselves in a calling were more willing to treat and care for patients with challenging conditions such as obesity, or nicotine or alcohol addiction. The lead researcher, John Yoon, commented: "For physicians, it may be that having a sense of calling to pursue personally fulfilling or socially significant work provides a strong enough motivator to persevere even in the face of challenges that can lead to burnout and job dissatisfaction."[8] An important characteristic of physicians experiencing medicine as a calling is seeking meaning and vocational fulfillment, particularly through relationships with patients; other professionals may experience medicine and relationships with patients (and colleagues) as depersonalized and tend to interpret challenging health conditions as a failure of patient responsibility.[9] How one views one's professional standing and experience is more than a matter of semantics: a sense of career as calling can have practical ramifications for patient care and for personal and professional commitment.

Still other understandings of the calling to medicine are deeply embedded within religious traditions of professional vocation. Reflecting the theology of the Catholic tradition, physician-ethicist Daniel Sulmasy comments, "Vocation, simply described, is a calling. It is God who calls us and calls us to be the person we have been created to be, to fulfill God's plan for us. It is what we in our deepest most central part of ourselves actually most desire. The match of those two is our vocation."[10] The "match," as Sulmasy phrases it, of divine plan and core personal meaning comprises the intrinsically related concepts of calling and vocation.

The etymology of vocation (*vocare* in Latin) means "to call." Historically, the theologies emerging in the Protestant Reformation rejected the specifically religious vocation of monastic life and interpreted calling and vocation as the role or occupation a person assumed in society. As developed by sociologist Max Weber, the transformational idea of calling is comprised of the view that "valuation of the fulfillment of duty in worldly affairs [is] the highest form of moral activity of which the individual could assume."[11] Two points stand out from this observation. Weber's attention to justifications for activity in the world is meant to differentiate the concept of calling from biblical—the call of Israel, or the call of a prophet to Israel—or ecclesiastical—the

---

8. Rasinski et al., "Sense of Calling," 1424.

9. Dik and Duffy, "Calling and Vocation at Work," 426–30.

10. Shorb, "Medicine as Vocation," lines 33–36; cf. Sulmasy, *Healer's Calling*, 5–20.

11. Weber, *Protestant Ethic*, 80.

monastic life—examples of serving God within the context of a religious community. A calling infuses worldly activity with the energy and commitment heretofore expressed in the religious setting. Secondly, calling is invested with ethical content; it is not a matter of moral indifference. Nor are duties in the world a matter of moral and religious indifference; action in the world expressed through a life task and one's position in the world are principal realms of the moral life. Through fulfilling familial, civic, and economic responsibilities, everyday activities (including marriage, parenting, education, work, and responsible citizenship) manifest and bear witness to values immanent within as well as transcendent beyond the temporal and material.

The religious understanding of calling and vocation as interpreted through the historical Christian tradition and embedded in my own faith tradition illuminate a moral structure and moral presuppositions of a calling that I contend are transferable to and embedded in understandings of calling in medicine. I delineate below four moral patterns of calling that are derived from the ethic of gift-response-responsibility-transformation and the principle of stewardship developed in chapter 3. In addition, this account of the moral features of calling reflects my own experiential insights of a personal calling as an educator and teacher.

Grace and Trust: In religious interpretation, a calling reflects an experience of divine grace or gift, with seemingly little attention to a person's moral action or works or their (lack of) social standing in the world. Persons who are responsive to a calling find an almost irresistible "pull" into not merely an episodic activity but a particular way of life. This means that a calling is experienced as much by the affections and by the transcendent dimensions of a person as by their cognitive capacities for rational decision-making. A person responsive to a calling is drawn into a compelling way of being-in-the-world. An aspect of calling may display a person as feeling more "chosen" than having "made a choice."

The concept of trust in a religious calling is embedded within the ethos of gift-responsiveness-responsibility-transformation. Trust is bestowed upon a person who is responsive to a calling and is thereby entrusted with responsibilities. The experience of a calling initiates a dialectic of trust-and-risk-taking. The bestowal of trust entails risk regarding expectations that the person will embody the virtue of trustworthiness. This requires both fidelity to the purposes of the calling and integrity in adhering to moral values and norms. As observed by philosopher Carolyn McCleod, trust can be "dangerous" for the trustee because they relinquish control to the person called over things that are of significant importance.[12] This dynamic is why the concept of trust is so crucial in the physician-patient relationship.

Agency and Responsibility: The risk-taking inherent to a calling involves reliance on others to exercise their moral agency and self-governance to carry out the entrusted expectations. Preparation, mentoring, and exemplification illustrate principles of responsible action, but ultimately the person called works out the application

12. McCleod, "Trust," para. 1.

of these responsibilities in specific contexts. The calling can thereby provide a moral tutorial for the person called: a discovery through responsible service of a self-in-transformation, a self that gives and forgives, mourns with and comforts others, and affirms dialogue rather than debate. This discovered self expands or enlarges a capacity to seek out the benefit of other persons in ways that include but extend beyond the physical realm of need.

Responsiveness to a calling requires the ongoing development of epistemic capacities to discern both what is happening in a specific situation and what kind of response is most "fitting."[13] The responsibilities of a calling are morally demanding, and in certain respects can be unique and distinctive, set apart from everyday responsibilities. A particular focus of responsibility in the interpretation of calling embedded in the stewardship principle emerges in the metaphor of "magnification."[14] A moral agent in a calling must hone attentiveness to the often neglected details of human need, and a seeing of other persons, society, and their relationships in a new and broader manner, thereby engaging the empathic imagination.

Community and Caring: Responsiveness to a calling situates persons within a small community with shared goals and common values, including an intermediate community such as a profession, wherein the shared purposes are constitutive of what is distinctive about the community or profession. The communal context for calling reinforces the fundamental experience of interdependency. A calling within a moral community should ideally be comprised of sharing responsibility and power with others. The human propensity for power, as exhibited in certain professional settings or as unrighteous dominion in the religious community, will not be eradicated, but can be mitigated through cultivation and expression of trusting relationships.

Within the moral community, however narrow or broad, moral responsiveness in a calling is directed towards caring for the interests and well-being of others relative to the interests of self. The actions exhibited by the Good Samaritan are paradigmatic ideals for the moral commitments of a calling. A calling of caring requires a different way of seeing or different perspective towards others, and especially towards the vulnerable members of a society, who are to be constructed as *imago Dei*. The basic subsistence needs of the poor, vulnerable, homeless, and hungry thereby receive preferential treatment. The experience of calling protects both vulnerable persons and vulnerable values, such as the equality of persons.

Witness and Re-storying: A calling is in part distinguished from careerism in that it involves commitment to a way of life or a way of being in the world rather than the performance of specific responsibilities of a position description. A calling thus is oriented more by the open-ended nature of covenantal commitment than by the details of a contractual relation. A person responsive to a calling may exemplify a different kind of standard of expectations, a higher standard of aspirational morality.

13. Niebuhr, *Responsible Self*, 60–68.
14. *Doctrine and Covenants* 84:33; 88:30.

One common illustration in the biblical accounts of calling is that fidelity to the responsibilities of the calling has primacy over pursuit of material welfare; the promise of providential care for material welfare means the calling is not sought out to rise in social class and wealth or political power.

A calling encompasses being and living out a witness to certain formative values, such as solidarity with others and healing commitments in medicine. This witness can be subversive and prophetic regarding the social order and the religious status quo insofar as those called to a pattern of life are often persons with very little social reputation. As stated in an early Christian epistle from Paul, the calling from God is issued to the weak, the lowly, the insignificant, and even the despised with regard to social status.[15] The called are generally not the elite, the rich, the powerful, the scholarly, or persons from the ruling class, but rather persons who have rather mundane occupations and who heretofore have lived their lives in relative obscurity. Responsiveness to a calling, then, is an occasion not only for personal transformation, but critical social witness as well.

These four patterns are discernable in understandings of medicine as a calling. The central moral claim in my interpretation is the embeddedness of a calling within the ethos of gift-responsiveness-responsibility-transformation. This enables us to see what is at stake, and what might be lost, were the concept of calling to be entirely subsumed into a careerism that so concerned Osler. This does not preclude any physician, regardless of whether they understand their professional role as a calling, a vocation, a profession, a career, or an occupation, from cultivating the skills, acquiring the knowledge, and developing the technical competence needed to become an excellent physician. It does imply that a background set of experiences, motivations, and commitments can influence a physician's sense of the scope of professional responsibilities and identity, including a calling to be a healer.

The language of calling and vocation remains relevant in discourse on medical professionalism. The Task Force of the Royal College of Physicians recently sought to identify the meaning and scope of professionalism in medicine. In discussing conceptual features of professionalism that should be retained for contemporary medicine, the Task Force characterized calling and vocation as concepts displaying a particular motivation for selecting medicine as a career: "The notion of a calling—choosing a career for strong personal reasons, a career that requires particular dedication to other human beings—[is] worth preserving" in the concept of professionalism.[16] The related concept of vocation, meanwhile, signifies "a passion and ethical commitment about a career in medicine."[17]

The report also incorporated the language of vocation in its concluding summary of medical professionalism: "Medicine is a vocation in which a doctor's knowledge,

15. 1 Cor 1:27–28.

16. Royal College, *Doctors in Society*, 18.

17. Royal College, *Doctors in Society*, 18.

clinical skills, and judgement are put in the service of protecting and restoring human well-being."[18] It is evident that the Royal College Task Force understands calling and vocation as particular and distinctive features of the broader notion of career, rather than as independent interpretations of a commitment to medicine. My contention is that just those characteristics of medicine the report is able to express best through its brief allusions to the language of calling and vocation—strong reasons, dedicated service to others, passion, judgement and discernment, and ethical commitments regarding human well-being—are precisely why medicine, while certainly a career, is more than a career, or employment, or a job within a business, in Osler's phrasing. It assumes the features of a calling or vocation with a particular kind of *telos*, that of healing.

The Bioethical Problematic of Healing

Although healing might, according to the "Physician's Charter," provide an orienting identity with broad application for members of the medical profession, scholarship in medicine and within bioethics literature often alludes to healing rather then rendering an exposition of its features. Physician Eric Cassell has observed on the elusive nature of medical healing: "What healing is, what healing actually does . . . is not described in the healing literature in a manner that will allow us to say that 'this is what healing does.'"[19] A recent acclaimed book, *Healing as Vocation: A Medical Professionalism Primer*, has indeed much to contribute to concepts of medical professionalism but very little to say about either healing or vocation, let alone their intrinsic connection.[20] An internet search on healing in medicine reveals very few conceptual expositions, but primarily associates healing with new-age or alternative and complementary methodologies: "Healing" is represented as carried out with cups and candles, or prayers and potions, or needles and nerves, or shamans and sacrifices, or massage and mindfulness.

In short, the language of healing and the concept of physician as healer in many respects seems to move away from medical science and mean a regression to an era when non-scientific superstitions reigned. The quasi-spiritualistic background of healing does not resonate with secularized medicine organized around replicable scientific methodologies. Healing seems to imply a phenomenon that cannot be empirically tested, a kind of "magical thinking" and practice that simply doesn't fit within the scientific and cultural demand for evidence-based medicine. David Barnard has phrased the point as follows: "the metaphor of medical progress [implies] emancipation from the bondage of religious belief and magical thinking."[21] Associations

18. Royal College, *Doctors in Society*, 45.
19. Cassell, *Nature of Healing*, 83.
20. Parsi and Sheehan, *Healing as Vocation*, 1–34.
21. Barnard, "Physician as Priest," 274–75.

of healing, meanwhile, signify abandonment of rationalistic, scientific medicine. Of course, if the threshold for professional acceptability is a rigorous standard of evidence-based practice, then a good deal of the treatments and procedures used in modern medicine would have to be discarded as well.

The scientific stigmatization of healing is no coincidence. The emergence of the self-image of medicine as an applied science in the early twentieth century ran contrary to the imprecision, absence of a scientific method, and enchantment of the world of nature historically conveyed in understandings that medicine was a healing profession. Cassell, who has eloquently argued for the revival of the healing character of contemporary medicine, finds the scientific-based methods of curing as distinct from healing processes that are beyond medical concern to be a fundamentally mistaken assumption at the basis of modern medicine. The distinction between rationalist science and the "magical thinking" attributed to ideas of healing, which underlies the conviction that patients who are cured are also healed, may reflect an incomplete understanding of the aims of medicine and an inadequate perspective on what medicine can be for patients.[22]

Bioethics has largely accepted the scientific paradigm of medicine, including its emancipation from religious belief and its associated critique of healing, as authoritative. In contemporary bioethical discourse, certain ends or goals have been established as constitutive of medicine as a practice, including respecting patient choice, curing disease, promoting health, preventing death, relieving pain, being present in suffering, and always expressing caring.[23] It is noteworthy that healing is omitted from these formative purposes. Contemporary conceptions of medical healing do not express the sense of a radical critique of the medical status quo; it seems that healing is peripheral to the purposes of medical professionalism. At best, healing is characterized as something "more" to which medicine can look upon as an ideal, but not something in the absence of which the medical care provided would be considered to have failed.

In articulating what a serious commitment to medicine as a profession of healing may entail, it is instructive to consider the patterns of healing and aspects of the healing process embedded in various biblical narratives that bear witness to healing. My contention is that, leaving aside the question of whether a scientific method, a religious or cultural approach, or even magical thinking is employed, there are significant conceptual convergences in the religious and the medical meanings of healing. These converging patterns provide insight regarding the meaning implicit in the claim that medicine comprises a healing profession.

22. Cassell, *Nature of Healing*, 69.
23. Hanson and Callahan, *Goals of Medicine*, 1–54.

Biblical Patterns of Healing

Jesus is distinguished by the Gospel writers from the very beginnings of his ministry for his powers of healing disease, sickness, and various kinds of infirmities. The narratives of healing are not a sideshow spectacle, but are integrated with his teaching, and bear witness to his divine calling. I will use as an illustration one of the more extensive narratives in which Jesus is reported to heal a man who was born lacking eyesight.[24] My analysis of the moral meaning of healing will build from this story into claims that have broader applicability.

This story is distinctive even within the gospel narratives of healing in that its narrative arc is generated by the man's experience of blindness from birth. This healing cannot then be a restorative encounter of health, but is necessarily transformative. The re-storying of the narrative begins not with the blind man, however, but with the followers of Jesus. Their inquiry of Jesus—"who sinned, this man or his parents, that he was born blind?"[25]—reveals a background narrative that diseases, physical impairments, or disabilities are consequences of human agency and its misuse. Disease or infirmity is situated within a narrative of *retributive justice*. It is a folk narrative of retribution that seems internally incoherent insofar as it requires some rationale for punishment of an innocent person: the disciples of Jesus seem willing to entertain the possibility that somehow, prior to his birth, the man sinned and thereby brought upon himself his blindness.

Jesus's reply to this inquiry is critical as a religious re-storying of disease, impairment, or disability. He disabuses his followers of the hubris of human responsibility and culpability, and thus also of the inclination to judge other persons for their good or ill health, with the simple observation, "neither . . . sinned." There are no grounds for judgment, for shunning or shaming, for constructing stigmas, or for exclusion of the ill and impaired from the community. A narrative of retribution is supplanted with a narrative in the biblical tradition of deliverance and rescue.

A second narrative then emerges: one of *witness*. The encounter between Jesus and the blind man is situated in the context of an unresolved dispute between Jesus and the community's religious leaders, the Pharisees, about the credibility of the witnesses to Jesus's teachings and ministry, and ultimately to the teaching and healing authority of Jesus. The various kinds of witnesses that Jesus claims attest to his authority necessarily threaten the legitimacy of the traditional and functional grounds of authority upon which the power and status of the religious and political elites rest. In this context of contested authority, Jesus informs his followers that, whatever the causal origins of the man's blindness, the occasion of his blindness will be a (further) manifestation or witness to "God's works." As related in the Gospel of Luke, the

24. John 9:1–12.
25. John 9:2.

prophetic statement of this messianic work and the responsibilities Jesus assumes in his ministry encompasses "recovery of sight to the blind."[26]

This discursive preface is followed by a very earthly and embodied encounter between Jesus and the blind man, the *healer's witnessing of the body*. Jesus spits on the ground, and from the saliva "makes mud," which is to say that this healing process makes use of the elements of the earth present at creation and out of which the human body has been formed. Jesus then applies the earthly substance with his fingers to the man's eyes. This anointing is a witness that healing is not a matter of magical thinking or magical wording, but rather involves the therapeutic power of touch.

The first words between Jesus and the blind man in this encounter are then spoken: Jesus instructs the man to wash in a nearby pool. The narrative is silent as to just how the man found the pool, whether he had assistance from others, or experienced some minimal vision on his own, let alone whether he actually could view the person who touched his eyes and gave him these instructions. It only reports that having performed the required washing, the man "came able to see." The re-storying now shifts from Jesus to the man himself and a narrative of *new identity*. Other persons who have known the man always and only as blind request his story: "How were your eyes opened?"

A third narrative, that of *prophetic witness*, emerges as the account relates that the man's experience of sight occurs on the holy day of the Sabbath. The social mores and religious law circumscribed the range of permissible activities on this day, including imposing restrictions on activity deemed to constitute labor or work. The story of a purported healing of a blind person is necessarily interpreted by the religious authorities as subversive of the religious order and their hierarchical control. The blind man is ultimately brought before the religious leaders who, against the backdrop of their controversy with Jesus about witnesses and authority, are depicted as having little alternative but to discredit the man's story and his character and offer a different narrative to maintain their credibility with the people: The person before them couldn't have been blind in the first place, or if he had been blind, his recovery of sight cannot have divine approval or authorization as it violates the religious law. The narrative initially presented the followers of Jesus as inquiring about the locus of sin that caused the blindness; ironically, the religious leaders insinuate that his recovery of sight must itself symbolize sinfulness. The leaders present a counter-narrative of *tradition* that locates their authority and identity with the tradition of Moses and the inviolability of the Sabbath: "We know that God has spoken to Moses, but as for this man, we do not know where he comes from." The irony increases as the counter-narrative presented by the religious leaders returns precisely to the original error of engaging in stigmatizing judgments of others.

The blind man who has received sight points out the internal incoherence of this counter-narrative to the religious leaders: Since vision is an unquestionably desirable

26. Luke 4:18–19.

feature of good health, it defies reason to contend that his new gift of sight would not warrant divine and popular approval. The blind man embodies the final prophetic witness and critique of authority, as he contends that were Jesus to not possess some authorized healing powers, he could do nothing, let alone provide healing to a person blind from his birth. For this testimonial, he is exiled from the community by the religious leaders.[27]

Although this is perhaps the most detailed account of healing in the numerous Gospel narratives, it is nonetheless illustrative of many of the biblical patterns of healing more generally. The patterns of encounter and interaction that comprise healing in the biblical narratives are embedded in some aspects of what healing seems to mean in contemporary medicine. Here I shall emphasize just five such connections: (1) making whole or wholeness; (2) restoring as re-storying; (3) authority for healing; (4) the embodied witness of healing; and (5) the social contexts and politics of healing.

Wholeness: The feature of healing as *wholeness* is intimated in Jesus's ironic comment to his religious skeptics: "Those who are well have no need of a physician, but those that are sick."[28] In several of the healing stories, the person healed is "made whole," and it is evident that wholeness includes but is not limited to recovery of physical health. The presupposition is that persons are more than just materialistic or biological beings; persons are embodied, but also transcend their corporeality. Wholeness can then encompass emotional or psychological well-being, social relationality, and the spiritual dimension of the person. Such a holistic account of the person is necessary for an understanding that, in modern medicine, patients may be cured but not necessarily healed; the healer considers not simply the bodily dysfunction but rather, as articulated by David Schenck and Larry Churchill in their ethnography of healers, addresses "the whole picture, looking at mind and body and soul."[29]

The conventional term for describing care in making whole that goes beyond the physical is "holistic." In certain circumstances of physical pain or existential suffering, a person can experience healing in an emotional, social, or spiritual sense, even if the physical being of the person remains afflicted, diseased, and sick. It is also embodied in the resiliency of persons who bear the burdens of chronic disease; curing or restoring to a former condition of health may not be possible, but healing can influence orientation and a quest for meaning through which a new self may be discovered. Making whole is often witnessed in the situatedness of dying within hospice care; even in encountering inevitable physical decline and imminent mortality, a terminally ill person can experience wholeness through embodied witness of caregivers to ensure they live out a full or complete life story.

Wholeness is embedded in the moral concept of integrity. The ministrations of medicine effect reintegration of the person's body, or reconstitution of their self, but

27. John 9:13–34.

28. Mark 2:17.

29. Schenck and Churchill, *Healers*, 57.

making whole also pertains to the healer. The healer's integrity is a matter of their moral character and commitment to their art and can perhaps be a pre-condition for the making whole of the patient. The biblical proverb "Physician, heal yourself"[30] continues to have resonance in some medical writings.[31] The proverb is suggestive of a necessity for healers to be persons of professional vocation who embody virtues of discernment, empathy, and compassion. The capacity to heal, or to possess healing powers, is correlated with the kind of physician in whom patients can confidently repose their trust.

Re-storying: An essential feature of healing as restoring wholeness is *re-storying*, that is, drawing on the narrative orientation of the human self, as well as others who are witnesses to healing, to construct a different narrative of the illness experience. As illustrated by the narrative healing of the blind man, persons who sought out or received the healing ministrations of Jesus had ultimately a different story to tell family, friends, the community, and a skeptical religious hierarchy, even if the person healed of a physical ailment did not immediately comprehend the entirety of their experience.

Re-storying and healing involve collaborative and communal, rather than paternalist and authoritarian, processes. As physician Lisa Sanders has written, "the right story has nearly miraculous powers of healing."[32] A narrative conception of healing requires a different set of professional skills and professional self-understanding than is presumed in an information disclosure and consent relational interpretation. The relational interaction is structured around a patient as a storyteller and a physician as an attentive witness and compassionate interpreter or translator; patient and healer collaborate to find a shared narrative that is authentic to the patient's experience and provides the clinical information needed by the physician for diagnosis and treatment. The patient's story simply cannot be heard as background noise to a template providing a disease diagnosis.

The physician as healer cultivates the capacity to hear the particular type of story told by the patient. A "good" illness story, Arthur Frank contends, is "the act of witness that says, implicitly or explicitly, 'I will tell you not what you want to hear but what I know to be true because I have lived it.'"[33] This kind of story is thus subversive of the stripped medical construct in which the patient is transformed from person into disembodied "case." Frank articulates three primary voices of narrative re-storying: restorative, chaos, and quest.[34] The patient's witness of their illness experience calls on professionals to also become witnesses through a retelling of the story. The process

---

30. Luke 4:23.

31. Schenck and Churchill, *Healers*, 73–86.

32. Sanders, *Every Patient Tells a Story*, 16.

33. Frank, *Wounded Storyteller*, 63.

34. Frank, *Wounded Storyteller*, 75–136.

of re-storying then bears a mutual invitation to finding and constructing meaning through the patient's ordeal.

Authority: It is striking how frequently the authority of Jesus to heal is challenged, even to the point of being accused of collusion with demonic powers; that many of the stories of healing occur on the Jewish Sabbath makes confrontation of some sort almost inevitable. His response to such accusations involves pointing out internal inconsistencies in the claims of his critics, providing re-interpretations of the tradition, and relying on several kinds of witnesses to the credibility and legitimacy of his authority. However, the biblical narratives do indicate that Jesus possesses a distinctive kind of authority, one that is noticeably different than the conventional religious teachers of the people.

To put the point in Weberian terms, Jesus possesses, or is possessed of, charismatic authority; the leaders who are both skeptical of Jesus and threatened by his actions are the repositories of tradition and possess authority based on the practices and rituals of the historical community. The central concern for my purposes here is not to resolve the dispute over authority, but rather to observe that both the narratives of healing as well as the counter-narratives presented by the detractors of Jesus attest to a consensus internal to the biblical tradition that healing requires some form of distinctive authorization.

The authority of physicians as physicians derives from processes of medical education, clinical training, and licensure that bestow socially-sanctioned and professionally-recognized authority on a physician to practice medicine. These processes manifest legal-rational and traditional forms of authority.[35] This includes a basis of scientific knowledge, technical expertise, and a commitment to the principles and responsibilities embedded in medical professionalism. Persons who avow charismatic authority in medicine are often dismissed historically and professionally as charlatans engaged in "magical thinking" and other forms of magic practice. Physician David Barnard observes that physicians possess a modified form of charismatic authority that stems from their intimate association with life and death, at least to an extent that the physician affirms the source of such authority, a "conscientious concern for the well-being of those for whom they care."[36]

An intriguing issue internal to the profession regarding the characteristics of the physician as healer is whether these characteristics are inherent to the legal-rational and traditional models of becoming a physician, or whether they are cultivated and acquired by special dedication or practices. Their ethnographic research leads Schenck and Churchill to contend for the latter view; they assert that it is important for researchers to explore "why some helping professionals learn to become healers, and why others never rise above the level of technical competence."[37] That is, the realm

35. Weber, "Politics as a Vocation," 78–79.
36. Barnard, "Physician as Priest," 273.
37. Schenck and Churchill, *Healers*, xv.

of healer and of physician are not co-extensive. It also follows from this point that engaging in a healing relationship is not restricted only to physicians. The community of healers is not defined solely by professionalism and professional authority. The range of healers could both be exclusive of some physicians, and inclusive of some non-physicians, such as nurses (or social workers, or clergy).

Witnessing the Body. As with the paradigmatic parable of the Samaritan, the Gospel narratives report Jesus as moved by compassion as he witnesses the pains and sufferings of others. Jesus is the first to notice the blind man suffering from his affliction, and thereby exemplifies empathic witness. Significantly, the healing process is frequently mediated by Jesus through an embodied encounter in which touch manifests healing. Jesus is portrayed as touching the afflicted body part of the sick person, including the eyes, hands, and face.

The embodied witness between the healer and patient holds great significance in contemporary medicine. Physician Danielle Ofri has written that the physical exam and touch is a distinguishing characteristic of the medical profession that sets medical practitioners apart from their counterparts in the business world. She contends, "there is clearly something special, perhaps even healing, about touch. There is a warmth of connection that supersedes anything intellectual, and that connection goes both ways in the doctor-patient relationship."[38]

The possibility of healing is often carried in the doctor's hands. Touch both expresses and cultivates trust between physician and patient. The vulnerability displayed by the patient and openness to the care-full touching of the physical exam offers transformation within the relationship. This is in part why many physician educators and physician-writers have expressed dismay about a too-heavy reliance on technological testing amidst the declining skills in the physical exam among the current cohort of medical practitioners. A relationship of transformative healing must be established through the body.[39]

Sanders has expressed criticism of what she calls an "interrogation" model of the physician-patient interaction, through which the patient's symptoms are related not through a story, but solicited in a series of questions to fit the medical template of "the chief complaint." And within the interrogation model, Sanders relates that an essential tool for physicians is using "only the barest bones of the original patient's story, stripped of all that is unique, personal, and specific, [and] reshaped by the doctor."[40] A deep tension emerges between the efficiency of the medical construct of the story and the embodied humanity of the patient and her or his story. A disembodied narrative cannot be a healing narrative.

A Politics of Healing. The political and institutional challenges to Jesus's healing reflect just how subversive the activity of healing persons who are sick can be. Healing

---

38. Ofri, "Not on the Doctor's Checklist," D5.

39. Schenck and Churchill, *Healers*, 51.

40. Sanders, *Every Patient Tells a Story*, 24.

was perceived as a threat to religious tradition, scholarly status, ritual requirement, and institutionalized authority. The healing stories thereby bear witness against a rigid status quo that has become preoccupied with the external observances of religiosity, such as in preserving the purity of Sabbath observance, to the extent that it neglects the purposes for which the religious law was given, including saving human life, healing from illness, and promoting practices of justice and mercy.

The healing narratives couple with parables such as that of the Good Samaritan to provide a profound prophetic witness and critique of moral hypocrisy, and in particular societal neglect of the vulnerable, the afflicted, and the wounded. The subversive and prophetic character of biblical healing patterns is an extension of the claim about the distinctive authority of the healer, whether as embodied in Jesus or through the healing powers he bestows upon some of his followers. Weber portrays charismatic authority as a creative and revolutionary force in human history precisely because of its iconoclastic nature that is not bound to traditional or even legal-rational patterns of authority.[41] The authority based on tradition or on legal-rational functionality is found inadequate for the needs of the community, and indeed frustrates the purposes for which the community had been formed. The iconoclasm of prophetic healing aims to not only critique societal practices, but also to literally embody the formative norms of the community for moral and social life, including hospitality and care for the wounded, the vulnerable, and the stranger. The moral witness embodied by the prophetic healer entails that healing encompasses not only a restorative understanding of "going back" to wholeness, but also going "forward" with a new understanding of what wholeness means.

Healing or wholeness of individuals must be situated within the broader politics of healing. Healing presupposes that the current order of the body, of nature, and even of the body politic is incomplete. The subversive nature of healing embedded within the formative biblical narratives presented not only a threat to the structures of economic, political, and religious power, but also promises of liberation for the socially outcast. Jesus's self-interpretation of his mission connects healing with deliverance of the oppressed and outcast, and the metaphors in the messianic moral witness have political connotations: "The Spirit of the Lord is upon me, because he has anointed me to bring good news to the poor. He has sent me to proclaim release to the captives, and recovery of sight to the blind, to let the oppressed go free."[42]

Healing as a sign of the kingdom was a very familiar Jewish tradition, and its in-breaking means a deliverance of the community from embedded structures of oppressive power, authority, and control, and the reformation of justice in the social order. The clear biblical connection between healing and liberation of the vulnerable should direct our attention to what are referred to as the social determinants of health. The biblical narratives of healing bear witness against social exclusion and access to

41. Weber, "Social Psychology," 295–96.
42. Luke 4:16–18.

care based on privilege.[43] Access to health care for millions in our society is impeded by political, economic, class, gender, and cultural barriers to health, and social, institutional, and professional structures of power.

Even if as an aspiration, healing bears witness against an industrial model of medicine and health care in which health care is understood as a mass-produced commodity that physicians deliver and patients and consumers receive or consume. Healing requires a medical culture that is conducive to relationship and community rather than an ethos of transactional provider-consumer relationships. Physician Victoria Sweet alludes to this background context in lamenting that, "in this day of efficient health care, no one ever gets even to see such a [healing] process."[44] A healing presence in medicine can be subversive to a profession that seems to follow the moral compass set by the law (contractual minimalism) and the marketplace (efficiency), and by the business ethos that, as consumers rely on the principle of personal self-determination, the customer's choice is beyond challenge. The question is whether medicine has become so reliant on external objectives and authorities that it is incapable of cultivating its own internal ethos and meaning. Something very significant about medical professionalism is thus being expressed and reclaimed in the assertion of the "Physician's Charter" that the core feature of professional identity is bound up with healing.[45]

Put another way, the biblical narratives of healing exhibit a profound critique and distrust of organized or institutionalized religion (one that has been carried over in much of contemporary American religiosity). This is partly attributable to the characteristic routinizing of charisma that transpires in the institutionalization of religion. Similarly, patient and societal dissatisfaction with the health care system is precisely that it is a system (or dysfunctional non-system in Cronkite's view), a corporate institution that—for all of, and perhaps because of, its marketing methods—is perceived to construe health care as a deliverable commodity with the consequence that impersonal transactions prevail in place of healing interactions. The critique of the impersonal exchange is reflected in the poster described in the vignette beginning this chapter that instructs clinicians to "Use my name, not my diagnosis." By contrast, in the phrasing of Peabody, "caring for" a patient is a form of healing, and assumes its own subversive manifestation insofar as both caring and healing presume a profoundly personalized relationship and commitment beyond curing and beyond practices dictated by the logic of efficiency.

A conception of healing as wholeness, and an understanding of wholeness as extending beyond the physical to encompass additional dimensions of the embodied self, must continue to be at the core of the meaning of healing. I have claimed a subversive role for healing in medicine in that it witnesses to an alternative set of values

---

43. Campbell, *Health as Liberation*, 103–24.

44. Sweet, *God's Hotel*, 179.

45. ABIM Foundation et al., "Medical Professionalism," 244.

and goals than are currently exemplified in models of medicine focused on consumer-ism, commodities, and cures. The trust necessary to any successful physician-patient relationship is cultivated by transforming powers of touch. It is also evident that re-storying and giving back the story to the patient is a key feature of the healing process. Finally, healing represents a commitment aligned with social justice and the equality of persons in their vulnerability.

Although the biblical narratives illuminate patterns of healing that can inform interpretations of healing in medical practice, one common aspect of healing is not immediately depicted: relationship. Strikingly, at least from the stories transmitted in the scriptural records, Jesus heals or makes whole people who are perfect strang-ers to him, or who have sought him out from his reputation. Any conversation or prior relationship is in the background, if not invisible, in the biblical narratives. This highlights the charismatic gift of healing in the narratives, but it stands in marked contrast to discourse about healing in modern medicine, within which healing is a process that occurs over the course of time as part of the essential relationship of physician and patient. As maintained by physician Eric Cassell: "healing occurs in the relationship—it is interpersonal—between the healer and the patient."[46] The healer in medicine is a guide and companion, bearing witness of core commitments to fidelity, non-abandonment, and presence so the patient does not, in the isolation and vulner-ability of their illness, journey alone to the dark places of their health condition.

Healing Relationship

The implicit presuppositions of healing in the literature of bioethics and medical humanities are focused on a relationship in which a physician brings to bear their knowledge of disease and the body, their technical competence in treatments, and their understanding of their patient as a person, not simply a disease entity. Since a disease or sickness affects not simply the body, but the entire self, the clinician bears responsibility for the health of the whole person. The vocation of a physician means placing the person at the center of medical concern, rather than a disease condition, medical science, or technological interventions. Healing requires comprehensive knowledge of the whole person, including their physical, emotional, psychological, social, and spiritual self. Cassell observes, "healers must learn as much about persons as they do about illness."[47]

Acquiring knowledge of the person required for healing them necessitates cul-tivating mutual trust in a covenantal form of relationship of open-ended duration. Through their ethnographies of healing, Schenck and Churchill identify a cluster of eight practically oriented relational healing skills. These skills provide insight into

---

46. Cassell, *Nature of Healing*, xvii.

47. Cassell, *Nature of Healing*, 2.

how clinicians can initiate and maintain relationships with "healing potential."[48] Given the historical roots of healing embedded in diverse spiritual tradition, the authors incorporate the general structure of rites of passage from anthropological accounts of religious experience to illuminate how the relational skills of healing can manifest transformed identities in the course of everyday clinical interactions.

A ritual of passage is a significant marker of fundamental thresholds and transitions in the course of a person's life, including birth, initiation into a (religious) community, puberty, marriage, and death, among others. The identity-confirming and identity-transforming processes embedded in such rituals have been characterized through a threefold structure of (a) separation, (b) passage or transition, and (c) reincorporation. The separation phase means the person leaves behind their former self, identity, or community, or way of life; as in the Exodus narrative, the Hebrew tribes discard their identity as slaves in bondage in a strange land. The transition or perilous passage reflects the liminal status of the person or community—they no longer identify with their former self, but they have yet to acquire the status of a new self or be accepted as a full member by a new community. This is manifest in the wandering of the Hebrew tribes in the desert wilderness prior to the covenant identity conferred on Sinai. The experience of liminality, of being "in between" identities, can be threatening or perilous. Liminal status customarily necessitates the presence of a guide or the experience of *communitas*, a community of those who share the experience of the passage so the person or community may find their way to a new status, identity, and communal relation. The final stage, that of reincorporation, means the person has acquired or received a new status or identity and has been welcomed into a new community (such as the community of adults, or new relationships embedded in a marriage). The Hebrew slaves become the people of Israel. This conferral of new identity is commonly signified by the bestowal of a new name, the wearing of new clothing, or some other markers of new identity. In addition to various rituals of transforming passages in religious communities, such as naming or confirmation, baptism, or bar or bat mitzvah ceremonies, a thin version of these elements of passage is embedded in university graduation and commencement ceremonies, as well as the white coat ceremony in medical education.

This basic structure in religious experience is adapted with some modifications by Schenck and Churchill to interpret how healing relationships are cultivated between patients and physicians. On their interpretation, patients are initiates undergoing a passage from the ordinary world of everyday life into the threatening and potentially perilous world of medicine and illness, a world the authors refer to as "the container." The container metaphor indicates the separate boundedness of the health care interaction and relationship from common experience in the everyday world. Within the liminal space of the container, certain activities which are not encountered or permitted in ordinary life occur that are of profound significance for the person

48. Schenck and Churchill, *Healers*, 36.

and for the relationship. These include intimate conversations about health issues and intimate physical contact (including the physician's witnessing of the body, touching of the body, and direct physical interventions in the patient's body). It is within what I designate as a "sanctuary of liminality" for the patient that the healing work or experience transpires and the healing relationship is confirmed.

In the medical container or liminal sanctuary, the clinician enacts several relational skills to foster trust in the relationship and in a healing process. These include what the authors designate as shorthand reminders, such as "be open and listen," "find something [about the patient] to like," "remove barriers," and "let the patient explain."[49] In particular, the physician as healer directs the relational skill of attentive listening to "listening for stories, for the narratives that give coherence to the lives of one's patients."[50] The exercise of these maxims in the medical container attests to the validity of Cassell's claim that the fundamental skill of healing is comprised of the capability of attentive listening as well as the significance of witness to the patient's story.[51] The dynamic of patient narrative and story and the physician's witness are necessary features of the re-storying process of healing.

As indicated, the experience of liminality is a perilous and threatening circumstance that typically invokes the experience of *communitas*. Schenck and Churchill contend that *communitas* is mediated in the liminal sanctuary through a powerful metaphor of "guide" that delineates the physician's presence and role for the patient. The guide metaphor has three specific implications.[52] The physician can guide the patient on their perilous passage because of their experiential familiarity with the landscape of disease, sickness, and mortality. The physician may not have specific knowledge of the landscape for a particular patient but they are familiar with the general contours and outlines of the transitional passage. Secondly, the physician can assume a mentoring role, at times mirroring the patient's narrative back to the patient, challenging their assumptions and sense of limitations, and collaborating in the re-storying process. A third feature of the guide metaphor involves the physician acting as a companion on the passage the patient is encountering, an exemplifying and embodied witness of the core commitments of fidelity, non-abandonment, and presence so the patient does not (as previously noted), in the isolation and vulnerability of their liminality, journey alone to dark places of their health condition. The implications of companionship for healing are eloquently expressed by one physician interviewee: "I think in order to really get to the point of healing, you have to love. You have to be compassionate, understanding, and willing to walk the wounded path with [the patient]."[53] The metaphor of "walking with" rather than "forging ahead" or "following

---

49. Schenck and Churchill, *Healers*, 31.

50. Schenck and Churchill, *Healers*, 12.

51. Cassell, *Nature of Healing*, 81–93.

52. Schenck and Churchill, *Healers*, 33–34.

53. Schenck and Churchill, *Healers*, 15.

behind" is an exemplary expression of *communitas* and the ethic of bearing witness as the physician is called to bear the burdens of the patient's woundedness.

The sanctuary of liminality is departed in the course of the end of the encounter to facilitate the patient's reincorporation by the community into everyday life. A question of importance in this transition is whether, consistent with the authors' appropriation of the rites of passage structure, the process of exit and reincorporation necessarily involves a change of status or identity. It would seem that, in particular situations of health crisis, such as diagnosis or treatment of serious illness, the patient's liminality is extended and prolonged, perhaps even to death. As expressed by Arthur Frank, some cancer patients may find that their exit from the medical container is simultaneous with an entrance into a remission society.[54] Alternatively, the patient may experience an end to their liminality and restoration to their familiar social place, but not necessarily a transformed status.

My claim is that there are two elements in the patient's experience of liminality that appear altered in significant and meaningful ways from traditional anthropological interpretations of rituals of passage. These elements represent a going forward towards wholeness. A first circumstance for the emergence of a new identity is intimated in Cassell's account of the inherent community of the relationship. He argues that, as the relationship unfolds, the healer's professional self "is forming a 'we' with the patient."[55] This "we-ness," which can be offensive and insulting in other non-intimate contexts, implies a collaborative coordination, a working together for common ends and purposes, as well as a sharing and merging of identities. The "we" of the relationship implies a new or emerging identity and bears witness to the patient that they have not been abandoned, nor are they entirely alone in their illness experience.

A second element of passages towards wholeness and healing reiterates the fundamental connection between wholeness and re-storying. On the basis of their ethnography, Schenck and Churchill maintain: "Patients can alter their sense of the meaning of their medical condition. So one way to think of healing would be to consider it as the acceptance of a new vision of one's own wholeness."[56] This vision, the exercise of the creative imagination embedded in the *imago Dei*, is really only possible with a healer's witnessing of the patient's story and a collaborative construction of a different narrative, a re-storying of the patient's experience. Insofar as meaning is constructed through some kind of narrative account, a discovery of a new perspective for the patient of being whole, of experiencing healing, entails revising some elements of the story, discarding other elements, and appropriating still other elements from other stories that are new for this particular patient.[57]

54. Frank, *Wounded Storyteller*, 8–13.

55. Cassell, *Nature of Healing*, 91.

56. Schenck and Churchill, *Healers*, 66.

57. Cassell, *Nature of Healing*, 91.

Schenck and Churchill observe, "Healing . . . [a]lways has to do with connections between people that make us whole and restore us to the deep sources of meaning for our lives."[58] This interpretation of healing in medicine doesn't presume an invariably successful, life-restoring, or life-saving medical outcome, or a medicalized narrative of restitution. It does imply that healing can encompass many life experiences and relationships, such as those experienced in family, friendships, or intermediate communities like those of religion; consequently, being a healer is not professionally restricted to those in the healing professions. Still, within medicine or nursing, healing will be experienced through a process of cultivating trust in relationship with a professional caregiver, who listens attentively, bears witness in the process of re-storying, and is present with and guides the perilous passages of the patient between health and sickness with compassion, solidarity, and fidelity.

Conclusion: Calling, Healing, and Covenant

My argument in this chapter is that the distinctive professional ethos of medicine, often expressed through the language of medicine as a healing profession, is partially shaped by concepts such as calling, vocation, and healing, which have meaningful resonance with the wisdom and practical witness of religious communities of moral discourse. In the course of a long process of secularization and institutionalization, which has included the emergence of a scientific paradigm as the dominant source for medical knowledge and understanding, and the rise of a marketplace model for enacting health care relationships, the influence of these concepts has diminished. In the absence of such enlivening and motivating concepts, medicine can become another career focused on transactional exchanges and manipulations to increase technical efficiency. I concur with the critique of instrumentalist medicine offered by bioethicists Lawrence Schneiderman, Nancy Jecker, and Albert Jonsen: "If the medical profession retreats to the position that it has no internal professional values and merely provides whatever patients, families, or insurers are willing to pay for, it can no longer claim to be a healing profession, that is, a group committed to healing and serving the sick. Instead, medicine becomes a commercial enterprise satisfying the desires of others."[59]

Physicians are more than mechanics with technical expertise; they are called to be healers. Although its precise nature is elusive, healing is comprised of patterns of caring that reflect restoring wholeness, re-storying meaning, embodied presence, and a relationship of bearing witness that goes beyond informational transactions to liminal transformations of identity for both healer and patient. The ethical wisdom of religious traditions is an important witness to this professional identity. This analysis of healing as a fundamental end of medicine provides the framework for the following chapter on covenantal relationships.

58. Schenck and Churchill, *Healers*, xiii.

59. Schneiderman et al., "Medical Futility," 669.

6

Covenantal Witness

Soon after being diagnosed with what ultimately would be terminal pancreatic cancer, Joseph Cardinal Bernardin spoke before the House of Delegates of the American Medical Association. In his address, Bernardin called on the medical profession to "renew its covenant" with patients and with society.[1] Bernardin argued: "The moral compass that guides physicians in meeting those obligations [to patients, the profession, and society] needs to be fully restored so that the covenant can be renewed."[2]

Bernardin's characterization of a covenantal relationship between society and medicine reflects a long tradition of situating the ethical commitments of medicine within a non-professional and even religious structure. The concept of covenantal relationship seems to have diminished significantly outside of religious traditions, most commonly supplanted by the secularized concept of social contract that draws on the metaphors of liberal political philosophy. On occasion, however, covenantal language reemerges. In the preceding chapter, I indicated that a task force on medical professionalism of the Royal College of Physicians invoked the language of calling and vocation as part of its understanding of medicine as a distinctive kind of career. The same organization initiated its analysis of medical professionalism by asserting that the success of medicine in achieving its basic purposes of relieving suffering, preventing disease, and treating illness "has been and remains founded upon a covenant between the medical profession and society."[3] The Royal College indicated a preference for articulating the relationship and mutual agreement as a "moral" contract rather than social contract on the grounds that moral contract presents a substantive

1. Bernardin, "Renewing the Covenant," 269.
2. Bernardin, "Renewing the Covenant," 272–73.
3. Royal College, *Doctors in Society*, 1.

ethical edge for medical professionalism.[4] The report also portrayed the relationship of a health care professional and patient as a "covenant of trust."[5]

The concept of covenant is invoked in discourse about medicine to mediate morally between different, although related, relationships. Both Bernardin and the Royal College of Physicians speak of two of those relationships: the macro relationship of the profession and society and the micro relationship of physician and patients. Two additional moral contexts of covenantal relations in medicine, which presume the meaningfulness of the basic social covenant, concern the moral commitments and identity of health care institutions, and the relationship between medical colleagues (a covenant with origins in the Hippocratic Oath). As expressed in one theological interpretation: "the language of covenant is the best model of the relationship between medical professionals and their patients as well as between medical professionals."[6] At the core of these claims is the idea that relationships within and about medicine and health care institutions are morally serious rather than morally neutral undertakings, structured, at least historically, by a vow, oath, or promise.

This chapter explores the moral meanings of covenantal commitments in medicine and health care. I offer an account of the moral structure and ethical content of a covenantal commitment, as rooted in the symbol of the *imago Dei*, and the resonance of this commitment for relationship and community in medicine. I will also examine the applicability of the moral structure of covenant for relationships of the medical profession with patients and the society. Both religious traditions and the medical profession, including health care institutions and individual physicians, assume the characteristics of an intermediate community in social and cultural life—that is, a community that mediates and interposes between the individual and the liberal state. A covenantal ethic and a covenantal community bear witness to core values embedded but often neglected in medicine, such as calling and healing delineated in the previous chapter as well as gift-based responsiveness, and also bear witness against the transactional interpretation of market-driven contractual medicine. The concept of covenant, like that of healing, has a very subversive character for the power structures of modern medicine. I begin with a discussion of the political narrative of social contract that informs interpretations of the medical profession.

Social Contract

Both medical professionals and bioethics scholars have recently tended to define the relationship of the medical profession to those outside of the profession, be it individual patients, patient populations, or the broader society, in contractual terms. The use of "moral contract" by the Royal College of Physicians is intended to be explicitly

4. Royal College, *Doctors in Society*, 17–18.

5. Royal College, *Doctors in Society*, 43.

6. Bouma et al., *Christian Faith*, 120.

critical of the moral neutrality and diminished ethical edge embedded in a social contract, a relational concept external to medicine and drawn from liberal political philosophy. Nonetheless, the concept of medicine as a profession is invariably connected to a contractual relationship with the society medicine is supposed to serve. Scholars in medicine have interpreted medical professionalism as comprising "the essence of the social contract" between medicine and the society.[7]

Physician Matthew Wynia contends that the origins of the social contract model within medicine occurred with the organization of the American Medical Association in 1847 and the promulgation of the original AMA Code of Ethics. The AMA Code is analogous to the Declaration of Independence insofar as it symbolically represents the commitments of a new form of association.[8] However, Wynia stresses that an ethics code does not imply an oath, vow, or promise. Although the contract is mediated through norms of reciprocity, it lacks the commitment to fidelity characteristic of calling and vocation. Furthermore, as William F. May has observed, the embedded moral relationship of the 1847 AMA Code was characterized more by professional philanthropy than of mutual contract: "The AMA viewed the patient and public as bound and indebted to the profession for its services but viewed the profession as accepting duties to the patient and public out of a noble conscience rather than a reciprocal sense of indebtedness."[9]

The social contract between the medical profession and society is organized according to the following parameters: In order to effectuate the delivery of health care through this professional association, society recognizes the profession's (a) monopoly regarding the use of medical knowledge, (b) autonomy in the practice of medicine to serve the best interests of patients, (c) self-regulatory supervision, and (d) methods for assurance of physician competence. In addition, the contract implies an obligation on the part of society to provide the profession with the fiscal and health care resources sufficient for it to accomplish its responsibilities to patients and to the society. The moral implications of the contractual understanding are reflected in just how close scholars Cruess and Cruess come to entitlement language in asserting that physicians and the profession "deserve" patient and public trust due to their knowledge, skills of practice, patterns of professional accountability and oversight, and in stewardship of societal resources.[10] The contractual understanding generates a different source for trust than a gift-based covenantal interpretation.

Contractual responsibilities for the profession are generated by a norm of reciprocity,[11] including physician professionalism based in the altruistic motive that physicians will put the interests of patients ahead of their own (a feature that recalls the

7. Cruess and Cruess, "Professionalism," 9.

8. Wynia, "Birth of Medical Professionalism," 25.

9. May, *Physician's Covenant*, 121.

10. Cruess and Cruess, "Professionalism," 17.

11. Cruess and Cruess, "Professionalism," 19.

commitment to service inherent in calling); social and professional exemplification of morality and integrity; a practice of transparency; and commitments to address social concerns relevant to a physician's expertise. In the interprofessional document "Medical Professionalism in the New Millennium" that I have previously cited, physicians who are oriented to their professional identity by the commitment of healing assume responsibilities for social justice in health care, including fair distribution of resources, eliminating discrimination, promoting cost-effective practice, and public advocacy to improve access to health care.[12] Reciprocity is clearly an important moral norm for social and professional interactions, but when embedded in a contractual self-understanding of professionalism, it gives moral primacy to transactional rather than transformational relationships within the profession, between physicians and patients, and between the profession and society.

Crises of identity and integrity experienced by the profession can be attributed to challenges to the norm of reciprocity and the embedded commitments of the contractual model. The social influence of the marketplace can diminish professional commitments to integrity, while government oversight and regulations (not to mention those from the insurance industry) infringe on professional autonomy. The issue of monopolistic authorization is challenged as members of other professions, not to mention patients, become increasingly knowledgeable about health, disease, treatments and pharmacology, and acquire treating responsibilities and medical knowledge. Correspondingly, society may well wonder, given historically diminished levels of physician affiliation with organized professional associations (including the American Medical Association), who in medicine is making and enforcing medicine's part of the contract? This may suggest that the social contract model of medicine, like the philosophical model from which it is appropriated, is a useful fiction.

It is somewhat of a puzzle that contemporary medicine would retrieve the contractual metaphor from liberal political philosophy to interpret the nature of its defining relationships. The liberal political tradition of social contractarianism as developed in Hobbes and Locke makes several presuppositions that, however well they serve in the realm of political life between moral strangers, do not seem coherent with the basic commitments and integrity of the medical profession. A social contract is necessary in the liberal philosophical tradition because of the inherent adversarial nature of human beings who are self-interested to the point that they cannot trust each other. The contractarian position also identifies the primary, if not exclusive, relationship of moral interest to be that between an individual and the state insofar as this relationship is held to generate the origins of social morality; various other relationships, such as within a family, or friendships, or various communities that are intermediaries between self and state, such as religious or professional communities, are of secondary or peripheral moral significance and derivative in moral content of the basic social contract between self and state.

12. ABIM Foundation et al., "Medical Professionalism," 243–46.

In the contractarian tradition, the authority as well as the limits of the state regarding oversight of individual actions is primarily mediated through the moral discourse of rights, a language that establishes protections to ensure respect and non-exploitation in the context of domineering political power and prevailing individualism and egoism. The social contract tradition also presumes that individuals are moral strangers, with no shared conception of the good life or the good society. Moral agents may be portrayed as "friendly" strangers insofar as they accept shared procedures to resolve conflict and manifest the minimal trust necessary for a cohesive society.[13] There is, however, no overarching societal *telos* that the society of strangers seeks to achieve.

The question then becomes just why the medical profession would want to stress its social situatedness through a relational model that presumes adversarial encounters, moral estrangement, power rather than partnership, and rights rather than responsibilities. Without some fairly discriminating and nuanced philosophical interpretation and professional application, all of these assumptions of the social contract paradigm push medicine precisely in the direction of legalism, moral minimalism, commercial primacy, individualism, and a distrust that permeates society as a whole. While the discourse of contract is congruent with both an increasing secularization of society and the professional autonomy of medicine, the contractual model neglects something of deep moral significance about persons and their orientation to relationship in professions and communities.

As displayed through the *imago Dei*, our basic human nature is creative, embodied, relational, and communal; this is manifested through our ongoing participation in families, friendships, education, voluntary associations, religious communities, and in professional societies, such as that instantiated in medicine. The liberal tradition of political philosophy gives rise to the contractual model emphasizing the relation of state and citizen, but persons are engaged in numerous relationships that serve as intermediating associations; indeed, the lives of most persons are much more oriented by involvement in these intermediate associations and communities than they are negotiating the citizen-state relationship. Theologian H. Richard Niebuhr puts the relational point this way:

> The fundamental form of human association . . . is not that contract society into which men enter as atomic individuals, making *partial* commitments to each other for the sake of gaining limited common ends or of maintaining certain laws; it is rather the face-to-face community in which unlimited commitments are the rule and in which every aspect of every self's existence is conditioned by membership in the interpersonal group.[14]

13. Childress, *Who Should Decide*, 48–49.

14. Niebuhr, *Responsible Self*, 73.

Niebuhr grants some social space for contractual relationships and the symbol of "man-the-citizen, living under law,"[15] but contract is not the fundamental form of association.

The contractual understanding can minimize not only the social and relational nature of persons, but also those characteristics constitutive of medicine as a profession. The profession cannot become a mere extension of an economic or political system without compromise to its identity and integrity; a definitive mark of a profession is autonomy and self-regulation. In Wynia's view, medicine must "maintain some distance from the state and market";[16] furthermore, "professional associations should serve, ideally, to moderate the potential negative effects of both markets and government regulation of health care."[17] Similarly, if the profession is situated in the liminal status of in-between self and state, and similarly situated relative to self and market, individual physicians as members of this intermediating profession can "serve as a bridge between ill people and their communities."[18] This requires resituating medicine with respect both to the state and society, to professional institutions, and to persons.

I do not contend that there is no room in medicine, let alone in the civic society, for contracts and the moral and legal protections provided by rights. Rights language has been a transformational rhetoric in the political realm, empowering revolutionaries against the oppressive power of despotic governments, and empowering minorities and the vulnerable against oppressive power of political, economic, and religious elites. Nonetheless, the emergence of rights discourse is always illustrative of a breakdown of patterns of conventional social order and power relationships. It is no surprise that when the emerging bioethics movement sought to challenge the paternalistic authority of medicine, the primary moral language was that of rights, primarily negative rights to noninterference, but also positive claims to information disclosure encompassed in rights to informed consent.

While rights language is very important, for example, in circumstances when religious liberty is in conflict with medical beneficence (e.g., conscientious objections), in an intermediate community directed by shared goals and common causes that unite persons in a moral relationship, we would think it very odd to have rights language permeate the air. Rights language is typically absent in the familial relationship, for example, whether between spouses or between parents and children, because its adversarial and power presuppositions are inimical to the purposes of the family relationship. Resort to the language of rights in such a setting emerges only when the relationship is fracturing, as in a divorce, custody disputes, domestic violence, and child abuse.

---

15. Niebuhr, *Responsible Self*, 51–54.
16. Wynia, "Birth of Medical Professionalism," 32.
17. Wynia, "Birth of Medical Professionalism," 32.
18. Wynia, "Birth of Medical Professionalism," 32.

As prominent as it is in medical and in bioethics discourse, the construction of social contract neglects the communal character of the person and the role of the medical profession as an intermediate community between the sovereign self and the sovereign state. It can skew the mediating influence of physician and professional in both a very individualist and a very minimalist direction. The spoken profession of the contract and its embedded values cultivate an attenuated trust of the public and of society in physicians. It is meaningful, then, that in both relationships between physician and patient, and between profession and society, the Royal College report deliberately eschewed contractarian language and appropriated covenantal language. While the physician-patient relationship is most commonly described by the Royal College in terms of a partnership metaphor, a concluding observation reinforces the moral nature of the relationship through both covenantal and *moral* contractual models: "Professionals, because of their covenant of trust with patients and their moral contract with society, are advocates for those they serve."[19] It seems important to consider the moral fittingness for medicine of a model of covenantal ethics.

The Moral Structure of Covenants

The Latin root of covenant, *convenire*, means a "coming together." That is, covenants presuppose relationship and community for a common purpose; the moral discourse of rights, by contrast, presupposes a "coming apart" or relational breakdown that contracts seek to prevent or forestall. Theologian Joseph Allen has expressed the intrinsic connection between covenant and community as follows: "A covenant model expresses the essential socialness of human life. It presupposes that every aspect of life is lived out of our belongingness with others in the human community."[20] Allen contends that covenant is the central relational model in the theological and moral witness of the biblical traditions and expresses an understanding of "God's character and action, as well as of human relationships under God."[21]

As delineated in my interpretation of the *imago Dei* (chapter 3), the biblical tradition contains numerous covenants; some of these portray a religious covenant between the deity and humanity, or what Allen designates as an "inclusive" covenant.[22] Inclusive covenants encompass the Noahide covenant, which mediates the relationship between God and the world, including nonhumans, and the divine promises made to the Hebraic patriarchs of prosperity, land, and unending posterity for their devotional fidelity. Inclusive covenants are "promissory" inasmuch as God both initiates the covenant and limits divine action with a promise, but does not impose covenantal obligations on the human parties.

19. Royal College, *Doctors in Society*, 43.
20. Allen, *Love and Conflict*, 46.
21. Allen, *Love and Conflict*, 46.
22. Allen, *Love and Conflict*, 39–41.

The promissory inclusive covenants contrast with the covenant of responsibility paradigmatically related in the Exodus narrative. Certain background conditions for the initiation of this particular covenantal relationship are embedded in the narrative: the covenantal commitment is preceded by an experience of circumstances of oppression or bondage, acts of deliverance, a journey or passage, and community memory. The moral meaning of the covenant of Israel is derived from and shaped by the prior, pre-covenantal history, which situates the covenantal moral commitment within the ethos of giftedness-response-responsibility-transformation. Giftedness is enacted through the deliverance of the slaves from oppression; responsiveness is manifested by the willingness of the people to bind themselves as a moral community to their deliverer; responsibility involves an acceptance of a way of life shaped by moral content and obligations, as well as a promise or witness to live in fidelity to the covenant over time; and slaves are transformed into a people called Israel that bear witness in the world through the ongoing living out of the covenantal responsibilities.

The religious or divine/human covenant provides a conceptual grounding and narrative resource for analogical reasoning in structuring human relationships as moral covenants. Of course, there are important moral differentiations between a religious and a moral covenant. Most obviously, the divine/human covenantal relationship, be it Noahide, Abrahamic, or Mosaic, is not marked by equality of status or power. This entails that the relationship is initiated by a divine gift, blessing, or grace. Other covenants in the biblical accounts, designated by Allen as "special covenants,"[23] are primarily moral in nature as they concern right relationships between human beings. Special or moral covenants morally mediate gifts and trust in human relationships such as marriage, parenting, and friendships, socially authoritative institutions, and at some historical junctures, relationships within as well as between nations.

The scope of moral covenantal responsibility is a pervasive issue given the limits of finitude and fallibility in human relationships. Insofar as covenants convene and bring persons together in community, it is important to ask towards who the covenant-directed responsibilities are to be assumed—that is, who is a member of the moral community. The Noahide covenant has been interpreted in Judaism, for example, to have universalized applicability, while the Mosaic covenants largely regulate conduct towards persons within the community of Israel, although certainly provision is made for care and hospitality towards strangers. Of course, this is the moral question implicit in the parable of the Good Samaritan. The scope of relationship-constituting covenants of marriage and friendship are generally confined to the relationship between the spouses or the friends, though they do not confer moral exemption from responsibilities towards others assumed on different grounds, be they covenantal or contractual.

As well as differences, it is possible to identify substantive ways in which religious and moral covenantal relationships correspond. As described previously, Bouma and

23. Allen, *Love and Conflict*, 41–45.

colleagues contend that human covenants are embedded in three characteristics that mirror the moral structure of religious covenants: (1) prior events or gifts that manifest personal vulnerability, (2) community creation within which identities of covenantal partners are shaped or transformed, and (3) an enduring quality over time that allows for the relationship to evolve in unspecifiable and unpredictable ways.[24] These features imply a shared moral logic and structure to a covenantal relationship, regardless of whether the relationship is situated within a religious context, a political context, a professional context (such as in medicine), or a context of intimates such as family and friendships. In these moral relationships, covenantal partners manifest patient commitment to the continuation of the relationship over time and circumstance and enact mutual capacity of caring response to the needs, be they physical, emotional, relational, or spiritual, of the covenantal partner.

A caveat attends this account of the basic normative logic of a covenantal relationship. As a descriptive matter, most agreements in contemporary society are contractual and transactional, and necessarily so. In large, impersonal, and bureaucratic societies, including institutionalized settings, in which the efficiencies of instrumentalized rationality are stressed and social interactions are generally between strangers who have yet to cultivate trust, an ethic of contract provides a necessary moral ground for the possibility of a cohesive society and transactional exchanges.

When a contractor comes to my home for some house renovations, I can expect to review a lengthy, small-print, legalized document, and formally ratify the agreement with my signature. This binds the contractor to perform the specified services and binds me to provide payment in exchange for those services. Similarly, the revocable living trust prepared for my estate planning by a trusts attorney required twenty-seven pages to delineate agreements, liabilities, immunities, and responsibilities of specific performance.

If I enter into an online agreement, such as use of a particular application for a mobile device, I can expect to click on a box that acknowledges I have read and accept the terms and conditions of the particular computer service; most often, of course, efficiency considerations mean I skip the reading portion. I assume some vulnerability as part of the cost of efficiency. The detailed and rather mind-numbing contractual disclosure statements of the service provider, which reflect both legal maximalism and moral minimalism, have become an occasion for satire. In one cartoon, a woman goes to greet a house guest, and upon opening the door encounters the visage and scythe of the Grim Reaper, whereupon her husband in a different room informs her, "why, yes, I did click 'do not accept'" the terms and conditions for a service for his computer program. This humorously highlights the enforceability provisions of almost all contracts, but also indicates the rigidity of a contractual relationship in which all contingencies are sought to be specified in advance.

24. Bouma et al., *Christian Faith*, 84.

Within my professional experience, my employment is structured clearly by a contractual understanding between myself and my educational institution. Even so, I hold to covenantal ideals and aspirations in my professional life and educational partnerships with students. I am a participant in a religious community and tradition that is organized by a moral logic of covenantal ethics. These covenantal relations mean that contracts and the reciprocity of rights and duties are insufficient for moral life and risk a sparse and diminished moral landscape. A morally diminished trust emerges in circumstances where a relationship that traditionally has been a matter of covenant is reduced to contractual and legalistic formalities, as when marriage is entered into only first upon the signing of a pre-nuptial agreement. The prospect of corrosion in the relationship is embedded in the very nature of the agreement.

In contrast to a contract, a covenant is not as formalized, is less legalistic, and is affirmed by a personalized promise rather than a rote signature. A covenant presumes a coming together for the cultivation and sharing of goods, the details of which cannot be specified in advance. It presumes a context of trust and the continuation of the relationship, even absent enforceability provisions. A covenant is thus more open-ended, mutually malleable, and expressive of trust than the transactional contract. In these respects, a covenant better accommodates the features of contingency and change and the necessity for flexibility within human experience, aspects that are especially relevant in health care settings.

The open-ended character of covenants does not push in the direction of libertarianism: it is possible to identify a moral logic, assumptions, and structure embedded in a covenantal relationship. This moral structure encompasses actions by which a covenant relationship is established, as well as those that perpetuate the relationship or delineate its termination. My exposition of the moral structure of a covenantal ethic is comprised of seven characteristics—giftedness, responsiveness, presence, fidelity, identity-bestowal and transformation, embodied entrustment, and renewal. This exposition situates covenant within the broader ethos of gift-response-responsibility-transformation. Following this exposition, I will examine the relevance of this moral structure for medicine as a profession and for healers in relationship with patients.

Elements of Covenantal Relationships

Giftedness

The partnership of a covenantal relationship is a matter of invitation rather than demand, and thereby symbolizes giving rather than merit, and grace and mercy rather than desert and justice. A covenant pertains in theological language more to grace than it does to law. This gift of grace can be constituted by the conditions necessary to our very being, such as the air we breathe, the love offered by the giver that culminates in the offering of self in a marriage relationship, or the trust, vulnerability, and psychic intimacy that theologian C. S. Lewis designated as the "naked personality" that characterizes a friendship.[25] A covenant presumes a gifted character to our experience in the sense that we have been chosen for the relationship rather than having done the choosing after the manner of an impartial and disembodied self engaged in deliberating between instrumental rational alternatives. Of course, this is why calling and vocation are central to the ethics of covenantal relationship. A covenant bears witness that not all our experience is a manifestation of self-determination and will-to-power, and that our relationships encompass both voluntary and involuntary relationships.

An ethos of gift and gratitude, a formative and transformative experience of giftedness, is prevalent, even if not primary, in the discourse of medicine and medical ethics. For example, Sir William Osler, in his classic 1889 *Aequanitmas* address to graduating medical students at the University of Pennsylvania, reminded his audience that "it is good to hark back to the olden days and gratefully to recall the men whose labours in the past have made the present possible."[26] The practices of the present and the expanding possibilities of the future are the legacy of previous generations of physicians. An ethos of giftedness is likewise embedded in the opening paragraphs of the classical Hippocratic Oath, in which the physician as healer acknowledges their gratitude and responsibility to their mentor or teacher through promising to teach the art of medicine to the male members of the mentor's family.

Within bioethics, William F. May counters what he refers to as "the conceit" of professional philanthropy, an idea that altruistic giving within the physician-patient relationship is initiated and comes entirely from the grace and good will of the physician, by illustrating that a fundamental gift relationship is at the moral foundations of medicine. May contends that the medical profession has less negotiated a contract with society than it has first been a recipient of many gifts from society, from mentors, and from individuals. These benefits include the commitment of resources and facilities for medical education, community support for institutions such as hospitals devoted to the provision of medical care, the granting of a monopoly over professional services, and the relatively high social esteem of the medical profession in an age of cynicism about authority.[27]

As presented here, the contractual model construes these necessary aspects of professional status to be part of the transactional exchange between the society and its delegation of authority for caring for the ill to the medical profession. These features are claims, even entitlements, that the profession has on the society in order for the profession to achieve the social good. However, this is, for May, its own kind of conceit: the foundational giftedness of the profession provides moral ground for understanding medicine and its relationship with society, and members of the profession in their relationships with patients, as covenantal rather than contractual. Similarly,

25. Lewis, *Four Loves*, 71.
26. Osler, "Aequanimitas," 9.
27. May, *Physician's Covenant*, 118–19.

Bernardin situated his account of the covenantal nature of medicine within prior actions that generate a form of moral indebtedness: "The power of modern medicine—of each and every doctor—is the result of centuries of science, clinical trial, and public and private investments . . . This faith [of people in medicine and in doctors] creates a social debt and is the basis of medicine's call—its vocation—to serve the common good."[28] The legacy of giftedness in medicine invites a different moral orientation in which professional integrity is not circumscribed by legal and moral minimalism.

This giftedness and indebtedness is explicitly acknowledged in the professional code of ethics of pharmacy. The first principle of the code entails "respect for the covenantal relationship between the patient and pharmacist," and a brief exposition of the principle grounds the moral obligations of the pharmacist in an ethic of giftedness and trust: "a pharmacist has moral obligations in response to the gift of trust received from society. In return for this gift, a pharmacist promises to help individuals achieve optimum benefit from their medications, to be committed to their welfare, and to maintain their trust."[29] It may seem rather ironic that this relationship is characterized as covenantal given that any individual patient is more likely to see their pharmacist in a commercial setting, such as a retail grocery chain or department store, and understand that they "pick up" a prescription from the pharmacist just as they would "pick up a few things" from the grocery. Nonetheless, this is an important illustration of professional recognition of prior gifts from the community, and an ethic constructed around the concepts of gift, responsiveness, and responsibility, in contrast to an ethic that generates professional responsibilities as a form of gratuitous philanthropic benevolence or even mutual contractual negotiation.

The element of giftedness is not only embedded in the social situatedness of medicine, but also emerges in formative features of the physician-patient relationship. In the context of the re-storying nature of healing, the metaphor of "giving back" is often invoked to portray physician interactions with patients and their illness narratives. The metaphor presupposes that the physician has first received something of indispensable value, moral as well as medical, from the patient's narrative witness to their vulnerability. Patients offer or donate their stories and their bodies to physicians in a manner that provides an opportunity to cultivate the physician's knowledge, skills, prudential wisdom, and practice in the course of caring for the patient.[30] In their ethnography of healing, Schenck and Churchill observe the phenomenon of "'gifting' back and forth" between the physician and patient as one of the marks of healing presence. As expressed by one of their physician interviewees: "[Patients] give me the gift of healing, and I give them back my presence."[31] When the profession acknowledges

---

28. Bernardin, "Renewing the Covenant," 270.

29. American Pharmacists Association, "Code of Ethics," Principle 1.

30. Gawande, *Complications*, 11–34.

31 Schenck and Churchill, *Healers*, 76–77.

the various gifts of the patients, physician responsibilities become a matter of respon-siveness that opens to the covenantal character of relationship.

Interpreting the relationship between society and the medical profession, and between individual physicians and patients, through contractual and transactional metaphors, diminishes the fabric of giftedness formative of both kinds of relation-ships. When the gift relationship is suppressed and displaced morally by a model of negotiation between mutually self-interested parties, the moral landscape of calling, healing, and trust is also placed in jeopardy. The offering and receipt of a gift or an unmerited benefit is not sufficient by itself; a covenantal partnership is instead embed-ded within several complementary features.

Responsiveness

"The human activities of healing, teaching, parenting . . . do not create—that is God's work—but from beginning to end, respond."[32] The bestowal of a gift offers a context for meaningful response; the implicit ethic is that of gift-response, grace-response, or call-response, rather than command-obedience, rights-demand, or contract-negoti-ation. The responsiveness embedded in a covenantal ethic and relationship does not refer to a kind of calculative form of reciprocity, or an instrumentalized exchange of services and payments, but rather typically signals "an incommensurability between the gift and any efforts to pay for it."[33]

Religious ethicist Paul Camenisch insightfully articulates the kind of moral re-sponsiveness to gift envisioned in a covenantal relationship. Camenisch contends that "gift both grounds and symbolizes a moral relation."[34] A gift may invite a new moral relationship, renew a relationship, or transform an existing relationship. The gift bears this potency because of embedded responsibilities, which is to say, at least part of the meaning of responsiveness is responsibility. This does not imply that offering the gift binds the receiver to an involuntary acceptance, but rather that when the agent exercises moral agency to accept the gift as a gift, responsiveness is an appropriate moral expectation. The mere proffering of a gift or unearned benefit does not restrict the moral agency of the recipient, nor does invitation to a covenantal relationship compromise respect for recipient agency for the gift or invitation by itself is not suf-ficient to establish relationship. Responsiveness is matter of agency and autonomy.[35]

In everyday experience of giftedness, responsiveness is manifested through a moral expectation that accepting a gift calls forth genuineness of appreciation in the recipient and a sincere expression of gratitude. The content of responsiveness is thereby shaped by gratefulness. Camenisch develops two further moral expectations

32. May, *Physician's Covenant*, 124.

33. Bouma et al., *Christian Faith*, 88.

34. Camenisch, "Gift and Gratitude," 3.

35. Allen, *Love and Conflict*, 19.

embedded in responsiveness and responsibility, which he designates as "grateful conduct" and "grateful use."[36] Grateful conduct refers to various actions performed to express the sentiment of gratitude, the nature of the gift, and the form of relationship. The scope of responsiveness can then range from verbalization of "thank you," the most common form of gracious response in everyday experience, to dedication to a way of life that honors and bears witness to the giver. This more profound commitment represents the kind of grateful conduct embedded in the biblical narratives of covenantal relation. Grateful use pertains to actions of the recipient in using, cultivating, and sharing the gift in ways that bear witness of fidelity to the intent of the giver as expressed through the gift. The range of possible actions that manifest grateful use is likewise contingent on the kind of gift and the implicit relationship and manifests a conceptual connection between responsiveness and the elements of stewardship delineated previously.

The quotation invoked to begin this section implies a moral equivalence of responsiveness in healing and in teaching (as well as in parenting). As I have previously situated my own professional vocation within a sensibility of both calling and gratitude, providing a short exposition of how responsiveness shapes my approach to teaching can help illuminate the larger conceptual point. My "call" within the teaching profession stems in part from responsiveness to the gifts of the pursuit of knowledge and the skills of interaction, as well as the virtues of patience and persistence, exemplified by numerous professors and mentors over the course of my education. These persons may have had academic careers, but they were fundamentally teachers and educators in the finest sense of those terms.

I have conceptualized my own commitment to teaching as an ethos of gift-responsiveness—that is, I have articulated a perennial aspiration to give to my students the kind of classes, the kind of education, I had received from my own professors. What I didn't fully appreciate as I started into the teaching vocation, and really not for some years thereafter, was how much the character of my teaching would also be shaped by the gifts I received from my students. The gifts of enthusiasm, of questioning that reveals both vulnerability and presents challenge, of consuming conversations, of words of appreciation, and ultimately of relationship, all manifest ways in which my students are teachers to me. In this respect as well, my teaching is characterized by responsiveness, by a "giving back."

I am also of the conviction that, just as I wasn't aware of this dynamic of gift and responsiveness as a student, my students for the most part are likewise in a different moral world from me. Indeed, the socialization processes of higher education and the marketing of the academy students are subjected to as they are recruited by different universities has cultivated an emphasis on education and knowledge as commodities, teachers as providers, and students as demanding consumers. The course syllabus is explicitly referred to as the "contract" between professor and student. Within

---

36. Camenisch, "Gift and Gratitude," 8–9.

this very thin moral world, I sometimes challenge my students to consider just how the professor-student relationship exhibits features of the Kantian maxim that we are never to treat others merely as means but always as ends-in-themselves. What, I inquire of them, would it mean for me to treat them merely as a means? And also, as an end? Their responses present interesting insights for me as to their expectations of professors in general, and of myself in particular. Those expectations do not reflect a covenantal relational dynamic, but rather one more compatible with a production-commodity-industry setting. However, this lack of shared vision doesn't make my teaching, or my learning, assume any less of a gift-responsive character. And, with certain students, or certain groups of students, the character of learning and teaching is inspired and oriented by a gift-relation. That may not generate an experience of a covenantal relation that perpetuates over time, but it provides a fuller, richer moral world than a production and commodity model, or a banking model of learning and education.

Responsible Presence

Although my students are not accustomed to thinking in covenantal terms about their relationships, when I inquire of them what differentiates a true friend from, for example, a Facebook friend, they customarily respond with a covenantal sentiment: the true friend is always present, will "always be there" in time of need. Presence is a form of bearing witness of solidarity with others in a covenant-created community. Presence is one form that responsibility assumes in the ethos of giftedness. A covenantal relationship is marked by virtues of presence, solidarity, and unwavering fidelity.

Presence in the midst of vulnerability is, in certain respects, a threshold test of covenantal commitment. In my own faith tradition, for example, persons manifest solidarity with and presence towards other persons through a covenantal promise or witness of responsibility to "mourn with those that mourn," be present to provide comfort, and "bear the burdens" experienced by others.[37] The others to whom one is present in a covenant of responsibility and solidarity are not defined by membership in community, but extend to the stranger, the wounded, and the vulnerable insofar as all persons bear the *imago Dei*.

A commitment of presence in vulnerability is especially significant in the context of medicine, as vulnerability to illness, adversity, or suffering is a characteristic feature that mediates the relationship of physician and patient. Although my account of healing stresses that vulnerability is intrinsic to the role of healer, it is the case as suggested by Bouma that "increased vulnerability of one party entails greater responsibility of the other."[38] The commitment of presence, to not only see the relationship through,

37. Mosiah 18:8–10.

38. Bouma et al., *Christian Faith*, 87.

but to see the covenantal partner through, healing lends itself to an ethic of witnessing care and non-abandonment of the patient.

For Bernardin, the commitment to presence and solidarity requires an additional responsibility of the profession and of physicians that pertains to the social dimensions of the medical covenant, namely, to ensure that patients are not abandoned by a fraying health care system. In particular, Bernardin claimed, "Physicians and the profession have a covenant with society to be advocates for the health needs of their communities and the nation."[39] It is possible that a covenantal ethic and a contractual ethic could generate similar moral conclusions despite diverse moral argumentation and rationales. In Bernardin's understanding, the medical covenant with society includes seeking to ensure access to health care as a basic human right and responsible stewardship of limited resources, a religiously-founded moral responsibility that he claims is preferable to the harsher language of rationing. Responsibility is manifested as presence to patients in the midst of their particularized vulnerability, solidarity with patients who are perennially vulnerable because of their social situatedness, and moral advocacy that bears witness of the need for social justice in health care distribution and bears witness against institutional and structural obstacles to access to a basic and guaranteed minimum of care for every person. The moral covenant requires a minimally just health care system.

Responsive Fidelity

In addition to presence and solidarity, covenantal responsibility is also specified as mutual fidelity, a promise of unwavering commitment between the relational partners over the course of time. The expectations of ongoing commitment were central to what Bernardin had in mind in characterizing medicine as a profession enacted through covenantal forms of relationships. His call for renewal of the medical covenant is based on promises of fidelity: "The covenant is a promise that the profession makes—a solemn promise—that it is and will remain true to its moral center."[40] This moral center for Bernardin is comprised of the physician-patient relationship: it is not just that the relationship manifests fidelity in the present, but as a covenant, the relationship must continue to display fidelity in an open, challenging, and unspecifiable future. The covenant is a kind of moral bedrock of non-abandonment when we experience our finitude, frailty, and contingency. The covenantal fidelity of the physician and of the profession is a responsive moral commitment that bears witness to patient and public trust in medicine's commitment to first promote the good of patients in their vulnerability. Thus, for Bernardin, "in individual terms, the covenant is the basis

---

39. Bernardin, "Renewing the Covenant," 273.
40. Bernardin, "Renewing the Covenant," 270.

on which patients trust their doctors. In social terms, the covenant is the ground for the public's continued respect and reliance on the profession of medicine."[41]

Since enacting complete fidelity over time is perhaps a moral ideal that cannot be realized fully by human participants, covenant accommodates renewal of the relationship. What a covenantal relationship seems much less accommodating towards, especially in contrast to a contractual understanding of relationships, is the cessation of the relationship, either because the terms have been fulfilled or the breaking of the relationship because the criteria of specific performance haven't been fulfilled. Covenant endures in a way that contract does not. The customary vows in the marriage covenant illustrate the permanence of the relationship through the ordeals of contingency that transpire in any relationship, be they sickness, poverty, or other forms of personal or relational adversity or suffering.

Mutual fidelity is an indispensable characteristic for healing. In the absence of the physician's unswerving commitment to keep promises to respect patient privacy and maintain confidentiality of patient information, the trust necessary to a successful relationship could never be cultivated. Moreover, it is likely that, in some instances, patients would be dissuaded from seeking out medical assistance. Having once accepted a patient into their care, physicians have made a moral promise of non-abandonment.

Mutuality in a covenantal relationship in medicine also means that patients are not "duty-free." Part of the covenantal fidelity of the patient is reflected in truthfulness with physicians. A very popular television medical drama of the past decade, *House M.D.*, developed its narrative arc in part around the diagnostic premise of the lead physician character that "everyone lies";[42] patients especially were no exception to this maxim. The physician's foundational assumption of mistrust warranted minimal attention to the patient's narrative and an immediate turn to testing technologies to confirm or rule out specific diagnoses; a patient's biological data were deemed more credible and reliable than the patient's story of their experience. If patients withhold relevant medical information due to embarrassment or fear of stigma, or physicians simply assume that everyone lies, the bond of trust upon which to create and maintain the relationship and to cultivate healing dissipates. When a patient has received a physician's recommendations for prevention or treatment and engaged in deliberation about alternative courses of action, fidelity entails at least a good faith effort on the part of the patient to consider the physician's recommendations, particularly when it comes to adopting lifestyle behaviors regarding nutrition, fitness, and rest, in the absence of which the patient may experience more serious illness.

A reliance on trust in the midst of vulnerability makes covenantal fidelity necessarily a risk-taking endeavor. The primary risk assumed is that one party will experience betrayal of trust and the relationship trust presumes, a moral failing expressed in our language of "breaking faith" with another. In the biblical tradition, rebellion

41. Bernardin, "Renewing the Covenant," 270.
42. Ruff and Barris, "Sound of One House," 84–87.

against the divine will comprises a broken covenant; we use language of brokenness in our relationships with significant others, such as breaking a marriage vow or promise, or betrayal in a friendship. While a covenantal commitment is premised on "giving back" in the relationship, a "going back" on a gift-initiated relational responsiveness is not a matter of moral indifference, but a substantive moral issue.

The feature of betrayal seems recurrent in the covenant of God with the people of Israel. The biblical narratives draw on analogies with a marriage relationship to interpret deviating from the covenant (through idolatry and neglect of the poor) as infidelity. The commitment of fidelity, the experience of vulnerability, and the reliance on trust implies why betrayal is the great vice that corrupts the relationship. This is God's constant charge delivered by prophetic witness against the people of Israel. The covenant is an expression of a community premised on trust, giftedness, reciprocity, and mutual care, and a betrayed, or broken, covenant symbolizes not simply rejection of responsibilities, but also of the identity, relationship, and worldview embedded in the covenant. A covenantal relationship expresses the same moral expectation about relational fidelity as Kant did: promises are *not* made to be broken. A covenant oriented by a healing witness is manifested by presence, solidarity, and non-abandonment that endures through the frailty and fallibility of the patient seeking healing.

Identity-Bestowal and Transformation

As with the structure of rites of passage associated with a healing relationship outlined in the preceding chapter, a central feature of a covenantal commitment is the bestowal and transformation of identity. In the biblical covenantal narratives, the assumption of new identity created by a covenantal commitment is commonly symbolized through name alteration: Abram becomes Abraham, Sarai becomes Sarah, and Jacob becomes Israel. Similarly, the covenantal binding together of marriage is witnessed by the joining of names or the assumption by one spouse of the name of the other.

Of course, nomenclature is but one symbol of acquiring and embodying a new identity, which reflects a deeper discovery of a new way of being-in-the-world and a transformed life or way of life. May contends of the covenant with Israel at Sinai, "these two aspects of covenant [gift and promise], taken together, alter the being of the covenanted people [of God] . . . so that fidelity to the covenant defines their subsequent life."[43] A covenantal commitment is not only identity-transforming with regard to past relationships, but is identity-constituting of new and present responsibilities in the expanded horizons of an open future. The altered or transformed sense of self and being in the world is similarly exemplified in the writings of St. Paul, for whom the covenant made by a Christian in responsiveness to the gift of salvation is embodied in the baptism ritual. Baptism bears witness to the biblical promise of deliverance from

---

43. May, *Physician's Covenant*, 115.

a bondage to sin, and finding a newness of life and liberating grace as a follower of Christ.[44] Every covenantal relationship involves some symbolic separation from or symbolic death of the old, some experience of incorporation so revitalizing it is as a new birth, and some experience of liminal wanderings in the transition in-between.

An important correspondence between external and internal forms of identity-alteration and transformation is displayed in covenant. A changing of names or a change of clothing are external, public, or visible forms of a covenantal commitment that reflect a deeper change in the core of the internal, private, and veiled self. This is in part why the healing commitment embedded in a covenantal relation of physician and patient is necessarily holistic; healing should have an impact on the entirety of a person affected by illness. The wholeness sought in healing extends beyond treatment for the external and visible body to the emotional, relational, or spiritual manifestations of the person.

A relationship between physician and patient that evolves into a healing interaction can bestow and transform identities. A particular physician is entrusted with intimate access to the person's embodied self in ways not true of other physicians. The interaction assumes a character of healing insofar as it is the occasion not only for medical treatments, but also for re-storying, embodied witness, and other elements of healing such that the identity of the person as patient—that is, as a passive agent that suffers, can be altered. A liminal status as patient in covenantal healing does not comprise the totality of a person's status and being in the everyday world.

Embodied Entrustment

The symbolism of responsive fidelity-borne witness through the body in a covenant is substantively different in moral meaning than the act of clicking on the computer box to signify contractual acceptance of the terms and conditions of the service provided. A covenantal relationship implies disclosure of a dimension of vulnerability to the other as trust supplants control as the medium of the relationship. Allen represents this feature of covenant through the metaphor of "entrustment" by which persons "place ourselves or something we value in the other's hands."[45] Allen's first example of entrustment is the quite literal way that patients place their embodied self "in the hands of doctors."[46]

This laying of hands in medicine is a process of identity-transformation and crossing of a threshold by the physician from strangeness to trusting partner. As exemplified in a physical examination, the laying-on of hands symbolizes the potent healing potential of trust; it is portrayed by Abraham Verghese as not merely having a utilitarian function of obtaining information, but as a potent symbol of commitment,

44. Rom 6:1–4.
45. Allen, *Love and Conflict*, 33.
46. Allen, *Love and Conflict*, 33.

presence, and trust: "in the case of the bedside exam, the transformation is the cementing of the doctor-patient relationship, a way of saying: 'I will see you through this illness. I will be with you through thick and thin.' It is paramount that doctors not forget the importance of this ritual."[47] The ritual incorporates the healer's witnessing of the body such that the interaction is altered from a transactional to a transformative encounter.

The practices identified by Schenck and Churchill in their ethnography of healing likewise display a ritualistic expression of embodied entrustment. A person who visits their physician crosses a threshold into the liminal space of the "container" or sanctuary of vulnerability and assumes a patient identity. The embodied vulnerability of the person in this experience of liminality is particularly prominent, and thus the patient has an inescapable need for trust as they place themselves in the caregiver's hands. The physician assumes different identities, including those of guide, mentor, and companion, which are more conducive to a trusting relationship than those conveyed by a competent and efficient technician or a contractual provider.

Renewal

As intimated by Bernardin in his prophetic call to the AMA delegates, covenants accommodate renewal. The possibilities of renewal, as contrasted with relational rupture, are significant insofar as living out the covenant in history can at best approximate but never achieve the ideal of relationship, and the relationship is necessarily open-ended, indeterminate, and shaped by contingency and human moral weakness. Just as the renewal of life in the spring season or a renewal of vows among married couples can bring new vitality and increased commitment in relationship, so the renewal of a covenant between profession and society and between physician and patient can provide reminders of the ultimate import of the relationship. The coming together that occurs in establishing a covenantal relation is not simply a one-time occurrence that forever lasts. The renewal of covenant presupposes a continual remembering of the covenantal promises and obligations and a returning to the binding ties of fidelity, presence, solidarity, and entrustment. The religious traditions emphasize this prospect of renewal in both retelling formative stories and in ritual enactments.

In the paradigmatic religious covenant of God with the people of Israel, the manner by which they are to shape their new life as a community begins with a call to remember the divine act of deliverance from slavery: "I am the Lord your God, who brought you out of the land of Egypt, out of the house of slavery."[48] The community-creating gift of deliverance is to be retold with each successive generation, a perpetual re-storying of how the community's identity was transformed and can continue to be renewed throughout the course of history.

47. Verghese, "Treat the Patient," para. 19.

48. Exod 20:2.

The community is thus situated in a historical and moral tradition, and its flourishing in large part is comprised of fidelity to its formative narrative and its historically embodied memory. This memory of giftedness is cultivated, this past moment is brought forward to the present, through the telling of stories, expressions of gratitude, and grateful conduct expressed through fidelity, presence, and solidarity. Israel receives frequent prophetic reminders of its grace and giftedness lest pride, conceit, and arrogance, and eventually betrayal, supplant gratitude and fidelity.

In human relationships, the processes of remembering and renewing provide resilience, fortitude, and resolution to sustain the commitment to a way of being and a way of living through covenantal aspirations. The responsibility of remembering applies not only to the initiating gift, but to the covenantal relation itself. The covenantal relation does not become a relic, but always permeates the present and thereby shapes the future. Just as promises are not made to be broken, so also a covenantal relation is not created to be forgotten.

In this regard, it is important to note that Bernardin's case for renewal of the medical covenant presupposes that the questions of professional identity and integrity are not simply imposed upon medicine from sources external to the profession, such as insurance or legal regulation and commercialization, but are also embedded in moral forgetfulness within medicine. He argued, "The age-old covenants between doctors and patient, between the profession and society, have been ignored or violated."[49] A prophetic call for renewal of covenant not only manifests changes in circumstance, but also is a necessity in contexts of moral crisis, when the very identity and integrity, the moral center, of the covenantal relationship is under threat.

The structures of delivery of care in contemporary medicine can diminish the covenantal aspect of remembering and renewal, indeed, to the point that the language of covenant is discarded in place of the political metaphor of contract, and the resonance of the concepts of calling and vocation are diminished to careerism. One of the most ethically problematic features of the drive within the health care industries to maximize efficiencies in the numbers of patients seen is that it fragments the memory of the individual patient as a person within and between physicians. It is a jolting and personal experience to learn that, in the absence of assistance from the medical record, the patient may well have been forgotten. After all, in previous interactions the patient is likely to have disclosed personal information and intimate stories, and displayed their emotional and physical vulnerabilities.

Patients are not in principle or practice abandoned by their caregivers; however, when patients and their narratives are forgotten and not remembered, and the story told by the "iPatient" of Verghese is the primary memory of the patient, a perception of depersonalization in the relationship most certainly intensifies. The moral core of covenant is further tested by delivery systems in which patient care is fragmented between specializations, and sometimes between practitioners within the same practice.

49. Bernardin, "Renewing the Covenant," 269.

For understandable reasons, patients may perceive that the commitment of fidelity to them is not being maintained.

Bernardin's prophetic call presented four realms within the covenantal status of medicine in need of ongoing restorative and renewing commitment, a renewal that seems an ever-present professional responsibility: (1) the moral compass of physicians must be reoriented to ensure the primacy of patients' interests; (2) professional technical competency must be complemented by holistic caring of physicians, including the physician assuming a role as guide in the processes of medical decision-making rather than functioning merely as a dispensary of technical information; (3) a restored and re-storying social commitment of "medicine's call—its vocation—to serve the common good" in responsive fidelity to the social investment in medicine; and (4) a revitalized assumption of advocacy roles by physicians for their patients in the face of covenant-compromising pressures of the marketplace, regulation, and administrative oversight, particularly as regards comprehensive reform of health care, and appropriate stewardship of increasingly limited resources.[50] Covenantal commitments to patients, fellow professionals, and society need renewing with each succeeding generational cohort of physicians. Indeed, for Bernardin, a principal professional responsibility of medicine is to train aspiring professionals to "live up to the moral responsibilities of a physician," which in turn requires medical educators themselves to be "living models of the virtuous physician."[51]

The current focus on professionalism in medicine represents a coordinated and formal effort to enact this responsibility, though professionalism is more commonly framed as derivative from a contractual than a covenantal context. Professionalism and mentoring situates responsibilities of new physicians to their teachers within a responsiveness to gift that is fundamental to a covenant within the profession.[52] It is significant that the "Physician's Charter" includes a principle of social justice and a responsibility of public advocacy as a defining moral feature of medical professionalism, thus expanding the scope of professionalism beyond the setting of clinical interactions.

Conclusion

It can surely be questioned whether medical relationships, including the relationship between profession and society and those between physician and patient, manifest the features of covenantal relationship delineated in this discussion. Ultimately, my claim is that medicine's status and integrity as a profession of healing requires the kind of professional commitment to society and to patients embedded in relationships oriented by the moral logic of covenant. The contractual metaphor and the discourse of

50. Bernardin, "Renewing the Covenant," 270.
51. Bernardin, "Renewing the Covenant," 272.
52. May, *Physician's Covenant*, 117.

rights, drawn from a political context of relationships between distrustful adversaries, provide a basis for a minimalistic professional morality, though very much influenced by legal considerations and defensive medicine. There are certainly realms within American health care in which a minimalist morality would be a welcome innovation, particularly with respect to provisions for a decent minimum in access to medical services.

The covenantal ethic and the contractual ethic may arrive at similar conclusions with regards to matters of justice and informed consent, but they clearly begin with different moral assumptions and presuppositions. A covenantal relationship embeds professional responsibilities within an ethos of giftedness and responsiveness and provides moral space for the concept of a calling to medicine and for medicine as a profession of healing, for medicine to bear witness to the experience of "healing, here." Understanding the covenantal dimensions of medicine also holds open the prospect of transformative possibilities promised by a healing witness rather than solely trans-actional exchanges. As challenged as such an ethic is by factors extrinsic to medicine, the clearest moral test of the covenantal ethic is the moral witness required by being with patients in the ordeals of suffering.

7

Being with Suffering

In Albert Camus's allegory *The Plague*, Dr. Rieux makes it clear to his colleague Tarrou that he has little patience for the theological abstractions and intellectualizing of Paneloux, the priest: "Paneloux is a man of learning, a scholar. He hasn't come in contact with death. That's why he can speak with such assurance of the truth—with a capital T." By contrast, healers who display compassionate presence in the midst of a patient's suffering acquire experiential insight and a practical imperative: "Every country priest who visits his parishioners and has heard a man gasping for breath on his deathbed thinks as I do. He'd try to relieve human suffering before trying to point out its excellence."[1]

This very pointed critique, which compressed Albert Camus's argument with Christianity into two sentences, presents several considerations for understanding the place of suffering in medicine and in bioethics. First, the intellectualized response to suffering is a common and often convenient path. Almost all religious traditions have developed a theodicy to provide explanations of evil, disease, adversity, pain and suffering, and catastrophe. Within some interpretative traditions, and particularly within the Christian tradition partially illustrated by Paneloux, the experience of suffering is placed within a more expansive narrative of meaning that bestows upon suffering some purpose, good, or redemptive value: the suffering and crucifixion of Jesus through which God brings about human redemption makes such a theodicy prominent within Christian understandings.

A second consideration is that any narrative or theodicy regarding meaningful or purposive suffering must be tested for coherence and comprehensiveness with human experience in the context of disease and death. It is one thing to learn about

---

1. Camus, *Plague*, 126.

suffering as a theological or even medical construct; it is quite another to learn to *be with* suffering as it is manifest among the ill and the dying. Being present as a witness to the sufferings of another person is at the core of healing practice; bearing the burdens and sharing in those sufferings is a central meaning of the virtue in both religious and medical traditions of compassion. Compassionate presence and a healing witness require experiences, perceptions, and practices distinctively different than those that may arise for the scholar. At the very least, awareness and being with the suffering of others is an occasion for acquiring intellectual humility.

Third, suffering (like pain) insists on a practical response and issues a *telic* demand to the physician, the caregiver, the healer, and the witness: "relieve" or "alleviate" the suffering. However, enacting the imperative to relieve suffering is seldom entirely clear, and certainly requires more than sermonizing. Indeed, in some circumstances, the suffering is so incessant and the demand so insistent that we may reflect that the person is "suffering a fate worse than death." The prospect of hastening death to alleviate suffering shadows many end-of-life discussions and has become publically visible in social and political advocacy of death with dignity.

A fourth issue that emerges particularly in our excessively medicalized society is comprised of a contrary path to intellectualizing suffering, and that is to medicalize suffering, or reduce suffering to a medical problem. The most prevalent discursive forms of this medical reductionism occur when the concepts of pain and suffering are used interchangeably: suffering is depicted as a form of pain, more intense and more extreme, but pain nonetheless. That position suggests that not only pain but also suffering are treatable by medical means. However, the experience of suffering inescapably raises questions as to whether there are aspects of experience that are related to embodiment, to disease, and to pain that fall beyond the domain of medical expertise. What suffering immediately calls for is compassion and presence, of "being with" suffering; medical interventions that aim to "do something about" suffering seem of secondary significance.

With these four considerations in mind, in this chapter I seek to extend the previous discussions of healing witness and covenantal relationship and assess their implications for bearing witness to suffering embodied by other persons as well as ourselves. This means balancing philosophical and ethical reflection on suffering with insights informed from the crucible of experiencing suffering. I begin with an explication of my assumptions about what it means to be with suffering.

Being with Suffering

Through the language of "being with suffering," I want to convey both an interpretation of an existential fact, that our experience of the human condition is marked and profoundly shaped by suffering, and a normative claim that there is a moral responsibility, exemplified in the ways of healers and the healing professions, to be present with, and embody compassion and empathy towards, persons who are suffering. It is particularly appropriate for a profession that claims identity through healing to understand one of its central ends or purposes to consist in the melioration or relief of suffering.

The interdependencies and intertwinings of human experience are a necessary aspect of being with suffering. Each person knows suffering not simply intellectually, but experientially. Each person can bear a particularized witness of the way that suffering shapes and defines their character, their life narrative, and their apprehension of meaning. It is very difficult, for reasons developed subsequently in the chapter, to share the personal experience of suffering, although important virtues in religious and medical traditions, such as compassion and empathy, as well as parental caring, seem to presume a reality to shared suffering. However, disclosing to another one's own experience of suffering so as to provide understanding is different than saying there is a core, common experience of suffering, which everyone regardless of the particularities of their life narrative has access to or experience of. The discourse of "being with suffering" implies the possibility of witnessing and sharing in suffering without requiring a common suffering experience or narrative.

Furthermore, each person is certainly a witness to the sufferings of other persons. We can run up against human finitude when inquiring why a person is undergoing the ordeal of suffering, but we can know that a person is experiencing suffering. Physician Eric Cassell puts the point simply: if we want to determine whether another person is suffering, we need only ask them.[2] We can know whether they are experiencing a profound loss of their wholeness, the ineradicable disruption of their narrative, or an emptiness of meaning, as forms of their suffering. We can also have some inkling, in part because of our own experience of suffering, that suffering presents us with a profound moral choice: to be callous or indifferent, to give voice to helplessness, or to be with another person in the midst of their suffering. That choice is portrayed narratively in the parable of the Good Samaritan (chapter 4). Witnessing another person suffering can move us to compassionate forms of bearing their onerous ordeal with them. Being with suffering is then one of the most profound ways in which we bear witness of our shared humanity and our covenantal commitment to a specific person.

I also contend that there is an interdependency and an intertwining of the experience of suffering with the experience of joy. At a more theoretical or philosophical level, we know the bitterness and anguish of suffering only through familiarity and experience of its contrary, the sweetness of joy. Buddhist teacher Joan Halifax, in the course of her experiencing the loss of her father, writes that her "heart broke open."[3] Even as we are right to be concerned about becoming callous to suffering or helpless before suffering, particularly in the healing professions, where witnessing suffering is

2. Cassell, *Nature of Suffering*, 42.

3. Halifax, *Being with Dying*, 52.

an everyday experience, at times being with suffering can open us up to the profound, the beautiful, or the joyful.

This intertwining of suffering with joy reflects what I contend is a dialectical dynamic of "undergoing" and "overcoming" in suffering. Suffering is often an experience of undergoing an ordeal, or being overwhelmed by the magnitude and intensity of some affliction, loss, or deprivation. In spatial metaphors, then, suffering seems to place us under, or to bring us low; this is why humility is such an essential virtue for being with suffering. However, personal resiliency and compassionate witness of others can transform undergoing to "overcoming," a resurfacing and re-storying emergence that finds expression in solace, consolation, new awareness, and even meaning. Overcoming the ordeal of suffering seems to presuppose an undergoing.

While I do not see suffering as an excellence to be praised in the way critiqued by Camus, I do claim that the crucible of suffering is frequently a teacher from whom we can acquire knowledge about ourselves, wisdom about life, and experience that becomes an invitation to empathy and fellow-feeling. This is certainly a presupposition of the concept of the wounded healer in medicine.[4] It is no coincidence in Camus's novel that, having critiqued Father Paneloux for extolling human suffering as a matter of divine presence, when Dr. Rieux is subsequently asked by Tarrou just who taught Rieux his sense of vocation, Rieux replies simply and concisely, "Suffering."[5]

Being with suffering requires discerning a narrative arc to experience and recognizing that our stories are bearers of meaning; suffering disrupts or renders incoherent that narrative and radically challenges the meaning and purpose embedded in the story. With respect to the dynamic of undergoing-overcoming, undergoing or being brought low by suffering may be reflected in a loss of voice and loss of narrative by which to communicate the experience; the possibility of overcoming suffering requires openness to what I have previously referred to as re-storying. There cannot be a restoring of wholeness to the person in the absence of re-storying; part of the moral responsibility of the person or community who bears witness with the sufferer is to offer resources that assist in the process of constructing a different story or a story with a different interpretation.

The appeal of various religious and spiritual traditions throughout history and culture resides in part in their capacity to be with and bear with the person that suffers. Religious communities embody practices of compassionate presence to the suffering and traditions of hospitality to the stranger or exile. They are repositories of experience and meaning informed and enacted through their own communal narrative traditions. The faith traditions cultivate theological reflection about what the experience of suffering entails for a belief or understanding of the divine presence, known as theodicies. Theodicies situate the experience of suffering within some grand and encompassing narrative of meaning, including but not limited to the punitive

4. Schenck and Churchill, *Healers*, 121.

5. Camus, *Plague*, 129.

narrative that Camus takes to task; alternatively, a theodicy can express that a meaning for suffering is beyond the limited capacities of finite human persons. These communities nonetheless make constitutive of their identity and integrity their capacity to be with and absorb the woundedness and suffering that afflicts human beings.

These reflections invite a different challenge presented by the normative responsibility of being with suffering, including those questions central to the ethics of virtue: what type of persons ought we to be so that we can be with suffering? What kinds of characteristics and virtues are required of physicians and nurses so that they can be healers with suffering persons? My experience has been that, because of the intense forms of vulnerability experienced by patients to whom they provide care, palliative-care physicians and nurses and other hospice professionals embody being with suffering. They are healers without curing. Persons and healers who are with suffering walk the path of suffering and loss of wholeness as companion, friend, and witness to the person suffering. Western culture has likewise acquired one formative narrative of suffering that answers these questions of virtue via negation—that is, we ought to avoid being (and doing) as the so-called friends of the biblical figure Job, who later referred to his companions as "worthless physicians" and as "miserable comforters."[6] Though the friends wove theodicies, they failed to be with Job in his suffering.

Being with Finitude and Fallibility

One of the foundational narratives in western culture on suffering, the story of Job is unique in the literature of the ancient world. Certainly, the infliction of pain from the gods is a recurrent theme in Greek mythology, as attested to by the myths of Prometheus or Sisyphus, among many others. These mythic characters have no option but to submit to the decrees of the gods whose mandates they have, in one form or another, violated. Job, however, is different. He cannot accept a divine being whose punishments or tests of commitment seem arbitrary and capricious. He seeks to situate his experience of ordeals of loss, dispossession, and suffering within a moral world in which justice is primary, a moral world to which even God is accountable.

While Hamlet may have contemplated the nobility of submissively suffering "the slings and arrows of outrageous Fortune,"[7] Job is quite unwilling to see his destiny determined by contingency and caprice. He seeks meaning and understanding, and thus poses a challenge to God, and to any monotheist religion, namely, that a world created and ordered by God ultimately must make sense.[8] Throughout the poem, Job hardly blesses the name of the Lord in the manner articulated in the first chapter. He questions, laments, pursues accountability, and requests that God be responsible to him by addressing his questions about the moral ordering of the world. And that is

6. Job 13:4; 16:2.

7. Shakespeare, *Hamlet*, 3.2.

8. Austin, *Re-reading Job*, 23.

precisely what the God who answers Job "out of the whirlwind"[9] does not do. God's answer to Job takes the form of question after question, not answers or accountability. The questions invite Job to responsibility and reflection on finitude. Through close attention to some of the features of the narrative, we can discern important aspects of the experience of suffering.

Following the introductory story in which Job is quite literally dispossessed of material goods, family, and his own health, the opening narrative concludes with a dramatic portrayal of how suffering *isolates* and *silences*. When Job's three friends—Eliphaz, Bildad, and Zophar—initially venture out to meet him, the narrative (perhaps ironically) emphasizes their intent of compassionate presence and witness: the friends seek not to engage in passing judgment but to "console and comfort him." As they approach Job however, the narrative indicates "they did not recognize him."[10] Job's ordeal has been so profound that, exemplified physically by the boils afflicting his body, he has become as a stranger to his friends.

This initial narrative also exemplifies just how a person experiencing suffering is *unable to find a voice* for their experience, or to give their suffering a narrative framing. A fragmented or fractured narrative, or a "loss of words," is one mark of a person experiencing suffering. Having finally approached Job, his friends "sat with him on the ground seven days and seven nights, and no one spoke a word to [Job], for they saw that his suffering was very great."[11] It is not without meaning that this witness of compassion, presence, and solidarity by the friends precedes any verbal utterance by anyone. The language of embodied presence provides a powerful witness to compassion, the narrative implies, more so than voice and verbal communication. "Being with" suffering is first a matter of bearing witness rather than action, being with the person suffering rather than doing something.

This point about the witness of being with suffering and the language of suffering is reinforced by what subsequently occurs. Once Job vocalizes his grief and loss, the silence of bearing witness to and being with suffering by the friends comes to an end, and they relentlessly contest his integrity, abandoning their pretense of non-judgmentalism. A dispute over integrity becomes a determinative feature of Job's story. Job is described by the narrator in the very first verse of the poem as a person who is perfect or without blame, upright, fears God, and avoids evil. These four characteristics comprise Job's integrity, and his exemplification of these virtues is attested to not only by the narrator, but by God in the pre-story as well.[12] The integrity-constituting characteristics of fear or reverence of God and avoiding evil are constructed subsequently in the narrative as the twin virtues of wisdom and understanding.[13] And Job bears

9. Job 38:1.
10. Job 2:11–12.
11. Job 2:13.
12. Job 1:1, 8.
13. Job 28:28.

a personal witness to his integrity: he depicts himself to be a deliverer to the poor, needy, and widowed, to be "eyes to the blind, and feet . . . to the lame."[14]

At one level, a presupposition of the suffering of Job is the perfect integrity of Job. After Job is dispossessed of his material wealth (which the story indicates is substantial) and many of his children are killed, God affirms that Job still "persists in his integrity."[15] In the course of his lamentation, Job both witnesses to his integrity and asks God to bear witness as well: "Let me be weighed in a just balance, and let God know my integrity."[16] And throughout the narrative, once they vocalize their views, Job's "miserable comforters" do their relentless best to erode his sense of self-identity and self-esteem through their unsubstantiated charges of Job's sins and his apparent blasphemies of God. Their entire explanatory narrative for Job's dispossession is that his integrity must have been compromised through his own actions—that is, they adopt a punitive narrative of the meaning for Job's suffering. Implicit in this trial over the integrity of Job is a further manifestation of suffering: *a threat or actual loss to the identity and integrity of self.*

Elihu, a person who enters the narrative near its completion, rejects the idea that Job has maintained his integrity, especially those aspects that represent wisdom (reverence of God) and understanding (avoiding evil). Elihu's observation is that "Job speaks without knowledge, his words are without insight."[17] This accusation seems to have merit, for when God finally bears witness to Job out of a whirlwind, Job is rebuked in the very first sentence of the divine response for his "words without knowledge."[18] However, this charge would seem to have validity only during the time that Job is experiencing his devastating losses. It would not seem to have explanatory power for *why* Job is suffering in the first place, and that *is* Job's question. Thus, there is a profound dissonance between personal experience and constructed narratives of suffering. In general, Job's friends are miserable comforters because they impose an *alien narrative* of sin and loss of integrity and a meaning of their own construction on his experience. They are not healers, for they do not receive, let alone give back, Job's own narrative witness.

The ordeal of suffering presented through the narrative of Job in part concerns the challenge of affirming and maintaining personal integrity even in the midst of profoundly disintegrating and disorienting experiences that silence, isolate, diminish voice, and invite an inauthentic form of re-storying. While Job bears witness to his moral integrity, he nonetheless acknowledges his physical, emotional, and relational *vulnerability*: He is no longer a whole person, and he resorts to metaphors of

14. Job 29:11–17.
15. Job 2:3.
16. Job 31:6.
17. Job 34:35.
18. Job 38:2.

brokenness and being "dashed . . . to pieces"[19] by his experience, metaphors that depict the personal depth of his suffering for those who seek to be witnesses rather than judges. Job experiences a shattering of self, an implosion of his world, and of his self in relationship to this world, and ultimately to the God who reigns in power and, presumably, justice over the cosmos.

However, lacking recourse to the punitive re-storying narrative offered to Job by his friends, his lamentation is that his experience of dispossession and disintegration seems inexplicable. Job and the comforters share the same basic theological premise: Persons who are innocent of blasphemy, idolatry, or various moral wrongs will be delivered from harm rather than having it inflicted upon them. Furthermore, Job and his comforters share a "law of the harvest" ethic: a person who lives by justice, integrity, and righteousness will experience a blessed and gifted life, including posterity, lands, and possessions, while a person who engages in wrong and harmful actions will be deprived of such blessings and experience some form of retributive repercussions.[20]

The wisdom dialogue between Job and his friends, which is comprised of seventeen discrete exchanges, presents no substantive challenge to this basic framework of a "harvest" theodicy and punitive narrative. The inadequacy of this structure ultimately reflects a further feature of suffering, a *quest for a re-storying narrative* that restores order and meaning. The dispute is not over the very general and abstract law of harvest principle of whether the innocent receive blessings and the evil experience affliction, but whether or not Job is just such an innocent person. The anomaly is how, in a cosmos in which God is worshiped as creator, sustainer, lawgiver, and covenant-maker who judges in justice, can persons like Job, who are distinguished by their integrity, experience the relational, familial, and existential losses and ordeals described in the story? Job's friends have a narrative to explain this suffering, a cause—alleged wrongs that are directly contrary to Job's perceived integrity—the effect of which is Job's punitive ordeal. However, the cause is experientially foreign to Job, and hence the proffered retributive narrative is alien; a new narrative must be constructed through re-storying that needs to take into account at least the inscrutable mysteriousness of the divine purpose.

When Eliphaz, for example, affirms that Job should "commit [his] cause" to God because God "wounds . . . but his hands heal,"[21] Job provides almost a verbatim refutation: God knows Job is not evil, and yet God "multiplies my wounds without cause."[22] Job maintains that he is part of the handiwork of creation, but contrary to his trust in the ultimate healing of divine presence, God instead breaks Job down.[23] In his perception of apparent betrayal, Job requires an answer of God, a desire that

19. Job 16:12.
20. Job 4:7–8.
21. Job 5:8, 18.
22. Job 9:17.
23. Job 5:8.

God be accountable to him (and to the humanity Job symbolically represents). He demands a different narrative than presented in the harvest ethic and the punitive story. Ultimately, of course, Job's quest for this narrative of divine accountability and for a causal explanation for his ordeals is revealed to betray a mistaken understanding of the nature of the divine. To draw on the framework of narratives formulated by Arthur Frank,[24] the story of Job begins as a form of restitution narrative, evolves readily into a chaos narrative, and is overlain with Job's quest narrative (a quest ultimately denied by the divine voice).

The narrative discloses that a further mark of suffering in a person consists in the *deprivation of a future* of possibilities. While it is not evident just what Job's aspirations once were, in the midst of his suffering, the devastation of his aspirations is now illustrated by metaphors of darkness, blackness, and absence of light. These portend what Job's future will be, and symbolically has already become: death. The symbolism of earth as devourer is potent; Job laments that he was conceived and born, and that he yet must remain among the living.

His comforters resort not to the language of consolation, compassion, or presence, but to that of condemnation and judgment. By contrast, when Job gives voice to his suffering, his is the discourse of lamentation. Lamentation in Hebrew poetry and Scripture is intensely personal; it is sorrowful, challenging, and realistic, but it is not self-pitying. The discourse of lamentation conveys a sense of abandonment and desertion, and even betrayal by others; Job's lamentation represents him as alone in the world, a stranger even in his own home. His grief, loss, and suffering have situated him in the condition of exile. *Exile and isolation* are further marks of a person being with their suffering. Abandoned by friends and remaining family, accused by the miserable comforters, without a narrative frame to comprehend his suffering, and lacking an explanatory response from God, Job may be physically alive, but his suffering manifests itself as a social, spiritual, and even existential death. Job speaks "in bitterness of soul,"[25] but he is not heard; only Job is with suffering.

Presence is the way in which we bear witness to the suffering and grief of others and express our compassion. It is not possible to fully enter into another's passion of suffering, just as it is not possible to fully enter into another's experience of pain or grief. Pragmatically, presence involves listening to the narrative of a broken world and the uprootedness of the person suffering and grief. This opens a path to healing; the person(s) bearing witness can be a companion on this journey, but the journey must itself be initiated by the person with suffering.

In the case of the comforters, rather than walking the path of woundedness and suffering with Job, they obstruct it by their accusations of wrongdoing, self-centeredness, and blasphemy, and indeed contribute to his burden of suffering. The friends may listen to Job's lamentations, but they do not hear his narrative or his supplication

24. Frank, *Wounded Storyteller*, 75–136.
25. Job 10:1.

for meaning, nor are they attentive to the profound depth of his suffering, which involves not simply loss and dispossession, but a narrative of inexplicability as well. Job employs a variation of a golden rule or reversibility ethic to indict his friends of callousness and indifference: he observes that, were his friends in an ordeal similar to his, even though Job could similarly accuse and chasten, he would instead use "the solace of my lips [to] assuage your pain."[26] It is part of the striking power of the narrative that it is Job, not the friends, who engages the empathic imagination.

When God finally answers his supplications, Job encounters an iconoclastic deity who shatters images of the self, perceptions of reality, and even interpretations of the divine. God answers Job out of a "whirlwind," a common biblical symbol of a theophany, but it is Job who is called to accountability by God. God's answering comes in the form of a remarkable series of nearly sixty questions that display the sovereignty and power of God in creating, ordering, and sustaining the natural world. Significantly, this litany of questions very seldom refers to man or to humanity, thereby signifying the smallness of humanity in relation to divine creativity. The litany of questions presents an anti-Genesis narrative, for among all the creative works performed by God from the foundations of the world, there is no mention of the creation of human beings. The concept of the insignificance of humanity relative to cosmos and bios, and the transience of human life, reveals a further dimension of suffering: Being with suffering induces humility as an antidote to *hubris*.

Despite bearing the image of God, there is little that human beings do to maintain the ordering of nature. The human capacity to ask questions that challenge the fairness or power of God as typified by Job is represented as simply lacking knowledge about the mysterious ways of the divine. Job is not the only person who wants the world and our experience, however mysterious it may seem, to make moral sense in some way. Within my own tradition, a world seemingly without an ultimate moral order and good simply is not compatible with the nature and character of the divine plan. Injustices and unfairness as well as ordeals of faithful commitment that otherwise seem capricious are incorporated within a pedagogical narrative. The first Latter-day Saint leader, Joseph Smith, was informed that, notwithstanding all his afflictions and travails, from loss of children to persecution from religious bigotry to incarceration without cause and ultimately to assassination by a mob, he was "not yet as Job," for he had not been abandoned by his friends. Instead, the ordeals of suffering would provide "experience, and be for [your] good."[27]

The LDS tradition thereby attributes a pedagogical purpose to the suffering of persons who live in covenantal fidelity but find themselves in a Job-like ordeal. Self-understanding, wisdom, and a variety of virtues are cultivated as a person continues to bear witness even in trials of faith. The divine ways may be mysterious in mortal life, but even if the precise pedagogical purpose for suffering may not be discovered

26. Job 16:4–6.

27. *Doctrine and Covenants* 122:7.

until the next life, the tradition affirms that there *is* an answer. However, the narrative of Job resists a pedagogical re-storying and resolution.

It is evident why Job is a biblical and cultural exemplar of a suffering narrative. The narrative presumes a clear sense of Job's wholeness and integrity, which initially is not disputed in the story, including by God. This integrity is threatened through Job's ordeals and dispossession, which are beyond his control, inexplicably imposed, beyond comprehension, and leave in their wake not wholeness but a self that is broken, alone, and abandoned. Despite Job's deepest efforts to resist the arbitrariness and capriciousness of life through affirming his integrity, his dispossession appears entirely beyond his control, the imposition of an inscrutable power or Other. The narrative provides insight into the soul-searing and emptying experience of the sufferer as do few other pieces in western literature.

The biblical narrative reiterates the limitations of intellectualized discourse about suffering and its causes or purposes for the person being with suffering. The punitive narrative of the friends discloses only that the purported comforters really do not know the person experiencing suffering, nor do they really know suffering. However, Job is not given an answer, just questions, from God about the purposiveness or justness of his ordeal, which works against a pedagogical narrative. Job's brokenness and woundedness, his being with his suffering, are themselves diminished relative to the grand cosmological unfolding he receives through the divine questioning. It seems to follow from these different responses to Job internal to the narrative that ill-informed discourse about suffering can itself be a source of suffering. The purposes human beings construct for suffering, be they punitive, pedagogical, or redemptive, may better reflect the human limits of epistemic finitude than apprehension of ultimate meanings. The narrative also illustrates that discourse about suffering can manifest a quite different experience than can be acquired through witnessing suffering or being with the sufferer as an embodied presence of human compassion.

These characteristics of being with suffering delineated in the Job narrative reveal just how substantial the responsibility contemporary medicine has assumed in articulating the relief of pain and suffering as one of its defining and distinctive purposes. The professionally and morally potent claim is that modern medicine can be more than either miserable comforters or metaphysical questioners to persons who experience suffering. At least one way that this professional responsibility has come to be understood is through medicalizing suffering or interpreting suffering as pain.

Medicalized Suffering

It is certainly reasonable to perceive a close interrelationship between pain, disease, and suffering. While it is not difficult to present examples in which a person experiences pain without suffering, or experiences suffering in the absence of pain, physical pain is frequently a source or cause of suffering. The language of suffering often arises in everyday, medical, and bioethics discourse, not in the context of the kind of existential catastrophe requiring a quest for metaphysical meaning as experienced by Job, but rather in reference to a person undergoing a difficult physical ordeal. For example, it is very common to speak of a person "suffering from" a particular medical condition, from something annoying but tolerable, such as "suffering from my allergies," to more chronic conditions, such as "suffering from diabetes," to potentially lethal diseases such as cancer or a heart ailment. This phrasing locates a source or context for a person's suffering, namely, an underlying disease condition that generates certain physiological symptoms. It is usually possible to construct a medicalized narrative for "suffering from," such as toxins in the air or the metastases of tumorous cells.

The encompassing medical narrative—you are suffering from such-and-such condition, this is why you are suffering, medicine can provide this prescription or that set of treatments to relieve your condition and alleviate your suffering—is one form in which the experience of suffering is subsumed under a medical or scientific explanation. However, this medicalized re-storying may often lack personal meaning, resonance, or healing potentiality for the person experiencing the condition. The medical narrative tends to be constructed as a composite story generalized from the experience of many persons that may not be particularized to the experience of the individual; it can then be questioned whether medicalized narratives reflect a way of being *with* the person in their suffering. It is still an intelligible question for a person who receives a cancer diagnosis to inquire "why me?" and, moreover, to wonder, "how can I find myself in this medical narrative?"

The limitations of the encompassing medical narrative are likewise implied in the common language among medical and nursing professionals of "physical suffering." The designation of suffering as physical gives suffering a locus within the physical body. This embodied place for suffering brings at least this form of suffering under the medical model. It follows that both suffering from and physical suffering ought to be susceptible to remedy from medical or pharmacological treatment and interventions in a manner similar to the experience of pain. However, physical suffering is not all-encompassing, and is implicitly, if not explicitly, contrasted with emotional, relational, spiritual, or even existential suffering. That is, a certain realm of suffering can be delineated as beyond, or potentially beyond, the realm of medicine and medical science. That clearly presents a challenge to the overarching narrative of scientific progress that promises both explication and relief from pain and suffering through advances of medicine and technology.

A method prevalent in common discourse to address this potential challenge to the science of medicine and to medicine's basic purposes is to conflate pain and suffering. This method is illustrated in Melanie Thernstrom's excellent book on chronic pain, *The Pain Chronicles*. Thernstrom begins her discussion by relying exclusively on the language of "pain" and then shifts without any inkling of difference to the language of "suffering."[28] Suffering is reduced to pain without remainder, and this conflation in turn makes not only pain and chronic pain but also suffering a medical problem that through research can eventually be domesticated and relieved. In her assertion that persons in chronic pain are "suffering from a lack of physical suffering,"[29] Thernstrom integrates the three approaches to medicalizing suffering I have delineated: suffering from, physical suffering, and suffering as (chronic) pain. Her claim is that a narrative generated by medical science doesn't (yet) have compelling explanatory power for a person with chronic back pain or migraine, and this unintelligibility itself becomes a source of suffering, even in the absence of physical suffering.

The presupposition on this analysis is that suffering as a form of pain has a physiological cause that in principle is discoverable as medical science advances in knowledge and continues to extend its domain over the human body. It is illustrative of this presupposition that among the many subtitles for *The Pain Chronicles* is "the science of suffering." Thernstrom's analysis of suffering as science reflects the progressivist impulse of modern western science that has led both proponents and critics to see its end to consist in mastery of the human condition.[30] The progressivist logic is that, in course of time, suffering can be rendered entirely scientifically explicable by a medical narrative and a fact-based scientific paradigm similar to that which is currently used for pain (though not yet for chronic pain). The same kind of progressivist appeal is embedded in Atul Gawande's laudatory assessment that the emergence of palliative care heralds "the scientific study of suffering."[31] This basic presupposition underlies Thernstrom's optimism that we no longer need to rely on metaphors, myths, narratives, or fruitless quests, such as undertaken by Job, to find some purpose or meaning to suffering; ultimately, scientific medicine will render chronic pain as well as suffering as malleable to medical treatment as tuberculosis was a century ago.

Although I am critical of Thernstrom's too-ready conflation of suffering as pain as illustrative of a broader conceptual problem, her chronicles of chronic pain nonetheless make a very substantial contribution to understanding the relationship of pain and suffering. Differentiating acute pain—which may be excruciating but of short duration—and chronic pain—which is often less intense or "sharp," but of long-term duration—is deeply resonant with the experience of millions of Americans.[32] A chronic disease and its accompanying continual pain surely is one source of suffering.

Thernstrom uses very telling metaphors to express the nature of chronic pain, for example, as a form of exile and banishment from the familiar; much as it may be longed-for, a person with chronic pain cannot return to their historical self-narrative. A medical narrative of restitution is inadequate for the experience of chronic pain.

28. Thernstrom, *Pain Chronicles*, 7.

29. Thernstrom, *Pain Chronicles*, 43.

30. McKenny, *To Relieve the Human Condition*, 25–38.

31. Gawande, *Being Mortal*, 142.

32. Institute of Medicine, *Relieving Pain in America*.

And, as delineated through the interpretation of the Job story, a threat to the integrity and intactness of the self is the core characteristic of suffering. Furthermore, treatment of chronic pain is frequently a trial-and-error proposition, and thus can be rather resistant to appropriation by the medical model and its reliance on replication and evidence-based outcomes. Thernstrom's numerous accounts of patients in chronic pain who engage in "doctor-shopping," as well as her own ordeal of chronic pain (alleviated in part through narrating her story as part of the chronicle), indicates that patients often find physicians lacking in compassion, and that the medical system is unresponsive to an experience that doesn't yet cohere with the medical narrative of pain and pathological physiology. This is to say that even the modern medical approach to chronic pain can exhibit characteristics of being a "miserable comforter." A contemporary challenge for medicine in the twenty-first century is precisely being with persons with chronic illness and pain.

Understanding Suffering

Although there are important interrelationships within reigning scientific paradigms between pain, chronic pain, and suffering, as physician Eric Cassell has cogently argued, pain and suffering are "distinctly different forms of distress."[33] The medicalization of suffering signifies not simply a conceptual problem, but also leads to inadequacies in the practicalities of caring for patients. Cassell makes his claim forcefully in *The Nature of Suffering and the Goals of Medicine*: "The test of a system of medicine should be its adequacy in the face of suffering; . . . [however], the central assumptions on which twentieth-century medicine is founded provide no basis for an understanding of suffering."[34]

These problematic assumptions are, for Cassell, rooted in a reductionist model of the biological and genetic sciences as enacted in contemporary medicine. Among other issues, the reductionist method leads medicine to focus on the disease manifested in the body, on pain as a symptom of the presence of disease, and to supplant healing with curing. This interpretation can give cogency to the common phrasing that a patient is "suffering from" a particular condition. However, Cassell contends that the biological reductionist vision blurs the primacy of the person in medicine, with profound implications for finding a place within a medical worldview for suffering: "[a]lthough bodies may experience nociception, bodies do not suffer. Only persons suffer."[35] Consequently, medicine must be more fully attentive to the many dimensions or aspects of a person for suffering to be understood, let alone for medicine to be with a person who is suffering. Otherwise, it is entirely possible that in the course of practical caregiving, the treatment of a disease condition will cause the person to suffer.

33. Cassell, "Pain and Suffering," 2283.
34. Cassell, *Nature of Suffering*, v.
35. Cassell, "Pain and Suffering," 2283.

Reductionist science has been abetted by reductionist philosophical accounts of the person, particularly those that have historically identified the self with the disembodied mind, as in the Cartesian ideal. This philosophical anthropology eclipses a need for inquiries into the experience of suffering, and Cassell draws out one profound implication of this commitment: "[A]s long as the mind-body dichotomy is accepted, suffering is either subjective and thus not truly 'real'—not within medicine's domain—or identified exclusively with bodily pain."[36] Notably, while *The Stanford Encyclopedia of Philosophy* has an extensive article on pain and its philosophical meanings, it has no entry on suffering. It seems as if suffering in itself merits no philosophical attention, a concept perhaps more at home in religious narratives that have been philosophically discredited; on this account, suffering becomes the experience of pain that is more intense and of longer duration. Furthermore, there is a political bite to Cassell's critique that has implications for bioethics insofar as much bioethical reflection is sourced in liberal political philosophy: "Considering persons as ahistorical, atomistic individuals, in which the body is separate from the mind, is not supported by a knowledge of suffering."[37] This is an epistemic claim that is grounded in the experience of persons who suffer and who bear witness to their suffering through their stories: suffering requires a richer and fuller account of a person than what science or philosophy, or the autonomous self as presumed in much bioethics writing, has presented. Hence, the paradox embedded in the goals of medicine: The medical vocation is comprised partly of the relief or melioration of suffering, but the medicalized narratives do not have space for a concept of suffering.

The reason for an insistence on a thick account of the human person becomes clear when Cassell formulates his definition of suffering: "Suffering is a specific state of severe distress induced by the loss of integrity, intactness, cohesiveness, or wholeness of the person, or by a threat the person believes will result in the dissolution of his or her integrity."[38] Though persons are identified with their bodies, they are not only bodies; hence, suffering cannot be equated with pain or portrayed as entirely consisting of physical suffering. The wholeness or integrity of a person can be threatened or lost through emotional distress or psychological ordeals, or relational disruptions, or (as in Job's case) a radical form of dispossession that challenges personal moral integrity, or forms of spiritual alienation or affliction. Suffering thereby does not presuppose or require the experience of physical pain, but rather the loss or threat of loss to self-identity and integrity that can manifest itself in numerous realms of a person's life.

Cassell's primary illustration of how the difference between bodily pain and suffering manifests itself is drawn, significantly, from a woman's experience in childbirth. There is little question that the pain experienced in childbirth, including the tearing of bodily tissues and the invasion of the body by various medical interventions, is the

36. Cassell, *Nature of Suffering*, 33.
37. Cassell, "Pain and Suffering," 2286.
38. Cassell, "Pain and Suffering," 2285.

most intensive experience of embodied pain. The pain can, of course, be alleviated to some degree with analgesics as well as breathing practices. However, in Cassell's view, such extreme pain should not be considered suffering, nor need it lead to suffering. There seem to be two distinguishing features in the context of childbirth (or at least, in many births): a woman's control over her body and relative control of the intensity of the birthing process and the purposiveness of the activity.[39] This purposiveness of giving birth and becoming a parent provides a narrative within which the woman can understand and give meaning to her experience. The birthing narrative entails that as the woman assumes a new identity, as mother, she retains and controls an important continuity in her wholeness as a person rather than experiencing a disruption or loss of her narrative coherence and integrity.

Cassell's reliance on the childbirth illustration to conceptually distinguish pain from suffering of course begs the question of whether the pain of childbirth becomes an experience of suffering when the woman loses control of the process (for example, a complicated delivery) or it lacks purpose for her (for example, the pregnancy was unwanted). He generally contends that people "suffer from" pain when "they feel out of control, when the pain is overwhelming, when the source of the pain is unknown, when the meaning of the pain is dire, or when the pain is apparently without end."[40] Certainly, some of these conditions apply in the case of complicated childbirth. They also, as Cassell acknowledges, are present in some circumstances of pain from a chronic illness, or the kinds of pain experience that Thernstrom chronicles. Recognizing these interrelationships of pain, chronic pain, and suffering doesn't collapse the concepts, but in fact supports a conceptual and pragmatic distinction between pain and suffering. Suffering may be relieved, even if the pain continues, through diagnosing a source of the pain, controlling its intensity, shifting its meaning, or anticipating its cessation.

The chronicity of experience nonetheless shifts in suffering in an important way: A person's sense of wholeness is reflected in part through their experience as a being in time that is demarcated into a past, a present, and an anticipation of a future. As persons are temporal beings, their coherence as a person is in part a function of being able to relate a coherent narrative about their life experience and their self-relationship through time. Suffering radically calls this temporality and narrative identity into question for the future becomes radically contingent; the future recedes as the present moment of suffering extends indefinitely. These phenomena underlay the suffering of Job. The loss of a future of open possibilities has as a consequence the inhibiting of a person's capability of telling the story of their suffering. The rupture (or threat of same) of the temporal is the context for the experience of what Arthur Frank

39. Cassell, "Pain and Suffering," 2285.

40. Cassell, *Nature of Suffering*, 35.

calls a "narrative wreck,"[41] in which self-conflict takes the place of self-coherence and integrity, and the self-narrative may be displaced by silence.

If childbirth in many, though certainly not all, cases exemplifies an experience of severe acute pain without suffering, the language of loss embedded in Cassell's definition of suffering points to a common illustration of an experience of profound suffering without pain, namely, grief over the death of a loved one. Although grief is certainly not without its physiological symptoms, the loss of relationship can be shattering of a person's wholeness and coherence, affecting every aspect of a person's life, including their capacities as storytellers. Living through the loss embeds the person in time and place. Bereaved persons are with suffering in undergoing an ordeal of transformative consequence, though it is seldom related to physical pain on the part of the mourner.

Cassell's interpretation of the distinctiveness of suffering relies in part on the question of meaning as rooted in his anthropology of the person. He contends that persons have "a transcendent dimension" or life of the spirit, by which he means an intense feeling of connection with "anything larger and more enduring than the person."[42] Cassell maintains that the medical profession seems oblivious to this aspect of the person; studies in recent literature on spirituality and health imply his impression is mistaken in certain respects.[43] Nonetheless, this transcendent dimension embedded in the *imago Dei* presupposes that persons are inherently meaning-making and meaning-sharing beings. Significantly, Thernstrom contends that scientific understanding and medical successes in pain relief and control have led to the conclusion that "pain is meaningless"—that is, there is no grand narrative of the purpose of pain.[44] By contrast, Cassell asserts that "meaning is essential to suffering."[45] That was certainly an assumption of Job.

Compassion and Suffering

Cassell's discussion is so compelling because the integrity and identity of medicine seem to ride on the question of how the profession addresses suffering: "The timeless goal of the relief of suffering remains the challenge to change and the enduring test of medicine's success."[46] His account creates complications for the medical profession in different ways. He is critical of scientific and philosophical assumptions about the person that have permeated medicine and tend to make suffering a subset of the question of relieving pain. However, having established that awareness of suffering is an

41. Frank, *Wounded Storyteller*, 55.

42. Cassell, *Nature of Suffering*, 41.

43. Cole et al., *Medical Humanities*, 314–26.

44. Thernstrom, *Pain Chronicles*, 119.

45. Cassell, "Pain and Suffering," 2287.

46. Cassell, *Nature of Suffering*, xv.

essential to the nature of the medical vocation, Cassell makes problematic the prospect of physicians carrying out the professional imperative to relieve suffering.

There is no generalized guidebook that physicians can rely on for recognizing or being with suffering. Suffering is as unique and as particular as each person. Hence, "[n]o one can know with certainty why another person suffers. One can know that someone is suffering, but not what it is about this specific person that leads to the suffering . . . What threatens the loss of wholeness of one person is not necessarily the same as that which jeopardizes another."[47] The claim of the unique individuality and particularity of suffering suggests an epistemic chasm between the physician and the person suffering to such an extent that the value and practical relevance of core virtues of the healer, such as sympathy, empathy, and compassion, seem diminished.

A way through this conceptual and practical impasse is suggested in the writings of bioethicist Warren T. Reich. Being with suffering is a matter of professional perplexity when the person suffering cannot find a voice or narrative by which to express their experience as suffering, or in Frank's phrasing, the person experiences "narrative wreck." Reich presents what he designates as "an experiential interpretation" of suffering and the corresponding response of compassion that is directed towards understanding "the sufferer's struggle to discover a voice that will express his or her search for the meaning of suffering."[48] Reich delineates three phases of this struggle of being with suffering, which illuminate a process by which the person moves from being silenced by suffering (or mute suffering) through a threshold of liminality (my phrase) in which suffering is expressed as lament, story, or interpretation, to a transforming experience of finding and accepting "the new voice of the suffering self."[49] My analysis here will focus on Reich's account of responsive being with suffering by "a compassionate other . . . that is devoted to sharing suffering and compassion."[50]

The initial phase of compassionate being with suffering by a caregiver is reflected in silent empathy and compassion. This dynamic of silent solidarity and bearing witness is the form of responsive presence displayed in the initial response of Job's friends as they find Job himself at a loss for words. They sit with him, speechless, but present for a week, with Job engrossed in his suffering. The silencing of the person witnessing suffering may reflect being overwhelmed in the presence of such anguish, but it also can communicate honor and respectful dignity for the person suffering, for "the silent word is spoken by one's entire presence."[51]

Being with the person in their suffering not only means respectful silence and presence, but is also a matter of place—that is, "an effort on the part of the caregiver to

47. Cassell, "Pain and Suffering," 2286.

48. Reich, "Speaking of Suffering," 86.

49. Reich, "Speaking of Suffering," 91.

50. Reich, "Speaking of Suffering," 91.

51. Reich, "Speaking of Suffering," 93.

place himself or herself where the suffering person is."[52] This placing reflects a "radical empathic position" in which the caregiver is beside the person, rather than behind or across from them. As C. S. Lewis observed in another context, being at the side of a person is a symbol of the intimate sharing and vulnerability displayed in friendship and companionship.[53] The empathic presence communicates a willingness to walk with the person through the woundedness of their experience.

A succeeding phase of being with the suffering person involves helping the person to find a language and voice for suffering that is authentic to their experience. Expressive compassion, as with expressive suffering, is the language of liminal transition, in that it seeks to invite connectedness in the face of loss of wholeness and integrity. The first form of expressive compassion is "the language of diagnosis itself."[54] As illustrated in various aspects of human experience, naming is a symbol of empowerment and control. The naming of the silence is thereby similar in form and content to Cassell's contention that providing information to a patient about their source of pain can be a way to the alleviation of their suffering. It must be noted, however, that resort to diagnostic language can risk medicalization.

A second form of expressive compassion is displayed through story as the compassionate caregiver "can assist in the reformulation of the story."[55] This language reflects the pattern of re-storying I have highlighted throughout my interpretation of the healing process of restoring wholeness. Re-storying requires attentive listening and empathetic entering into the narrative of the suffering person, including both the former narrative that is now broken or wrecked and the emerging narrative of suffering. As noted previously, the story of Job is ultimately a quest narrative that emerges out of a chaos narrative, but the inattentive comforters of Job focus only on restitution themes.

A third form of expressive compassion is what Reich refers to as "the translational statement, which converts the sufferer's experience into comprehensible words."[56] In those painfully reflective moments in my mother's ongoing ordeal with the physical and other limitations of her stroke, she would utter remarks such as "you don't understand what this is like," and occasionally, "no one understands." One mode of response of compassionate being with suffering can acknowledge the reality of personal epistemic and experiential finitude and the isolation, loneliness, and sense of betrayal out of which such a remark is voiced. A compassionate witness also invites a relation with a person who can be with suffering and who can offer a bond of connection and presence, perhaps even of solidarity.

---

52. Reich, "Speaking of Suffering," 93.
53. Lewis, *Four Loves*, 66–67.
54. Reich, "Speaking of Suffering," 93.
55. Reich, "Speaking of Suffering," 94.
56. Reich, "Speaking of Suffering," 95.

Expressive compassion can also involve interpretative statements, which differ from translational statements in that interpretation seeks to "enhance intellectual understanding"[57] or broaden the understanding of the person suffering. This can be a risky mode of compassionate utterance, for an external interpretation of the person's experience of suffering may come across as insensitive or inattentive, impose an alien narrative, and cannot be effective unless "appropriated as the internal interpretation of the sufferer."[58] The interpretive statement risks the imposition of an alien narrative that led to Job's exasperation with his friends as miserable comforters, no longer with him in suffering.

Just as the person suffering enters a final phase of identifying with a new sense of self and story, the compassionate caregiver also experiences a profound change in identity, in voice, in integrity, and in story. The experience of identity-transformation means that being with suffering ultimately reflects the covenantal commitment of bearing witness: a transformation of a physician or caregiver into the identity of witness and compassionate healer who walks the path of woundedness as a companion and friend with the person suffering. Reich portrays the identity-transforming process experienced by the caregiver as analogous to "conversion"[59] as the experience of being with suffering invites and reinforces a deeper commitment to be a person of compassion.

Bearing Witness of Suffering

This exploration of religious, medical, philosophical, and ethical narratives and accounts of suffering is suggestive of several ways through which being with suffering witnesses to a fundamental human responsibility to bear the suffering of other persons and also illuminates the distinctive professional commitment to alleviate suffering. Suffering is an experience of profound isolation, a form of contraction of self to a point that a person suffering may perceive that "no one" is able to understand or empathize with their experience. Suffering can make a person feel as though they are exiled from those interactions and relationships that have formed their everyday experience, that they are not only alone but in the hells of unremitting loneliness. C. S. Lewis relates that in the midst of his deep grief over the loss of his spouse he felt as though he were a social outcast residing in a colony of lepers.[60] The person with suffering experiences a contraction of the temporal; a future of possibility—life plans to fulfill, relationships to cultivate, and aspirations to achieve—are eclipsed by the prolongation of the present ordeal of suffering. This is why the chronic nature of some illnesses is a cause of substantial suffering: the ordeal seems literally without end.

57. Reich, "Speaking of Suffering," 97.
58. Reich, "Speaking of Suffering," 97.
59. Reich, "Speaking of Suffering," 98.
60. Lewis, *Grief Observed*, 10–11.

The melioration of suffering is thus in part comprised by compassionate presence, an embodied witness that the suffering person is not abandoned by the moral community of medicine or by familial caregivers. The physician can discover a calling to bear witness through the patient's story of illness and suffering. Presence is a witness and reminder to the person of their inherent dignity and value. Moral communities of witnesses share in bearing the burdens, wounds, and mourning of the person suffering by absorbing the suffering into their common life and narrative extended over time. Presence does not mean the caregivers understand the particularized ordeal of the person's suffering, but it conveys experiential knowledge of suffering and its isolation. Presence is a witness that though we do not understand the meaning of all experiences, there is an inescapable depth and transformative power to compassion. Compassionate presence is a necessary feature of being with suffering.

As powerfully illustrated in literature as varied as the story of Job or *The Plague*, suffering is marked by the loss of a voice capable of articulating a coherent narrative of life. A person experiencing suffering may not lose their voice; they may, as portrayed in Edvard Munch's "The Scream" or in Tolstoy's character of Ivan Ilyich, indeed be screaming, but the person is not able to give voice to a narrative that makes sense or gives coherence to this experience. When the person expresses that "no one" understands, the referent of "no one" includes themselves. Suffering that is expressed in the discourse of lamentations may be heard by comforters as protest or anguish heard as rebellion.

A moral community and profession that makes a commitment to be with suffering conveys that the silences imposed by suffering do not comprise the final words. A constitutive feature of the witness of compassionate presence is assisting the person suffering in a search to find language, to find an authentic voice, which expresses their ordeal. The risk inherent in the role of compassionate witness is becoming a "miserable comforter" by substituting one's own language and story for that of the person in the hells of suffering. In speaking of their suffering, the sufferer in fact seeks commonality with a person who by their listening will become a witness in healing. The narrativelessness of suffering invites the community to bear witness to a narrative re-storying that brings coherence out from the experience of chaos. This does not mean what Frank refers to as "narrative surrender" to a medicalized or scientific story.[61] It rather entails a mutual commitment to restoring wholeness through re-storying. The process of re-storying, a core element of healing, is a necessary mark of being with suffering.

In Tolstoy's novel, *The Death of Ivan Ilyich*, the protagonist Ivan Ilyich has an inner dialogue characterized by his incessant query as to the purpose of his suffering, to which at one point an inner voice replies, "There is no reason [for the torments]. They just are."[62] The coming apart of the self, its disintegrating identity, is necessarily associ-

61. Frank, *Wounded Storyteller*, 6.
62. Tolstoy, *Death of Ivan Ilyich*, 100.

ated with a loss of meaning. The person who questions, as Ilyich did, what they did that made this happen to them, finds the torment of suffering to consist in the fragility of the "I" and the "me" and the world of the self on the verge of disintegrating. The answer to the question may not seem discernable in the throes of suffering. Suffering is not a medical or a moral problem to be solved, but a condition of our mortality to be lived through. Being with suffering can mean coming to acceptance of the "just are" characteristics of suffering.

The healer's witness of being with suffering means having the courage and integrity to be present when the sufferer experiences abandonment even in the darkest nights of the soul. While walking the wounded path between the dialectical dynamics of isolation and presence, loss of voice and narrative re-storying, undergoing and overcoming suffering, breaking down and breaking open, being with suffering means a witness of faithful companionship as a person suffering seeks to find their way to purposiveness and meaning. That walk sometimes takes the person and their companion through the valley of the shadow of death.

PART THREE

Bearing Mortality

8

Dying Well

I was working late in my office on a chilly and rainy fall evening when my intellectual focus was disrupted by my cell phone. My sister was on the other end, and after our mutual greeting, she got straight to the point of her call: "Court, I'm calling with a message you've been dreading receiving for the past twelve years." As the words lingered momentarily, I quickly raced through several possible scenarios about a dreaded message twelve years in the making: had something happened to my sister? Was there a relationship problem somewhere in our extended family?

I simply was not prepared for the actual message my sister delivered: "I wanted to tell you that our mother passed away in the hospital about fifteen minutes ago." I was immediately both stunned and emotional. My sister and I had exchanged emails just a couple of hours previously, discussing arrangements for my mother's home health care. We had been told by a hospital nurse earlier in the day that our mother would shortly be discharged after a two-day hospital stay accompanied by instructions for rehabilitation. We had been seeking clarity from her attending physician on her post-discharge plan of care. How was her dying the same evening even within the realm of possibility? I could not hold back the tears as I recognized that my mother had died alone, with no loved ones or family members to accompany her on her final mortal journey.

I had visited my mother the week previously, and though it was clear she was experiencing the physical infirmities and disabilities of fourteen years of life following a severe cerebral hemorrhage (as related in chapter 1), her mind remained alert and sharp as ever. We had discussed the results of her medical tests following a short episode of facial paralysis in which she was unable to speak. The initial diagnosis she had received was a small TIA—or a "mini-stroke," as the hospital physician described it—but various blood tests and imaging scans revealed nothing unusual. She had returned home the same day, and though rather fatigued from the ordeal, including the "bumpy ride" in the emergency vehicle to the hospital, she was otherwise the same mother I had known for the previous fourteen years. At the end of my visit, I gave my mother a kiss on her aged and wrinkled face, we exchanged expressions of love, and I left for the airport.

Within a few days, the ordeal repeated itself: my mother experienced facial paralysis upon waking for the day, and an inability to form or vocalize words. An EMT team again transported my mother to the nearby hospital emergency room, during which time she regained her ability to speak. More tests, the same blood, CT, and MRI imaging scans as the previous week, with again no apparent abnormalities detected. The admitting physician did not think this was a TIA, but the recurrence of the symptoms was troubling, and she wanted my mother to stay in the hospital for observation for a short period of time. This proposal did not go over well with my mother, but eventually she relented, which was taken by staff to be authorization for staying in the hospital.

At this juncture, an oasis of humanity in the midst of a depersonalized institutional setting emerged. A different physician contacted my sister, indicating that he was reticent to discharge our mother to her home without a more structured and higher level of care than could be provided by her home health aides. He recommended that my sister read the best-selling book by physician Atul Gawande, *Being Mortal*, to gain some insight into the likely course of our mother's remaining life and the conversations we needed to have as family regarding her home and hospital care. The physician then made a specific recommendation for hospice care. My sister was surprised by the recommendation, and, being aware that hospice is typically utilized in situations where death is certain and relatively near in time, asked whether the physician believed our mother was nearing death (and, unspoken, if there would be time for the family to gather as families have always done). The physician replied that, while one could never be certain in these kinds of matters, he was confident she was not close to death. The recommendation for hospice would mean that the care my mother needed, including rest and transport, could be provided without necessitating ongoing frequent trips to the hospital should some so-far-as-yet unexplained symptom occur. The physician had reviewed the prospect of home hospice care with my mother, and true to character, she replied, "I'm not ready for that." All the same, my mother agreed to stay in the hospital through the weekend, and the physician indicated that he would communicate the in-home hospice proposal to my mother's primary physician in anticipation of a conversation between my two siblings, myself, the physician, and a social worker on the ensuing Monday.

My sister was calling to initiate that conversation, which never occurred. What had transpired over the final two days of my mother's life is perhaps best situated by a critique of medical callousness presented by Gawande. Gawande acknowledges the importance of the dying role for both the dying person and the significant relationships in their lives: "People want to share memories, pass on wisdoms and keepsakes, settle relationships, establish their legacies, make peace with God, and ensure that those who are left behind will be okay." He then proceeds to a biting indictment of technological society and of medicine: "the way we deny people this role, out of obtuseness and neglect, is cause for everlasting shame. Over and over, we in medicine inflict deep gouges at the end of people's lives and then stand oblivious to the harm done."[1]

I doubt I will ever understand the reasons my mother, myself, and my family members were denied precisely these meaningful moments of mortality by insensitive members of the medical and nursing professions, and by the depersonalization and fragmentation of a large health care institution. My mother's sister, likewise uninformed by the medical staff about my mother's condition through the course of the day, arrived at the hospital within minutes after she died. When my sister called the hospital some five minutes after that, a male nurse answered my sister's inquiry by saying, "KC? Oh, she passed away a few minutes ago. There's a person here named L, do you want to talk to her?"

Conversations that we had been promised would happen between the attending physician and the physician on call over the weekend never happened. Conversations that we had been promised would happen between us and the attending physician (the reason for my sister's persistence in calling) never happened. Was it really so hard for anyone providing care for my mother to pick up a phone and call someone in the family? Or perhaps I should first ask, was anyone in the hospital providing care? Or, did anyone care enough to see beyond the problem of a tired elderly woman who didn't want to be in a hospital bed, but who was not recovering from many maladies? Why was caring so hard?

As much as it pains me to compose this, my mother did not die well. She died in a hospital bed, quite possibly the last place on earth she would have wanted to spend her final days in mortality. She died without anyone from her family present, her children, her grandchildren she'd seen a day earlier, her siblings. She died alone, and I mean that literally: not only was no member of her family present to say good-bye, no one was in the hospital room with her. She died without anyone of significance in her life knowing, even as she was treated as a person of no significance by those who did know. All of these wounding circumstances of her dying were entirely avoidable with some basic communication. Perhaps not surprisingly, given the indifference displayed by the medical and nursing staff, there was never any expression of condolences from the medical or hospital staff; no statement like "I'm sorry for your loss." My mother was a lost patient to them.

---

1. Gawande, *Being Mortal*, 249.

The story of my mother's dying, and dying poorly, sets the context for my explorations of what it means to die well. You'll excuse me if my experience has made me a bit cynical regarding the marketing discourse about and supposed commitment to compassionate and quality care at the end of life provided by contemporary health care professionals and institutions. The hospital in which my mother died markets itself on "providing high-quality healthcare" imbued with "a tradition of caring and healing [that] will never fade." Perhaps end-of-life care doesn't fit within this tradition, perhaps it is not "healthcare." The general question of dying well nonetheless insists upon our attention: one of those questions of mortality that bioethics once thought it important to address.[2]

In his discourse "At a Graveside," Christian philosopher Soren Kierkegaard articulated a profound insight on the meaningfulness of our mortality: "To die is indeed the lot of every human being and thus is a very mediocre art, but to be able to die well is indeed the highest wisdom of life."[3] The first part of Kierkegaard's observation, that mortality is a universal given of the human condition, does not necessarily sit comfortably in the mindset of many persons in the modern era. We are continually portrayed or self-portrayed as embodying a denial of death and as engaging in various strategies to evade or delay its ominous onset, including fitness, diet, related programs of health and lifestyle wellness, and aging management. Numerous medical interventions, from vaccinations to life-extending technologies and organ transplantation, promise longevity coupled with aspirations for a substantially compressed period of morbidity and decline.[4] The appropriate application of these technologies has posed profound ethical questions for medicine from the very beginnings of the era of contemporary bioethics.

It is nonetheless the second portion of Kierkegaard's claim that has more stunning implications: dying well manifests the acquisition of the highest wisdom of life. This clearly is not meant to imply that one only learns wisdom during one's dying, after it is too late to change the course of one's life. Instead, Kierkegaard intends that we acquire this life wisdom over the course of our lives in order that we experience both a full life and a good, peaceful, dignified dying. This transpires in part through a meditative personal confrontation with one's mortality while alive and healthy, what Kierkegaard refers to as "earnestness."[5] This is not an easy task precisely because of the modern ethos of death denial and evasion, an increasing reliance on ever more effective life-prolonging medical technologies, and quite candidly, a kind of professional state of being callous and uncaring. In certain respects, aspirations for longevity have supplanted wisdom in our cultural, medical, and personal encounters with mortality. Likewise, this has substantial ethical implications for medical practice.

2. Ramsey, "Indignity of 'Death with Dignity,'" 209–22; Kass, "Averting One's Eyes," 67–80.

3. Kierkegaard, "At a Graveside," 76.

4. Emanuel, "Why I Hope to Die at 75," 76.

5. Kierkegaard, "At a Graveside," 94–96.

This chapter is devoted to bearing witness to an understanding of "dying well," and to professional aspirations of caring and healing, in the context of cultural evasions, medical technologies, and the realities of personal callousness and institutionalized indifference. Few recent writers have pursued these kinds of questions more relentlessly than Gawande. I want to begin my exploration by considering the professional, ethical, and existential issues he addresses in *Being Mortal* as a way to sort out differences between the "mediocre art" of dying, the experience of dying poorly when caregivers do not care, and our hopes for dying well.

The Medical Culture of Dying

Gawande's analysis of modern dying begins, as does that of so many other authors, with reference to Leo Tolstoy's *The Death of Ivan Ilyich*. Gawande's medical school education on mortality and death consisted of a sole session of a weekly seminar in which he and his colleagues took up the meaning of Tolstoy's novella for their medical training. The anguish that Ivan Ilyich experienced in his dying was attributed by the seminar students to "a failure of character and culture."[6] Ilyich's physicians as well as his family were insensitive to his sufferings and perpetrated the deception that so tormented Ilyich. The seminar participants contrasted this callousness with the "honesty and kindness [that are] basic responsibilities of a modern doctor."[7] And Ilyich (and Tolstoy) had the misfortune to live in a rather primitive, pre-scientific era of medicine. Clearly, in the twenty-first century, Ilyich's condition would have been diagnosed, and medications or treatments would have cured him, restoring him to his career, relationships, and family. So much for medical meditations on mortality: modern medicine ends the story before it begins.

Two features of the medicalized culture of dying are worth identifying from Gawande's initial encounter with the construction of mortality in medical culture. First, Ilyich's dying is taken to be the paradigm case of the bad or awful dying process (itself a problematic interpretation). Perhaps we are not as a culture or a profession clear about what comprises dying well, but we do have clear illustrations, even in literature, of the kind of dying we wish to avoid. Secondly, although Gawande and his physician cohort were quite confident about the virtues central to a physician's moral character and integrity, it is not at all evident that they embodied these virtues in their own practice. Gawande observes that he and his classmates were most concerned with knowledge, scientific knowledge about the body and its pathologies, and medical knowledge about how to diagnose and treat. The capacity for empathic presence, honesty, and kindness was taken for granted, or perhaps deemed a secondary skill relative to curing disease.

6. Gawande, *Being Mortal*, 2.

7. Gawande, *Being Mortal*, 3.

Yet, as Gawande initially encounters his own seriously ill patients, he quickly recognizes that this devotion to the sciences failed to prepare him for the care required by the dying. Gawande finds that in the treatment and care for one dying patient, he and his team were actually "worse" than Ilyich's physicians; they had provided ever more invasive treatments that essentially inflicted new forms of physical torture without any "acknowledgement or comfort or guidance" about the person's impending mortality.[8] Empathy, compassion, kindness, and witnessing presence are not so easy to come by, after all. Something else is involved in the medical understanding of mortality than failures of character and culture.

Medicalization and Uninteresting Patients. Obstacles to dying well and to compassionate presence by caring healers are encountered long before the actual onset of the dying process. Gawande situates his discussion of the issues dying poses for medicine within a cultural and professional narrative about aging, frailty, and dependency as decline. Dying well presupposes consideration of how fully we have lived prior to experiencing the inevitable declines and debilities of aging, and whether we have found meaning and purpose in these years: that is, whether we can answer the question "what makes life worth living when we are old and frail and unable to care for ourselves?"[9] My mother would have answered that question with reference to her family, her grandchildren and great-grandchildren, and her passion for reading. All of this was denied her in her dying, for biomedical science, technology, medicine, and institutionalized health care constitute their own character-shaping culture, and this culture has medicalized both aging and dying. Mortality has become a medical experience managed by members of the health care professions, and the locus of control of the dying process resides not with patients or their families, but rather in the "imperatives of medicine, technology, and strangers."[10] Similarly, aging and debility are, like pain and suffering, constructed as medical problems that should be malleable to medical remedies, even as the language of medicine dictates institutional priorities of safety and survival in the context of aging.[11] The humanity and the ethics of both aging and dying well have been supplanted by impersonal forces, institutional priorities, and medicalized cultures.

It is in perceiving that the medical culture of dying carries over to issues that first emerge in the medical culture of aging that Gawande again finds wisdom in Tolstoy's story of Ivan Ilyich. Tolstoy's novel is less about dying and death and more about living authentically rather than falsely even in the midst of diminishing health. This possibility requires a culture of caring that is denied Ilyich; Tolstoy's novel thereby reveals "the chasm of perspective between those who have to contend with life's

---

8. Gawande, *Being Mortal*, 6.

9. Gawande, *Being Mortal*, 92.

10. Gawande, *Being Mortal*, 9.

11. Gawande, *Being Mortal*, 79–110.

fragility and those who don't."[12] This epistemological chasm of empathy underlies the medical problematic of suffering discussed in chapter 7; in the context of the elderly population, fragmented perspectives culminate in a context of care that is increasingly institutionalized and veiled from public view, as well as a realistic perception of fear of abandonment by the elderly and dying. As aging inevitably evolves into dying, the experiential chasm becomes more pronounced and displays that, despite enormous technological advances over the past century, society's culture of aging and the medical culture of dying have really achieved little moral progress. Gawande contends, "This simple but profound service—to grasp a fading man's need for everyday comforts, for companionship, for help achieving his modest aims—is the thing that is so devastatingly lacking more than a century later [than Tolstoy]."[13] Had my mother's physicians read that passage from the book they recommended my sister read? Would these good words have made any caring difference?

Gawande rightfully presents a stinging indictment of the medicalization of aging and dying. Treating aging, debility, and mortality as medical concerns has been a failed experiment in social engineering. It has failed because society has placed "our fates in the hands of people [medical professionals] valued more for their technical prowess than for their understanding of human needs."[14] In this culture of medicalization of the human condition, the physician increasingly assumes a role analogous to a technician or mechanic rather than healer; the human body is professionally constructed as a complex and worn-out machine to be fixed and repaired, incidental rather than intrinsic to personal identity. Ultimately, Gawande writes that "those of us in medicine . . . often regard the patient on the downhill as *uninteresting* unless he or she has a discrete problem we can fix."[15] Neither aging nor dying are fixable problems, however, so to avoid being neglected or perceived as uninteresting, a person needs to avoid becoming an elderly patient with a serious condition. Perhaps these constructions explain the neglect and inattention towards my mother from the medical and nursing staff. She was an "uninteresting" patient to her professional caregivers and the health care institution with its philosophical façade.

The American Immortal. The intrinsic intertwining of cultural and professional inadequacy with respect to both aging and dying attested to by Gawande is likewise reflected in the writings of physician Ezekiel J. Emanuel.[16] Emanuel contends that aspirations for longevity must be situated within what he calls a rich and complete life. This completeness to life is inclusive of, though not limited to, love, relationships and posterity; personal achievements in a vocation or career; and conveying a meaningful legacy and memories to children and grandchildren, all the while experiencing

12. Gawande, *Being Mortal*, 99.

13. Gawande, *Being Mortal*, 100.

14. Gawande, *Being Mortal*, 128.

15. Gawande, *Being Mortal*, 29; my italics.

16. Emanuel, "Why I Hope to Die at 75," 74–81.

minimal physical or mental limitations. Within this understanding, dying well means a life well-lived and shaped by wisdom, relationship, and meaning, such that though death is an occasion for sadness and grief, it is not a tragic occurrence.

In contrast to the interrelationship of a complete life and dying well, Emanuel develops his own cultural indictment of social processes and a characteristic self-image embedded in the culture that he designates as "the American immortal."[17] An ideal type, the American immortal engages in various health-enhancing dietary, fitness, and lifestyle activities for the instrumentalized purpose of endless life extension. The immortal's expectations are not solely with longevity, but rather with perpetuating the health and purposiveness of middle-age into "the golden years." Healthy living and preventive medical care will compress morbidity into a short span rather than a protracted and lengthy period; consequently, the aspirations embedded in the character of the American immortal are that we will live increasingly longer lives and then die with minimal debility and decline. Although Emanuel does not delve deeply into the cultural context, he describes this perspective as a "quintessentially" American idea, as it symbolizes embedded cultural narratives regarding progress, optimism, individualism, and most notably, freedom from contingency. In this self-image, dying well will mean hardly dying at all.

Emanuel argues that the aspirations of this cultural type are a fantasy, a kind of magical thinking, because the empirical evidence of the past quarter century simply does not bear out the validity of the compressed morbidity thesis. He draws an even sharper distinction than Gawande on the intertwining of aging and dying, claiming that "health care hasn't slowed the aging process so much as it has slowed the dying process."[18] This elongated dying is increasingly marked by chronic illness and debility, as represented by the higher incidence of stroke, dementia, and Alzheimer's in the population, thereby diminishing the meaning and possibility of dying well. The ideology of the American immortal is furthermore enacted at a societal level; it not only propels continual biomedical research and advances that medicalize aging, but substantially increases health care costs and distorts or misorders priorities for health care services. One evident result of this misordering is less funding for research, treatments, and rehabilitation for chronic disabling conditions such as stroke. My mother's experience of a very prolonged period of debility of nearly fifteen years is not the cultural norm, but neither was she an outlier.

Emanuel likewise shares with Gawande the view that the cultural and medical problematic of dying and death is not initiated by the onset of the dying process, but rather reflects deeply rooted cultural perspectives that shape a person over a lifetime. An understanding of dying well is necessarily shaped by constructed narratives of living well, including the story of aging that precedes dying. However, the life narrative constructed by the American immortal evades a serious grappling with the core

17. Emanuel, "Why I Hope to Die at 75," 76.

18. Emanuel, "Why I Hope to Die at 75," 77.

existential questions of our nature, identity, purpose, and meaning, and instead defers throughout life to an "easy, socially acceptable agnosticism."[19] The life story of the immortal is constructed within a disenchanted world immune from matters of meaning. The earnestness of confronting and living with mortality that Kierkegaard articulated as a necessary condition of dying well eludes the worldview of the immortal.

Significantly, Emanuel seeks to escape the influence of the immortal ideology for his own life. He establishes a biological age (seventy-five) after which he claims he personally will refuse any preventive procedures (such as a colonoscopy or a flu shot), decline any life-extending medical treatments, and accept only palliative and comfort care. In so doing, he acknowledges but also seeks to evade the experience of an extended morbidity. In particular, his refusal of life-prolonging treatments after he achieves the age threshold is intended to avoid bequeathing a legacy to children and grandchildren in which "memories of vitality will be crowded out by the agonies of decline."[20] Emanuel observes a constriction of self as a person ages, including a narrowing of ambitions and expectations. This is partly due to the limits of neurological plasticity, and also to diminishing communal involvement and support beyond one's immediate familial relations. Space likewise contracts, as an aging person's world may no longer encompass an active professional or engaged communal life, but concerns mobility within a neighborhood, and eventually within one's home, a sitting chair or wheelchair, and ultimately confinement to one's bed. This biological and social reality impedes the hope of providing lasting memories to significant others and children in prime of life. The ultimate tragedy for Emanuel is not death, but an elongated dying process that is marked by frailty rather than vivacity. The protracted duration of dying obstructs dying well.

Emanuel's biological threshold of seventy-five is intertwined with a biographical narrative that encompasses a complete life. Yet, as Gawande observes, determining when a person is dying has now become a professional puzzle for which medicine has no clear answers. Gawande maintains that, in the context of life-prolonging possibilities of technology, he is unclear just "what the word 'dying' means anymore. In the past few decades, medical science has rendered obsolete centuries of experience, tradition, and language about our mortality and created a new difficulty for mankind: how to die."[21]

What Matters. As Gawande formulates the issue, the central difficulty for the medical profession with respect to both aging and dying well is that it imbibes in a form of professional agnosticism that parallels the social and personal agnosticism that Emanuel maintains so characterizes the immortalizing fantasies. "The problem with medicine and the institutions it has spawned for the care of the sick and the old," Gawande maintains, "is not that they have had an incorrect view of what makes

19. Emanuel, "Why I Hope to Die at 75," 81.
20. Emanuel, "Why I Hope to Die at 75," 79.
21. Gawande, *Being Mortal*, 158.

life significant. The problem is that they have had almost no view at all."[22] If the profession gives negligible attention to the question of a meaningful life, it follows that choices regarding end-of-life care that raise such a question become problematic if not dilemmatic.

The question of the scope of medicine's expertise as technical but not as a witness to existential meaning is certainly not a new issue. Sociologist Max Weber framed the issue in the early part of the twentieth century in the advent of the era of scientific medicine: "Whether life is worthwhile living and when—this question is not asked by medicine. Natural science gives us an answer to the question of what we must do if we wish to master life technically. It leaves aside, or assumes for its purposes, whether we should and do wish to master life technically, and whether it ultimately makes sense to do so."[23] The medicalizing cultures of aging and dying instantiate what Weber designated as a "disenchanted world"[24] in which questions of meaning, including the meaning of a life in the shadow of death, cannot even be raised let alone answered. The difficulty is that as beings embodying the *imago Dei* we necessarily engage in a quest for a life of meaning and purpose, which is inclusive of a desire for dying well.

The technical mastery of medicine regarding life-extension and dying prolongation manifests the paradigm of instrumental rationality and its methods of efficiency and effectiveness. This entails that medical institutions and hospitals may well foster a neglect on those matters that would be most meaningful to persons under their care who are approaching the end of their life. As suggested by the mission statement of the hospital in which my mother died, a commitment to "excellent health care" for patients may not encompass the provision of health care to patients who are "uninteresting" in the way Gawande suggests or who are actually dying. In the absence of some substantive professional vision about dying well, the practical gap is filled by the directives of technology, professional ethos, and culture: "we fall back on the default, and the default is: Do Something. Fix Something."[25] These directives disclose the workings not only of the so-called technological imperative that if an intervention can be done, it will be done, but also a presumption of success: In the case of serious illness, some medical intervention will pull the patient through their ordeal and deliver them from death, at least until the next crisis. In a culture in which medicine is valued for its technical efficiencies and instrumentalized rationality, aging, dying, and death seem to be anomalies, contradictions that threaten professional self-understanding. As Gawande articulates the point, "nothing is more threatening to who you think you are than a patient with a problem you cannot solve."[26] That was the kind of patient my mother

---

22. Gawande, *Being Mortal*, 128.

23. Weber, "Science as a Vocation," 144.

24. Weber, "Science as a Vocation," 139, 155.

25. Gawande, *Being Mortal*, 174.

26. Gawande, *Being Mortal*, 8.

presented to various physicians, nurses, therapists, and home health aides; the threat to professional identity can be avoided by evading the patient.

Re-storying and Relationship

The metaphors relied on by several physician-authors are revealing of how medicine's technical prowess comes to be enacted and why it seems to fail for cultivating a culture of dying well. Medicine's identity is bound not to healing in this discourse, but rather to its technological proficiency at solving problems or puzzles presented by bodily pathology. This is manifested in the training of medical education in which dying is approached as "a set of medical problems to be solved."[27] As physician Sherwin Nuland articulated in his award-winning book *How We Die*, "the solution of The Riddle of . . . disease" is a more compelling challenge for physicians than the advancement of patient benefit: "It is The Riddle that drives our most highly skilled and the most dedicated of our physicians."[28] The professional preoccupation with the puzzle or riddle amenable to solution means the patient disappears or becomes "uninteresting."

An embedded assumption of the puzzle metaphor is that, given enough time, financial investment, scientific study, research investigations, and professional and public patience, the riddle or puzzle can in fact be solved. The scientific basis of medical knowledge is designed to provide answers or solutions to an array of diagnostic and prognostic perplexities. The application of this knowledge in medical treatments that provide cures, or at the very least, in the case of chronic illness or aging, provide a way for managing that which cannot be cured forms the basis for the narrative of continued medical progress. The medical encounter with dying, however, betrays the model of puzzle/solution as inadequate and even insensitive. Dying cannot be constructed as a problem that can be solved when it is a permanent and inescapable feature of human experience.

The philosophical concept that Gawande ultimately relies on for developing an ethic of care when cure is not possible is that of autonomy, though he invests it with a narrative valence that distinguishes it from the bioethical principle of respect for self-determination. Gawande draws on the philosopher Ronald Dworkin to contend that, in the midst of various physical limitations and personal ordeals, "we want to retain the autonomy—the freedom to be the authors of our lives."[29] He subsequently specifies the concept of autonomy to be a matter of "remain[ing] the writers of our own story" and of retaining "the freedom to shape our lives in ways consistent with our character and loyalties."[30] While we have minimal control over many of the circumstances of

27. Byock, *Dying Well*, 35.
28. Nuland, *How We Die*, 249.
29. Gawande, *Being Mortal*, 140.
30. Gawande, *Being Mortal*, 140–41.

life, including aging and our mortality, "be[ing] the author of your life means getting to control what you do with the [circumstances]."[31]

The construction of self as an author and life as a narrative provides a context for infusing the narrative with a personal quest for meaning and purpose independent of the medicalizing culture. This interpretation of self as author of a life narrative moves very much in the direction of Kierkegaard's virtue of earnestness and thus expresses a more demanding encounter with mortality than contentment with the comfortable agnosticism appropriated by the ideology of the American immortal. In Gawande's view, "[l]ife is meaningful because it is a story. A story has a sense of a whole, and its arc is determined by the significant moments, the ones where something happens."[32] Dying well is thereby comprised in part through articulating a cohesive narrative of life and embodying that story and its constituent values in the context of professional and familial pressures to compromise personal integrity or to re-story one's self in an inauthentic manner. Dying well should reflect an authenticity about how a person lived.

However, the medical culture of dying is not driven by an authorial interpretation and narrative, but is instead embedded within a professionally and ethically problematic account of the profession. Already informed by technical and puzzle models, Gawande descriptively situates conversations regarding the end of life between patient and physician within a contractor and consumerist model of interaction rather than a partnership or covenantal model: medical interactions are increasingly cast as "a retail relationship. The doctor is the technical expert. The patient is the consumer."[33] The retail relationship emphasizes physician identity only as a technical expert who provides information so the patient can make decisions about the means necessary to achieve their own goals. Relating generalized technical knowledge entails knowing less about the particular patient. This becomes especially problematic when the patient has not made an assessment about their own goals for end-of-life care, or the issue of goals does not surface in physician-patient conversation.

Gawande observes that the increasingly prevalent retail relationship can be effective when there are clear choices and clear patient preferences. However, these conditions seldom prevail in circumstances of end-of-life care. The consumerist or retail model of relationship is not conducive to cultivating the trust necessary to engage difficult conversations or to provide a comfortable context for disclosing ambiguities and uncertainties relative to prognoses. It reinscribes in medicine the ethics of strangers and transactional interactions delineated in the contractual understanding of relationships. The ethical implication of the retail model is that the patient not only has a right to refuse or request medical interventions at the end of life, including physician aid-in-dying, but that their request, whatever it is, is *morally right* as well.

31. Gawande, *Being Mortal*, 210.

32. Gawande, *Being Mortal*, 238.

33. Gawande, *Being Mortal*, 200.

Yet, even though it may seem that there is no moral appeal in a transactional retail relationship beyond patient self-determination, other narratives from the profession, the market, and the culture work to supplant the patient's authorship of the story, thus undermining rather than affirming patient choice. The retail relationship inscribes the dichotomy between facts and values into medicine and reflects the thinnest version of autonomy of the independent self such that the patient's story is narrated through the idiom of the marketplace.

The retail model of medicine is a conceptual extension of the contractual and consumerist accounts of medical transactions delineated in my discussions on healing and covenant. The model may be descriptively illuminating, but normatively misrepresents the character of relationships between physicians and patients in end of life care. The question then becomes what might be some constructive and fitting understandings. Gawande's writing suggests the presence of at least five primary interpretations of the physician embedded in the medical culture of dying. In addition to the retailer model, Gawande presents the physician as a *general* in a militaristic model, the puzzle-seeking *technician* of the mechanical, fix-it approach to the human body, the *rescuer* of the heroic narrative, and the *parent* who may engage in deceptions or evasions to avoid destroying hope in the narrative of medicine's relentless progress. Not one of these images of professional self-identity is especially compatible with the normative interpretation Gawande proposes for the patient experience: the *author* in quest of the autonomy and authenticity necessary to write their own story. These contesting interpretations of the physician, as well as the correlated roles of the patient embedded in them, no less present obstacles to ensuring that the patient can experience a dying authentic to their values and integrity.

The prospect for conflict or misinterpretation between the five models of the physician and the authorship model of the patient's experience is not conducive to a converging caregiving dynamic. This provides the philosophical, professional, and cultural context for Gawande's penetrating exploration of medicine's responsibility to the dying. His wrenching discussion is framed by the tragic story of Sara Monopoli, a young (thirty-four years old) woman diagnosed with an inoperable lung cancer while in the final weeks of pregnancy with her first child.[34] Ms. Monopoli's story is tragic in several respects, but for Gawande's purposes, Monopoli provides a cautionary example of medical overreaching: Ms. Monopoli did not retain the kind of autonomy to write her own story and be the author of her life in the time remaining to her and her family following her diagnosis. What clearly took over the patient's story were professional narratives of rescue and militarism. These narratives were complemented with the "seemingly unstoppable momentum of medical treatment,"[35] which necessitated evasions and deceptions characteristic of a paternalist model and fatiguing medical treatments characteristic of the technical and instrumental model.

34. Gawande, *Being Mortal*, 149–90.
35. Gawande, *Being Mortal*, 165.

All of these physician identities seeking to treat Ms. Monopoli's cancer worked to preclude conversations, not only between physician and patient and family, but also within the family. The imperatives of treatment and technology meant that Mr. and Ms. Monopoli simply were not able to have a conversation about how they wished to share the remaining months of Sara's life. After all, thirty-four-year-old women with no prior history of predisposing conditions are not supposed to contract lung cancer right as they are to give birth to their first child. The cultural and medical story of "fighting the battle" against cancer, and the medical commitment to ensure a restitution narrative, did not provide a place for alternative stories that may have in turn provided space and time for meaningful conversations. The question, really, is why? What obstacles are embedded in medical culture, and in the culture as a whole, that inhibit self-storying and re-storying in the dying process?

Despite more than a quarter century of public policies promoting discussion about patient preferences at the end-of-life through advance directives and other methods, Gawande implies that the medicalization of dying perpetuates the approach of denial and evasion. He portrays a medical profession whose members are very uncomfortable in conveying the likely bleak realities of prognoses to patients. Physicians may rely on euphemisms of various kinds that provide patients with reassurance, but they are reticent to disclose the patient's actual survival chances, let alone the prospects for recovery to a condition of a quality life as may be dictated by the conventional restitution narrative.[36] Empirical studies disclose that physicians tend to err in their prognostic disclosures on the side of survival by a factor of five.[37] Patients then live and die under the illusion fostered by the rescue and military narratives that medical interventions are more effective in delaying death than is actually the case.

Alternatively, physicians suppress the prospect of more pessimistic diagnoses: physicians may accompany the American immortal in indulging in fantasy and magical thinking in some of the more difficult and anguishing situations. Even Gawande concedes that he engaged in speculative fantasy in conversations with Sara Monopoli and her husband, raising the fallacious prospect that an experimental drug could be effective against both her lung cancer and a newly developed thyroid cancer. He contends that "discussing a fantasy is easier" than realistic conversations about the dying process and the anticipated outcome of death.[38] Professional evasion and reassurance is thus bought through cultivating false or misleading hopes on the part of patients and families.

The illusions of hope are perpetuated by the longtail phenomenon—that is, the willingness of patients and physicians to believe that this particular patient will be the person that is the outlier or exception that survives long past the expected prognosis.[39]

36. Frank, *Wounded Storyteller*, 75–96.

37. Gawande, *Being Mortal*, 167.

38. Gawande, *Being Mortal*, 169.

39. Byock, *Dying Well*, 65.

Gawande concedes that "there is almost always a long tail of possibility" for survival;[40] however, the evasive medical narratives of dying proceed as though everyone, not just an occasional fortunate survivor, will experience increased longevity. "The trouble," he contends, "is that we've built our medical system and culture around the long tail," a foundation that functions "as the medical equivalent of dispensing lottery tickets."[41] Although conversations about end-of-life preferences are increasing in frequency, these often occur so late in the process that they have a negligible influence on the patient's and family's experience of dying. Evasion, illusion, fantasy, and poor communication patterns about dying and death lead to situations in which physicians violate the commitment of *primum non nocere* and inflict the "deep gouges" on patients and families that I referenced in the dying of my mother.

Mortal Responsibilities. Gawande portrays the challenges for professionals, institutions, patients, and families about end-of-life care as partly attributable to an "unresolved argument about what the function of medicine really is";[42] or as I have framed the point in my discussion of medicine as a healing profession, the core issue revolves around the narrative ends and purposes of medicine. The militaristic "fight" against death and disease may suffice in some situations, but it is inadequate, and can even be unethical, when the battle cannot be won. A more nuanced and complex account of the physician's responsibility and identity is embedded in the medical culture of dying, though Gawande does not name it. Significantly, this more complex understanding of the profession and of the physician underscores the covenantal interpretation of physician-healers as *witness* and *guide*: "our responsibility in medicine is to deal with human beings as they are. People die only once. They have no experience to draw on. They need doctors and nurses who are willing to have the hard discussions and say what they have seen."[43] Physicians and nurses have a professional and moral responsibility to give voice to their experience, acting as truthful witnesses and providing the companionship of a faithful guide. Everyone will die, but no one should die alone in the strangeness of a hospital bed.

A very compelling account of professional identity as witness and guide is presented and embodied in the anguishing posthumous memoir of neurosurgeon Paul Kalanithi, *When Breath Becomes Air*. In engaging in conversations with patients about their end-of-life prognosis, physicians assume a burden of what Kalanithi provocatively phrases as a "mortal responsibility."[44] The assumption of both a moral and a mortal responsibility, including responsibility for inevitable failures, cannot be undertaken by a professional in a retail or consumer-based relationship. Rather, it requires a covenantal partnership and relationship in which the physician embodies a wit-

40. Gawande, *Being Mortal*, 171.
41. Gawande, *Being Mortal*, 171.
42. Gawande, *Being Mortal*, 187.
43. Gawande, *Being Mortal*, 188.
44. Kalanithi, *When Breath Becomes Air*, 114, 151.

ness and promise of non-abandonment. Hence, for Kalanithi, the ritual of informed consent becomes "an opportunity to forge a covenant with a suffering compatriot: *Here we are together, and here are the ways through—I promise to guide you, as best I can, to the other side.*"[45] Kalanithi experiences this covenantal commitment and the shared burden of mortal responsibility as both a physician treating terminal patients and as a patient with a terminal diagnosis of lung cancer.

The professional responsibility of witnessing and being with dying is no less paramount than being with suffering. Three primary patterns of responsive being with dying can be developed: conversations designed to elicit patient priorities; re-storying the experiences and decisions of dying persons within a meaningful narrative of their life; and discerning models of dying well, as exemplified in hospice and palliative care, that can be integrated more broadly in medical practice. The mortal responsibility of witnessing, covenantal companionship, and guide is, in my analysis, carried out on different (albeit intersecting) levels. There are practical considerations about what should be done in certain complex circumstances of end-of-life care; professional considerations about the roles medicine can and should play that are compatible with its narrative purposes and commitments to patients; and structural and institutional issues regarding the reforms necessary for medicine and health care institutions to become moral communities with the courage to confront mortality and incorporate end-of-life care within their institutional missions rather than hide dying and death behind evasive marketing missions.

Conversations. Gawande remains committed to the indispensability of having difficult conversations about end-of-life care, notwithstanding politicized objections about "death panels." Empirical research attests that patients who have substantive discussions with their physicians about options and preferences with respect to end-of-life care experience a more peaceful dying process and diminished family anguish; there are no second-guessing regrets about trying the next alternative. Rather than embodying the more domineering professional roles at the end of life such as fighter, rescuer, or parent, a physician should direct their professional responsibilities towards interpretation, collaboration, and guidance. A physician must do more than provide information about options, as though choices about treatments and about dying were similar to choices in a consumer retail store. The physician's mortal responsibility means bearing witness to the patient of their experience, especially when the practical implications of patient values are unclear. The physician as healer guides the patient in constructing or re-storying their choices in light of their priorities.

The commitment to conversations as part of dying well is reflected through the educational efforts of the Conversation Project that Gawande helped to initiate.[46] This program provides educational materials for persons facing the end of their life, as well for as their relatives, about how to begin and structure a conversation on the values and

45. Kalanithi, *When Breath Becomes Air*, 88.
46. Visit their website at https://theconversationproject.org/.

priorities of the person for end-of-life care, and specific choices about life-sustaining treatment. The process begins with a question that Gawande ultimately found his way to in caring for his patients as well as his own father: "What matters to me at the end of life is . . . ?" The responses to that query will vary by each person, of course, but can provide direction about the nature of medical interventions the person seeks or wishes to decline. Developing a conversation around this question can mean addressing more specific matters, such as the level of the person's understanding of their condition and alternative treatments; the level of involvement in decision-making the person wishes to assume; the balance the person seeks between longevity and quality of life; the person's fears regarding under-treatment or over-treatment; and the roles and presence of loved ones in the dying process.

The process of articulating a narrative of a meaningful life requires a fundamental recognition that persons approaching the end of their life have priorities beside longevity, and that the "American immortal" critiqued by Emanuel is indeed merely caricature. Seriously ill patients who are authors of their story express core needs that take primacy over life-extension, including fulfillment in family relationships, mental awareness, minimizing pain, avoiding being a burden to their significant others, achieving a sense of completion about their lives, and hoping that the ending of the journey of life has mattered. Save for relieving pain and suffering, these needs are for the most part relational matters and issues of meaning, not medical issues or questions, which is why medical management of aging, dying, and death can be so profoundly alienating. This leads to the core question for Gawande regarding structural and institutional changes: "How can we build a health care system that will actually help people achieve what is important to them at the end of their lives?"[47]

Part of the response to this question involves appropriating understandings of dying embedded in palliative and hospice care programs. I have been profoundly influenced and moved by the hospice discourse of "being a witness" and "companioning in the journey" of a dying patient. Hospice can represent a new ideal for how to die in the context of modernist evasions and medical battles against death; indeed, hospice symbolizes a retrieval of the *ars moriendi*, or "art of dying," for our era.[48] The central issues that patients in partnership with their physicians need to engage as they deliberate about end-of-life matters may be adapted from palliative care contexts: the dying person's understanding of their current health condition and prognosis; the person's fears as their dying process unfolds; the patient's goals should their condition worsen; and, the trade-offs persons are willing to make (and what is non-negotiable) so they can achieve completeness to their life narrative. Delayed conversations about such questions tend to mean later admissions to hospice care programs devoted to improving the quality of remaining life. Coordinating and integrating hospice and palliative care into the continuum of care available for seriously ill patients seems a

---

47. Gawande, *Being Mortal*, 155.
48. Gawande, *Being Mortal*, 165.

moral imperative that can provide resistance to cultural and technological imperatives that insist on continuing treatment.

This makes for a very compelling approach to the end-of-life and to dying well. A plan based on values, educational resources, an approach to conversations, and exemplary models in a community of care is an important start, but actually implementing this in practice creates its own challenges. For reasons I do not understand, my mother's dying was marked by a complete void of conversation between her primary physician, herself, and our family, and failures to assume mortal responsibility occurred at the three levels of practical, professional, and structural responsiveness. I find it tragically ironic that the on-call physician recommended that my sister read *Being Mortal* to give her some understanding of what might lie ahead for my mother. A reading recommendation took the place of what really needed to happen: a conversation. My mother died before my sister was able to obtain the book.

The Wisdom of Hope

Hope is an essential characteristic and virtue for dying well. Hope in general pertains to an expectation of a promise or a goal that is yet to be but can be achieved in the future. On some accounts, death is an ending to future achievements and accomplishments, and so hope can seem vacuous. The object of hope must be reframed in the setting of dying from the question of whether one will die to the how and the circumstances of dying—that is, towards those matters over which a dying patient can exert influence, control, and authorship of their narrative. The reconceptualizing of hope presupposes a pattern of truthful disclosure of information, or what Kalanithi refers to as "accuracy that preserves hope,"[49] rather than paternalistically protecting the patient from prognoses that may be considered to "take away hope." Medical practices, technologies, and patterns of communication can converge to create false or illusory hopes for recovery in dying patients and their families.

Preserving hope sometimes seems to function as an overriding imperative for professionals in end-of-life care. Ira Byock, a prominent physician in the emergence of palliative care and hospice programs, observed that his father's physician rationalized nondisclosure of the father's terminal prognosis on the grounds that "a doctor must not destroy hope. I know what I'm doing."[50] Byock questions the trade-offs this imperative of not destroying hope, as rooted in a concept of not harming, seems to demand, including a compromise of truthfulness, respect for patient choices, and allowing space for the patient's narrative. In this instance, the physician's paternalistic pretensions generated and perpetuated false or fantasy hope—that is, an expectation of a medicalized narrative of restitution, a recovery of health and a restoring to one's former mode of life—when there was no good medical reason to support that

49. Kalanithi, *When Breath Becomes Air*, 95.
50. Byock, *Dying Well*, 10.

expectation, and substantial evidence to indicate that Byock's father was indeed at the end of his life. When patients or their families are portrayed as "clinging to hope," or "hoping against hope," it is often this illusory hope that is presumed; if there were some medical grounds for thinking that further interventions could be effective, the patient and family would receive some hopeful assurance from that evidence. Persons clinging to hope are clearly in a condition of heightened vulnerability and sensitivity to words and actions, or their omission.

The longtail phenomenon delineated previously illustrates circumstances in which a person with a terminal diagnosis observes empirical evidence that the duration of life post-diagnosis is variable rather than uniform, and that some individuals survive numerous years beyond the median.[51] A statistical hope for a longer survival duration is thus not necessarily empirically unfounded or baseless, though statistical hope may also be accompanied with an expectation of a healthy life free of disease complications in the intervening years. Gawande's caveat about the "lottery ticket" nature of either the far right end of the longtail or a life of full health prior to death is therefore applicable to statistically-generated hopes. An assumption by either the physician or the patient that a particular patient might win the lottery and beat the odds is a recipe for evasions.

When discussion shifts from hopes for continued longevity to the circumstances of dying, however, there are objects of hope that seem very reasonable expectations. The aim can be to provide patients who are irreversibly dying with "the best possible day."[52] The integration of palliative care in the dying process can actualize a hope to be *relatively free of pain in order to maintain relational presence* and connection. Preserving such a hope is a mortal responsibility of medicine; once the goals of medicine are expanded beyond the narrow construction of fighting the enemy of death, relieving pain and meliorating suffering are core purposes of the healing arts.

The rights possessed by terminally ill patients in all states to refuse medical treatment points to another hope within reason: *freedom from unnecessary attempts to prolong life unduly* or from disproportionate burdens to the patient. Ideally, decisions to enact this hope and exercise the legal right to stop or forego interventions will come subsequent to collaborative conversations between the patient, family members, and the physician or other professional staff. These conversations should assure patients that the care they receive will be of the highest quality, and that the dying process will avoid those kinds of situations patients have observed or read about, and to which they have responded, "I don't want to be like that at the end." The promises embedded in the mortal responsibilities of medicine should be recognized as an expression of covenantal commitment.

The fidelity and identity of the healer is comprised in part by a commitment of witness and presence to the dying person. This commitment addresses the profound

51. Gould, "Median Isn't the Message," 1–4.
52. Gawande, "Best Possible Day," paras. 10–14.

hope of all persons, especially those in institutionalized settings conducive to strangeness and unfamiliarity; namely, that they will have companionship and not have to traverse one of the primary thresholds of life alone. In *How We Die*, Nuland presents two related dimensions of this hope: The first aspect is constituted by a promise by health care professionals that the patient *will not be physically alone* while dying. A second aspect of this commitment is expressed through "the promise of spiritual companionship,"[53] which largely, though not exclusively, falls to family, friends, spiritual leaders, and occasionally, the healer. The anguish experienced over my mother's dying was that neither of these forms of hope and promise were fulfilled, and at least the first promise was callously disregarded by the professional staff.

The witness of companionship underlies why so many hospice workers say they find it a privilege to be with a patient in their dying process. It informs as well the self-referential construct within the hospice community that hospice staff are "midwives" to the dying: the midwife metaphor does not presume an after-death birth metaphysic, but rather is intended to convey the profound bonds of compassionate companionship and presence experienced in the passage from mortality. The professional caregiver can know about the person while the spiritual companion knows the person.

Dying well bears witness to a life of meaning. Nuland contends that a hope "we can all achieve . . . resides in the meaning of what our lives have been."[54] An aspiration for meaning is a central response of Nuland to the expressed hope of dying persons, and formally advocated by right-to-die advocates, for a *dignified death*. A dignified death is not a matter of conferral by a legal statute, but rather is comprised of a life well-lived. Nuland argues: "The dignity that we seek in dying must be found in the dignity with which we have lived our lives. . . . The art of dying is the art of living."[55] The claim makes a critique that the state or advocates of policy legalization should not make a pretentious assumption about what comprises a good or a dignified death; in the context of a liberal political ethos that is agnostic about the good life, and the good society, a good death cannot be legislatively prescribed. The hope for dignity entails some form of coherence and *authenticity* between personal ideals and values enacted over the course of one's life, which is inclusive of, not separate from, their dying. A dignified death is not a statutory conferral, but rather enacts authorship over the ending of a life narrative that reflects on, and is consonant with, the values by which one has lived out their life.

There are then some forms of hope, including comfort, covenant, companionship, presence, dignity, authenticity, and legacy, that are intrinsic to the highest wisdom that comprises dying well. Such wisdom can help us differentiate between reasonable hopes and illusory hopes. Furthermore, the wisdom of hope differentiates between

---

53. Nuland, *How We Die*, 243.

54. Nuland, *How We Die*, 242.

55. Nuland, *How We Die*, 268.

hopes with which medicine can assist in the realization and hopes that should not be medicalized. For example, an aspiration and hope I have commonly heard expressed by elderly populations as well as college-age students is "I [hope I] will be remembered" or "I want to be remembered for the way I lived." While we have substantial control over the way we live, whether we are remembered, how, and for what, is really beyond our control. Even survivors do not entirely control the nature or content of memory. The central concern of memory and legacy with respect to end-of-life care is that physicians honor the life of the dying person such that memories of the dying process do not obscure or eviscerate memories of the life well-lived. Medicine has a mortal responsibility to honor the values by which the dying person lived out their life.

An Art of Dying

We had reached a point in my mother's ongoing hospitalizations where an on-call physician had made a recommendation for hospice care. We never had the follow-up conversations to initiate that process. As I have witnessed the deep commitment and embodiment of care, empathy, presence, and companionship by hospice staff, I retain some confidence that, had the transition to a hospice program been achieved, my mother would have had the experience of dying well. I thus want to conclude this chapter by proposing what that experience could have been, and ethically *should have been*, through an analysis of Byock's pioneering writing on palliative and hospice care programs.

Byock maintains that the culture of dying in the United States is suffused with a "plague of dying badly."[56] As with other authors, Byock situates the catalysts for bad dying and the obstacles to dying well in social and cultural realties, which subsequently manifest in medical culture, including medical education, the entrenchment of curative medicine, and financial pressures. Ultimately, however, our cultural plague of bad dying is set within a broader cultural reality in which a failure of empathic and moral imagination culminates in pervasive violations of the ethic of non-harm and non-abandonment: "underlying the mistreatment and needless misery of the dying is that America, as a culture, has no positive vision and no sense of direction with regard to life's end."[57] Byock concurs with Gawande and Emanuel that medicine has appropriated an agnosticism about the human good that, however comforting it may be experienced during most of life, can be wrenching when mortality inevitably intrudes upon practical decision-making.

My own sense is that we tend to proceed by a method of *via negativa*. We have a pretty clear idea of the kind of dying or death we wish to avoid—that is, a dying in excessive, uncontrolled pain, alone and abandoned in our relationships, or deprived

---

56. Byock, "Physician-Assisted Suicide," 1.

57. Byock, *Dying Well*, 244.

of ways of communication by speech and touch in our sustaining relationships, and thereby experiencing a disintegration of not only our body, but also of those values and hopes that have helped define the narrative arc to life. We are not perhaps as direction-less as Byock suggests, although the direction is comprised of "away from" a dying characterized by these features. This "away from" is insufficient to generate the kind of positive vision that Byock asserts is needed to transform the experience of dying.

Through his experiences as a hospice physician, Byock rejects the concept of the "good death," which he maintains tends to be articulated in terms of negation, or what a person wishes to avoid, in favor of the more process-oriented and growth-affirming language of "dying well."[58] "The concept of dying well," he argues, offers a "realistic and affirmative goal for life's end," comprised of "an understanding of dying as a part of full, even healthy living, and towards accepting care for the dying as a valuable part of the life of the community."[59] Dying well is embedded with a sense of directionality and purposiveness we can move toward. Hospice care embodies this distinctive approach because death is no longer understood and feared as the enemy to be fought, but rather is a presumed outcome. The moral realities and mortal responsibilities for caregiving at the end of life are dedicated to aiding the dying person in living fully and living well during the remainder of life.

Byock seeks to de-professionalize, de-medicalize, de-institutionalize, and de-mystify dying and death. Responsibility for caring for the dying ultimately lies with communities; the dying person, family members, and the community should avoid delegating important responsibilities to strangers, to the medical profession, and organizing institutions. Part of what has gone wrong in the broader culture's denial and defiance of death is precisely the evolution of dying and death into a problem of medical management. Dying persons and their families have many basic needs that must be met, but only one is uniquely medical: the control of physical symptoms, including pain. Other needs for physical, emotional, or spiritual care, companionship, and recognition as a person, rather than a burden, a problem, or a puzzle, are "broader than the scope of medicine."[60]

Byock's affirmative vision for dying well focuses on four features. The first two features of comfort and companionship are the foundational bedrock and necessary conditions for the realization of the other two features, relationship completion and finding meaning.

Comfort: The physical comfort of the dying patient falls in the domain of medicine and requires palliative care and relief of pain, and melioration of patient suffering. On Byock's view, physical distress or "physical suffering can *always* be alleviated."[61]

58. Byock, *Dying Well*, 32.
59. Byock, *Dying Well*, 246.
60. Byock, *Dying Well*, 247.
61. Byock, *Dying Well*, xiv.

This is an indispensable consideration given that the public portrayal and perception of the dying process is often marked by what dying patients and their families want to avoid: debility, diminished capacities, and pain. The editorial board of *The New York Times* recently commended the legalization of physician-assisted death on the grounds that most dying persons in the United States face "dismal choices" and "excruciating pain."[62] Palliative medicine and hospice care are best positioned to address patient pain and physical distress and to be demonstrably and invariably effective.

Companionship: The presence of others, both family and friends, and professionals, who genuinely care for the dying person and are willing to be with them and bear their ordeal in compassionate witness to the person's significance and the meaningfulness of their relationships, is a core feature of dying well. The physician's witness of non-abandonment is a critical ethical commitment. Byock's commitment of presence is voiced more as a member of a compassionate community of care: "We will be with you. We will bear witness to your pain and your sorrows, your disappointments and your triumphs; we will listen to the stories of your life and [we] will remember the story of your passing."[63] If isolation, deprivation, and abandonment are among the greatest fears of dying persons, and presence, witness, and recognition are among their greatest needs, it is surely within the capacity of a caring moral community, including health care professionals, to ensure that no person dies alone.

As the foundational features of comfort and companionship are established, it becomes possible for persons to experience dying not as painful, irreversible decline and loss, but as an occasion for profound personal development. Byock identifies two particular realms in which this development can occur: relationship and meaning. He contends: "When people are relatively comfortable and know that they are not going to be abandoned, they frequently find ways to strengthen bonds with people they love, and to create moments of profound meaning in their final passage."[64] Removing the obstacles the medical culture of dying presents to the cultivation of relationships and for dying persons to be the authors of their stories can transform what Gawande describes as medicine's source of "everlasting shame" into a passage for healing.

Byock embeds "developmental landmarks" in his affirmative vision of dying well that can sustain and extend a dying person's sense of relationship and meaning.[65] These achievements can enrich the person's own life and the lives of others who find it to be a privilege to be witnesses. The "landmarks that underlie dying well" are comprised of verbal expression and actions that reflect forgiveness and reconciliation, gratitude and thankfulness, love and caring, and "saying good-bye."[66]

62. Editorial Board, "Aid-in-Dying Movement," paras. 3, 6.

63. Byock, *Dying Well*, 246.

64. Byock, *Dying Well*, xiv.

65. Byock, *Dying Well*, 33.

66. Byock, *Dying Well*, 166.

Relationship: The achievement of relational landmarks encompasses the dying person's experience of love for self and for others and the completion of relationships in such a manner that "there is nothing left unsaid or undone."[67] Byock engages the dying person in an exercise of contemplating and imagining their imminent death, a process that echoes Kierkegaard's recommendations for cultivating earnestness. In one encounter with a hospice patient who had heretofore experienced tension with family members, Byock asked the patient to "look beyond denial" by considering the following concerns: "What would be going through your mind as you lay dying? What would be left undone? Is there anything you haven't done or said to someone important?"[68]

Byock also invites family members to engage in an imaginative prospective reflection about an occasion of a future retrospective review of the dying process of their relative. This searching (and potentially painful) mode of reflection is prompted by such questions as "Was there anything else we should have done? Did we seize every opportunity, take every action, for a peaceful loving end?" This imaginative process can help families ensure completion to the relationship rather than feeling regrets after the death.[69] Initiating such processes in advance can ensure that families and other caregivers respond affirmatively to these questions.

Meaning: The developmental landmarks of meaning include a person's acceptance of their mortality and the finality of their life and cultivating a new or transformed sense of self. Byock contends that this is a narrative endeavor insofar as it involves the sharing of stories between the generations, mutual affection, and time spent together in joy and in sadness, all of which can create a lasting legacy. It includes expectations and hopes on the part of the dying person to participate in meaningful milestones, such as being present for a school graduation or a wedding, or interacting with a new grandchild: "a person may consciously or unconsciously decide to stay alive for an anniversary, Christmas, or another special holiday, or to complete an important relationship."[70]

Byock contends that landmarks of meaning for some dying persons move beyond the worldly and interpersonal and approach the realm of mystery and the transcendent. Such growth develops from within a person, within the experience of their dying; the prospect of death facilitates emergence of a transformed self. The context for a transcendent landmark of meaning is characteristically accompanied by some form of spiritual practice, such as meditation, prayer, or musical ritual.[71]

The particularities of individual patients preclude the possibility of formulating a philosophically or conceptually normative approach to dying well, such as the

67. Byock, *Dying Well*, 120.

68. Byock, *Dying Well*, 163.

69. Byock, *Dying Well*, 120.

70. Byock, *Dying Well*, 235.

71. Otterman, "In Hospices and Homes," paras. 8–12.

still-influential "stages" of dying model. Companionship and relationship completion may for some persons be peripheral to a quest for meaning through the dying experience. In reflecting on the experience of one patient who engaged in "defiance of death" to the point that sedation to unconsciousness was used as a last resort, Byock contends, "dying well is fundamentally about people experiencing something that has meaning and value for them."[72]

Conclusion

This has been a wrenching chapter to write and to return to, recollecting the sentence where my writing broke off and was not completed when I received the phone call from my sister. I have said that my mother died poorly. It's hard to escape that conclusion, though to the best of our knowledge, she was not in pain in those final hours on that final day. I am not sure, though, that being free of pain encompasses entirely the concept of comfort. I would have liked to have engaged in the imaginative processes Byock invites prospectively rather than experience the searing pain retrospectively. Ultimately, dying well is now more than a warm, fuzzy concept for me, but has assumed the character of a moral imperative to which I must bear witness.

72. Byock, *Dying Well*, 217.

9

Medical-Assisted Dying
and the Soul of Medicine

Ira Byock's account of the plague of dying badly in American culture, discussed in the preceding chapter, has a very immediate practical implication: advocacy movements to legalize physician-assisted death. Legalization of physician prescriptions to hasten the death of terminally ill patients is the tempting professional recourse to resolve the problem of bad dying.

This approach to medical management of the dying process is made explicit in a recent issue of the prominent news journal *The Economist*, which featured a cover story entitled "The Right to Die."[1] The feature story situated the nature and scope of this right in the context of debates over legalization of what was designated as "doctor-assisted dying," using the widely-publicized story of Brittany Maynard as its illustrative patient. Ms. Maynard, a twenty-nine-year-old married woman, was diagnosed with terminal brain cancer in the winter of 2014. She and her spouse, Dan Diaz, moved from California to Oregon to have access to a physician-prescribed medication to end her life as permitted by the statutory provisions of Oregon's Death with Dignity law. Ms. Maynard ingested the life-ending medication on November 1, 2014.[2] Her story had a catalytic effect on advocacy movements to legalize physician-prescribed medications to end life in other states, including California, which adopted an "End of Life Option Act" in 2015 that sanctioned physician-assisted death.

The legalization of physician-assisted death, initiated through the Oregon statute in 1997, clearly represented an important first step in recognizing an extensive scope of the right to die. Though the Oregon Death with Dignity law is frequently portrayed

1. "Right to Die," para. 9.
2. "Final Certainty," para. 16.

as a model for legalizing physician assistance in dying in numerous other states, an accompanying editorial in *The Economist* argued that physician-assisted dying confers insufficient recognition on the right to die. The anonymous authors of the editorial asserted that "we would go further" than the Oregon law and advanced a case for expanding the practices legally warranted by the right to die to allow for physician administration or provision of lethal medication to (1) persons who are physically incapacitated and cannot self-administer prescribed drugs; (2) persons who are suffering from a chronic, but non-terminal, condition; (3) persons experiencing mental pain or suffering; and (4) children facing an imminent death from a terminal condition.[3] This rather stunning expansion marks an important legal, professional, and ethical transition from legalizing physician-assisted death to legalizing what is now referred to as "medical-assisted death" or "medical aid in dying." The language reflects the pervasive trend to medicalize the dying experience. The model jurisdiction for medical-assisted death is not Oregon, but Belgium and the Netherlands, and more recently Canada.

In this chapter, I want to make the case that expanding the right to die along the lines of the European or Canadian models to include physician-administered euthanasia for terminal or chronically ill patients, or patients experiencing suffering in the absence of a terminal condition, would be (1) a moral mistake, (2) contrary to professional integrity, and (3) misguided public policy. Given that there is not societal or professional consensus about the practices permitted in the Oregon model of physician-assisted death, it is premature to advocate rights to euthanasia especially as a remedy for the plague of bad dying. I first present a brief account of the social construction of the right to die, and then indicate how arguments expanding the scope of such a right presume moral equivalence between the negative right to forego medical treatment and the positive right to request physician assistance to hasten death. I direct attention to the value-laden shifts in language, as illustrated in the nomenclature of "medical-assisted death," that renders invisible the moral commitments and professional responsibilities of the physician as healer. I conclude with arguments against proposals to legalize physician-administered euthanasia rooted in covenantal concepts of relationship, healing, and solidarity.

Constructing the "Right to Die"

The concept of the right to die seems at first glance to be a very puzzling moral and legal claim. Rights are justifiable claims against others requiring their nonintervention (a "negative" right) or their assistance (a "positive" right). We appeal to our rights as grounds for preventing other persons or institutions from depriving us of an important interest. A philosophical correlation exists between rights and duties; an appeal to a right represents a claim that some others have a duty. A valid moral right means

3. "Right to Die," para. 9.

that others have moral duties to refrain from intervening with our decisions or our actions, or to assist us in achieving our ends. However, ultimately no person or medical technology will prevent us from experiencing dying and death. Hence, the philosophical puzzle: How can we have a right to something that will happen no matter what we or anyone else does?

In one of the initial bioethical analyses of the right to die, philosopher Hans Jonas attested to the "exceedingly odd" nature of this right. Jonas attributed the philosophical construction of the right to die to the emergence of life-prolonging medical technologies: "medical technology . . . can still put off the terminal event of death beyond the point where the patient himself may value the life thus prolonged, or even is still capable of any valuing at all."[4] The philosophical basis for the right to die provides a specific rationale for the right to refuse treatment, but Jonas presciently acknowledged that more "worrisome cases are those of the more or less captive, such as the hospitalized patient with terminal illness, whose helplessness necessarily casts others in the role of accessories to realizing his option for death."[5]

The language of the right to die in bioethics and popular discourse points to two primary considerations: the circumstances of dying and decision-making authority regarding choices to continue or refuse life-sustaining medical technology. It manifests a moral objection to the impersonal, protracted, and painful circumstances of modern dying that diminish personal dignity—that is, just those circumstances Byock has in mind in designating our era as defined by the "plague of dying badly."[6] The bioethical construction of the right to die symbolizes that in the perception of patients, proxies, and advocates of patient rights, it is now more difficult to die in a manner consonant with the patient's values. *That* is the fundamental deprivation that right to die discourse seeks to rectify.

This account of the construction of the right to die clearly does not settle matters regarding the situations in which such a right is relevant, nor does it resolve the normative moral and legal question of what should be decided. However, the account does affirm not only a critique of the circumstances of bad dying, but also a normative claim regarding who should have authority to make decisions about end-of-life care and treatments. The right to die reposes decision-making authority and control over end-of-life care and choices in the autonomous patient, whose values and preferences can constrain the impact of the undesired circumstances of dying. I wish to briefly develop the discussion of the circumstances of dying before turning more directly to the moral, professional, and legal arguments on the patient as decision-making authority over end-of-life choices, including choices to hasten death by a medication or requesting administration of a lethal medication.

4. Jonas, "Right to Die," 31.

5. Jonas, "Right to Die," 36.

6. Byock, "Physician-Assisted Suicide," paras. 3, 6.

Why It Is Harder to Die

In *Being Mortal*, physician Atul Gawande draws on a variety of patient narratives to highlight some reasons for why it has in fact become more difficult for many patients to die relative to prior eras of medicine.[7] Ironically, some influences are attributable to the successes of medicine rather than medical failures. The causes of death in the twenty-first century are significantly different than a century previously. The majority of persons who died in generations prior to World War II experienced death from infectious disease, such as polio, influenza, or tuberculosis. Various antibiotics, including penicillin, have significantly altered the general patterns of disease etiology in the population such that nearly 90 percent of persons currently living will die from a chronic ailment, such as heart disease, cancer, lung and pulmonary diseases, diabetes, and Alzheimer's disease.

The implications of this shift for personal and cultural experience of the dying process are profound. The chronicity of both disease and the dying process references a ubiquitous pattern in which many people are diagnosed of their terminal condition several years before they actually die. Such persons experience a period of gradual decline in health, with accompanying co-morbidities, which limits their physical well-being and social interactions, and thus diminishes quality of life. This period of prolonged morbidity is a fearsome prospect for leading bioethics scholars and physicians, as illustrated by physician Ezekiel Emanuel's provocative essay regarding foregoing further life-sustaining treatments after a certain biographical life span has been reached.[8] The concept of the right to die then reflects profound concerns to avoid a protracted dying process. Indeed, the fear of protracted dying has supplanted the fear of death as the more meaningful worry about mortality in the contemporary period. It should then be no surprise that fears regarding deprivation of an accustomed and desired pattern of living is a significant consideration in the debate about legalizing physician-assisted dying and euthanasia; according to data compiled over two decades from the Oregon Health Authority, physicians report that about 89 percent of patients who request a prescription from a physician to hasten their death express a concern that they are "less able to engage in activities making life enjoyable."[9]

A contributing factor to the lengthening chronicity of disease and dying is the research development and successful clinical application of innovative biomedical technologies. As illustrated by numerous precedent-setting legal cases, biomedical technology can prolong biological life for what may be seen or experienced as an indefinite period of time.[10] Advances in technologies such as pacemakers, chemotherapy, or transplantation can provide proportionate benefits for several years, but

---

7. Gawande, *Being Mortal*, 149–90.

8. Emanuel, "Why I Hope to Die at 75," 74–81.

9. Oregon Health Authority, "Oregon Death with Dignity Act," 10.

10. Filene, *In the Arms of Others*, 11–93.

at some point the wrenching question of when to stop treatment and rely on comfort care must be addressed. The professional recourse in the absence of clear direction from the patient is "do something,"[11] and while there is almost always something else medicine can do, continued technological interventions mean it may no longer be clear, even for physicians, just when a person is actually irreversibly dying.

Prompted in part by the logistics of access to life-sustaining technologies, in part by the economics of health care delivery, the dying process has become increasingly institutionalized and medicalized. Although in the past two decades, an increasing number of deaths in this country occurred in a patient's home and in hospice settings, it remains the case that a majority of deaths occur in institutionalized settings, such as hospitals, nursing homes, assisted care facilities, or in-patient hospice facilities. The displacement of dying to institutions means that terminally ill persons experience dying as a profoundly alienating experience. They receive treatment from strangers in a setting where the presence of technology is pervasive, and nearly everything from food to time is unfamiliar and disjointed from their life narrative, including control over their choices. Institutionalized settings of care disempower the patient by instituting numerous "little" deaths prior to the end of life, including loss of mobility, diminished choice over clothing, eating, and medication, and restricted hours for the welcoming presence of members of a caring community. Persons such as my mother do not want to spend their final days on a schedule established for institutional conveniences.

Perhaps most significantly, end-of-life care can entail a constant series of choices about medical treatments for which there has been inadequate preparation and little communication between patient, family, and physician. Ideals of shared decision-making often fail to address the realities of difficult choices in circumstances of uncertainty. Gawande's analysis indicates that physicians evade hard conversations and are excessively optimistic about the patient's prognosis, and duration and quality of life, even in the presence of a terminal condition.[12] For many patients, dying is constructed as beyond their control and not simply because of an irreversible biological process. The chronicity of modern dying is complemented by control by institutions, technologies, and professionals, meaning that death is medicalized and medically managed. This background explains why patients and their advocates make recourse to the language of a right to die to retain some control and influence over the circumstances of dying and about decision-making authority. Through the appeal to the right to die, the dying process and death are brought into the realm of choice; how and when to die becomes the purview of patient autonomy.

11. Gawande, *Being Mortal*, 174.

12. Gawande, *Being Mortal*, 167–68.

Theses of Moral Equivalence

The arguments to expand the right to die articulated in *The Economist* seem stunning in both scope and breadth, but they essentially extend an evolving moral logic in historical reasoning about the right to die. In the formative years of the bioethics movement and through important legal cases, right-to-die discourse reflected a moral claim concerning a patient's right to forego medical treatments at the end of life. This claim was primarily derived from two major ethical principles: respect for personal autonomy and professional duties of beneficence to relieve pain and suffering. The principle of patient self-determination encompasses commitments to respect patient choices to be free of unwanted bodily-invasive treatments while beneficence imposes a professional responsibility to minimize or remove burdensome treatments, whether these consist of respirators, feeding tubes, or antibiotics.

The ethical arguments of autonomy, bodily integrity, beneficence, and compassion established moral and legal patient rights to forego life-sustaining treatments. Many bioethics scholars did not deem it to be a large philosophical or moral leap to rely on the same cluster of principles and values to support legalizing physician-prescribed medications to hasten the death of a terminally ill patient. At the policy level, advocates of the Oregon Death with Dignity Act contended they were not creating a new right in their efforts to legalize physician-assisted death but rather were building on rights already embedded in the law.[13] The proponents contended that the right to die as a liberty to forego medical treatments was philosophically and ethically equivalent to the right to die as a liberty of a terminally ill patient to request a hastened death through physician-prescribed medication. This latter right has sometimes been formulated as a right to death with dignity. The claim of moral and legal equivalence is now recognized in statutes and legal decisions in seven US states—California, Colorado, Hawai'i, Montana, Oregon, Vermont, and Washington—as well as the District of Columbia. The number of jurisdictions will inevitably become larger as legislation modeled after such precedents is introduced in numerous other states.

The contemporary question presumed in the argumentation in *The Economist*, with which numerous bioethics scholars concur, is whether there is also a philosophical and ethical equivalence between the rights to die either through foregoing treatment or by requesting a medication to end life and the right to die constructed as a liberty of a terminally or chronically ill patient to request physician-administered euthanasia on grounds of respect for autonomy or relieving pain and suffering (or both). Legalization advocates have long argued that a person's ability to exercise their right to die should not be contingent on their physical capacity to enact the right—for example, persons with ALS should not have their access to a physician's means of hastening death restricted simply because they are incapable of the motor movements necessary to self-administer a lethal medication. The legal requirement of patient

13. Campbell, "Ten Years," 33–46.

self-administration of the medication stipulated in the statutes is critiqued as morally arbitrary and even discriminatory. Similarly, insofar as beneficence manifests a central purpose of medicine to alleviate patient pain and suffering, legalization advocates argue that it is difficult to justify distinctions drawn in state statutes between persons with terminal disease and chronic disease, and between physical pain and mental suffering.

The moral logic of the principles of patient self-determination and physician beneficence is one form arguments assume for not only legalizing physician-prescribed medications to terminally ill patients, as recognized in the US jurisdictions, but to also legitimate a practice of physician-administered euthanasia as recognized in some European countries and Canada. Expanding the scope of the right to die beyond physician prescriptions to hasten death simply articulates the embedded moral precedents of appeals to autonomy and beneficence supporting physician-administered euthanasia, even though the laws in almost all jurisdictions have not yet arrived there. On the equivalence interpretation, the ethical argument is effectively resolved through precedent; what remains to be addressed are pragmatic considerations of changing laws and policy.

To be sure, extending the moral logic of the right to die beyond patient refusal of medical treatments to encompass physician assistance in hastening the death of terminally ill patients and physician-administered euthanasia for terminal and non-terminal patients has been anticipated with apprehension by other scholars and ethicists for decades. I have already noted how this question obliquely emerged in the foundational formulation of the right to die of Hans Jonas. Writing some years later, when the concept of the right to die had culminated in a basis for legal rights to forego medical treatment, including refusing medical feeding tubes, one of the pioneers of bioethics, Daniel Callahan, objected to then-incipient proposals for legalizing physician assistance in hastened death on the grounds that the moral justification for legalization reflected a "boundless logic."[14] Callahan presciently recognized that once the moral rationale of respecting autonomy, physician beneficence, and physician compassion was deemed philosophically and professionally sufficient for legalizing physician actions to prescribe a lethal dose of medication to terminally ill patients, there would be no reason in principle to not allow life-ending medication to patients who suffered in the absence of a terminal illness or to restrict access to patients whose autonomy resided more in decision-making than physical capacities.

More recently, Supreme Court Justice Neil Gorsuch made a similar argument (prior to his appointment) in his critique of legalization proposals. Gorsuch acknowledged the moral force of principles designed to protect individual choices, but questioned the seemingly limitless logic of unfettered autonomy. If respect for personal autonomy is understood to be the primary or exclusive consideration in moral choice in a liberal political society, Gorsuch asserted that citizens will be compelled to

14. Callahan, *Troubled Dream of Life*, 107.

concede that it is arbitrary to legalize physician assistance in hastening death through prescribed medications while prohibiting physician-administered euthanasia: "a strict adherence to the harm and neutrality principles would tend toward a right to euthanasia as well as assisted suicide."[15] The moral logic of autonomy by itself contains no rationale for permitting one practice in medicine but not the other.

The implications of the thesis of moral equivalence can be illustrated with reference to an amendment proposed to the Oregon Death with Dignity Act in the 2017 Oregon legislative session. As noted, the Oregon Act currently permits physicians to write a prescription for life-ending medication for qualified terminally ill patients—that is, it reflects the first thesis of moral equivalence between the right to forego medical life support and the right to request a prescription to hasten death. A legislative amendment designated as SB 893 sought to remedy those provisions in the Oregon statute that have been a post-legalization concern in bioethics scholarship and in advocacy organizations, namely, that a person's choice to hasten death through a medication prescribed by a physician is voided in the advent of loss of physical (self-administration) or mental capacity (impaired judgment).

The ethical critique of these restrictive provisions was put forcefully by a cohort of bioethicists in a statement submitted to the Oregon legislature as to why SB 893 should be adopted as an amendment to the Oregon law: "While those of us in Oregon enjoy a legally secured right to self-deliverance, if we wait too long and lose either the ability to ingest the drug or to understand the significance of doing so, we forfeit the chance to end a waning life at the time and in the manner of our choice. We may be compelled to suffer a lingering and grievous death it would have been reasonable to avoid."[16] That is, a provision interpreted for two decades as a safeguard for patient autonomy and for reasonable policy regulation has under the force of the expanding logic of the right to die (or "right of self-deliverance") become construed as internally contradictory and inconsistent with the law's purported objective of ensuring patient choice at the end of life.

The remedy proposed by SB 893 for this inadequate and paternalistic protection against compulsion from a bad dying involved rewording the statute following the precedents of advanced directive legislation developed for circumstances of foregoing treatment. The thesis of moral and policy equivalence is clearly embedded in this proposal. A terminally ill patient who sought to obtain physician assistance in dying would be permitted to appoint an "expressly identified agent . . . authorized to assist with the procedures for ending a patient's life."[17] The rationale underlying this modification is that loss of capacities, physical or mental, should be no more an obstacle to obtaining physician assistance in hastened dying than they would be to cessation of treatment under a relevant advance directive. A person who planned for

---

15. Gorsuch, *Future of Assisted Suicide*, 95.

16. Dr. Kenneth Kipnis, email correspondence on March 1, 2017.

17. 79th Oregon Legislative Assembly, "Senate Bill 893," 1.

end-of-life choices through formulating an advance directive and appointing a health care representative but subsequently lost decision-making capacity could have their autonomy extended through a surrogate decision-maker.[18] Insofar as there is moral equivalence between allowing patients to die following treatment refusal and death hastened from physician assistance, the principle of fair treatment entails that the concept of extended autonomy should be applicable whenever a patient experiences compromised physical capacities and impaired judgment.

Proponents of the SB 893 amendment claimed that, in its current form, Oregon's pioneering law legalizing physician-assisted death insufficiently guarantees respect for personal self-determination, is exclusionary of persons with compromised capacities, and fails to encompass the full range of potential medical situations for which terminally ill patients might request a hastened death. The boundless logic of self-determination is manifested in a further proposal in the amendment that moved well beyond the current law: The designated agent would be empowered to both "collect medications . . . and administer medications to the patient in the manner prescribed by the attending physician" in accord with stipulations in the person's advance directive.[19]

Significantly, the moral logic of respect for autonomy and compassionate beneficence in the amendment would extend assistance in hastening death, not only to a euthanasia procedure in the absence of a patient's ability for self-administration, but even beyond physician-administered euthanasia. The procedures required to end life need not be directly overseen by a physician, but can become a responsibility of the expressly identified agent designated in a person's advance directive. The use of the language of "agency" and the procedural mechanism of appropriating the precedent of advance directive legislation indicate the proposed modifications to the current statute are deemed not only consistent with but also required by respect for patient choice.

The SB 893 amendment to the Oregon Death with Dignity Act did not pass in the most recent legislative session, though I am confident that a variation will be reintroduced in each subsequent session. When the Act was originally proposed in 1993, restrictions on patient participation were designed to assure the public that a groundbreaking practice of physician-assisted death could be carried out according to a reasonable regulatory scheme. The Act intended to establish a middle ground to encourage professional responsibility for developing "best practices" instead of either supplanting medical judgment by legislative micro-management or allowing for a medical practice without any professional or public accountability. The central argument for emendation is that such provisions have become burdensome, arbitrary, and unfair obstacles for some patients. The thesis of moral equivalence indicates that these patients, who have legally-established rights to die through foregoing life-sustaining treatment and through physician-prescribed medication, have an equally valid right

18. Veatch, *Basics of Bioethics*, 101–2.

19. 79th Oregon Legislative Assembly, "Senate Bill 893," 2.

to die via physician-administered euthanasia or by designated-agent euthanasia. The claim of proponents is that it is legalistic and paternalistic to deny patients their rights based on compromised physical ability or mental capacity. The question is then whether the Oregon model of legislation should be revised or supplanted by something like the approach adopted in Canada in 2016.

A Case for Medical-Assisted Dying

In a recent essay, legal scholar Thaddeus Mason Pope maintains that the safeguards embedded in statutes legalizing physician assistance in dying can become obstacles for patients to have access to what Pope designates as "medical aid in dying."[20] Pope intimates that moral arguments, legal precedents, and sound clinical practices should lead jurisdictions in the United States to follow the path of end-of-life options set out most recently by Canada. Before examining his proposals for areas of legal reform, it is first important to consider the moral, political, and rhetorical work that is achieved by the value-laden nomenclature of "medical-assisted dying" or "medical aid in dying."

The debates in Oregon about what to call the process when a physician writes a prescription to hasten the death of terminally ill patient reflect a long-standing polarization. Advocates of the Oregon Death with Dignity Act recognized through focus-group studies that using the language of "physician-assisted suicide" or "euthanasia" to refer to this process was likely to spell its demise before Oregon voters (as had been the case with similar measures in Washington and California in the early 1990s).[21] The language selected by legalization advocates, death with dignity, was clearly as value-laden and politically potent as the language of "suicide." The language of dignity conveyed a meaningful aspiration for both patient choice and as much patient control of the circumstances of dying as was possible; the phrasing also rhetorically diminished the role of physician participation. The content of a dignified death was otherwise unspecified. The political implications of death-with-dignity language are especially clear: who would not be willing to support a dignified death? Notably, in its annual public reports on the prevalence of the practice, the State of Oregon has shifted its language from "legalized physician-assisted suicide" to its current usage of "death with dignity." That does not itself reflect a change in formal state position from neutrality to support, but rather conveys an evolving discourse in which requests of terminally ill patients for a medication from their physician to end life have become normalized within the medical profession and within broader civic discourse.

The practical ramifications of language have been especially perplexing and contested within hospice communities, a significant consideration insofar as over 90 percent of Oregon patients and over 75 percent of Washington patients who request a prescription under the death with dignity statutes are enrolled in hospice care. During

---

20. Pope, "Medical Aid in Dying," paras. 1–4.
21. Jones, *Liberalism's Troubled Search*, 76–86.

the past decade, I engaged in two studies on the policies regarding legalized physician-assisted death of hospice programs in both Oregon and Washington. I found that there was no consensus among hospice programs on what to call the practice or what patients were making requests for, but instead a veritable moral Babel: for some hospices, especially those with religious affiliations, the language of "physician-assisted suicide" was retained, while a plurality of hospices affirmed the indispensable role of the physician but softened any social stigma by discarding "suicide" language in favor of "dying" or "death," as in "physician-assisted death" or "physician aid in dying." Still other programs utilized language that placed more attention on the patient's actions, such as "patient self-administration" or "patient requests for hastened death," a construction that diminishes the role of the physician. And, some hospice programs deferred to the titles of the respective state statutes, referring to the practice under its statutory construct of "death with dignity act."[22]

I first encountered advocacy of the language of medical-assisted dying as part of a community hospice ethics committee subsequent to my research. Committee members were deliberating on a proposal to replace the language of "physician-assisted death" then used in the hospice's policies and procedures with more fitting terminology reflective of the hospice's non-judgmental and neutral stance. The hospice staff was concerned that the language of "death" was too final and did not reflect the objective of hospice philosophy to improve the quality of the dying experience for all its patients. Hospice staff members on the committee maintained that as hospice provides holistic care to all patients, including patients requesting medication from a physician to end their lives, the policy misrepresented hospice caregiving in focusing attention on the assistance of a "physician."

As the sole ethicist on the hospice ethics committee, I indicated to the committee members that, based on their critiques, perhaps the more appropriate phrasing for the practice was "hospice-assisted dying." As I anticipated, that phrasing did not prevail given long-standing hospice sensitivities about being known as "the place one goes to die." What gained more traction among the committee was a proposal from a member who also served in an advisory capacity with the national legalization advocacy organization, Compassion & Choices, namely, "medical-assisted dying." The intent of this language at the time was only to refer to what was legal under Oregon law—that is, physician-prescribed medications to hasten death. While recognizing that medical assistance in this practice is of a broader nature, including matters of information disclosure and palliative care measures, I argued against adoption of this phrasing, since it obscures the fact that nothing can happen in this process without two physicians agreeing to participate, the law itself does not require any other forms of medical or health care-based assistance, and the phrasing implies a medicalization of the dying experience, which is directly contrary to the philosophy of hospice care. My contention was that it was important to recognize physicians as the professionals

22. Campbell, "Meanings of Physician-Assisted Death," 223–49.

with primary professional experience and legal responsibility for enacting a patient request, and that including this in the phrase affirmed physician accountability. I also wanted to affirm the integrity of hospice philosophy and its goals regarding quality end-of-life care.

In the intervening years, the language of "medical-assisted dying" or "medical aid in dying" has evolved in bioethics discourse, if not in more common parlance or legal provisions, into a catchall phrase for all the kinds of practices delineated previously as part of the social construction of the positive right to die. Medical-assisted dying doesn't include the negative rights to forego medical life support and rely on palliative care, but the phrase does imply that rights to have a physician write a prescription to hasten the death of a terminally ill patient are conceptually and morally equivalent to rights of terminally ill or chronically ill patients to have a physician (or designated agent) to administer lethal medication to end life. The language of medical aid in dying, especially as represented in Pope's analysis, subordinates the role of the physician to broader purposes of medicine, and hence elides professional ethics and calling. It also converges into one constructed concept a range of practices that arguably suppress important ethical, professional, and legal distinctions.

Whether the language of physician-assisted death, death with dignity, or medical-assisted dying is adopted, both pragmatic and principled professional and policy concerns underlay Oregon's decision in 1994 to authorize physician-prescribed medications to end life and simultaneously retain a legal prohibition on physician-administered euthanasia. It is not entirely a surprise that some twenty years into the legalization experience, a more expanded scope of autonomy rights finds its way into a proposal for a legislative amendment. Nor is it a surprise that such an expansion would receive support from bioethicists, many of whom have argued in their writings and in legal briefs that commitments to the principles of respect for autonomy and beneficence permit voluntary euthanasia and non-voluntary euthanasia, albeit under the supervision of compassionate medical personnel. My point, however, is that these kinds of expansions need to be argued for rather than assumed or obscured by conceptual construction.

With this conceptual caveat, let me examine the kinds of burdens Pope asserts patients are experiencing under the current regime of death with dignity statutes, as well as the expansions of patient rights he proposes in his advocacy of medical-assisted dying. In particular, he contends the following four provisions originally enacted as safeguards should be rescinded as they have now become obstacles to patient choice and access.

Age restrictions. Pope argues that current statutory provisions mandating that a person must be at least eighteen years old to make a lawful request for medical assistance in dying are unduly restrictive and should be changed to allow mature minors to make such decisions. This would make access to medical-assisted dying consistent with laws in some jurisdictions that allow mature minors to make determinations about continuing or foregoing life-sustaining medical treatment. Implicit in this expansion of age threshold is not only a claim about the maturity required to make a meaningful life-or-death health care decision, but also a thesis of moral equivalence between treatment withdrawals and hastened deaths.

Capacity. Pope contends that current statutory provisions permitting access to a life-ending medication by persons assessed by physicians to have decision-making capacity are exclusionary for "patients who have no other exit option."[23] This echoes the claim made in the Oregon SB 893 legislative amendment. Expanding patient eligibility criteria to include persons who may suffer from diminished capacity from circumstances such as advanced dementia incurred over the course of their illness and who no longer can exercise capacity at the time when they would otherwise request medical-assisted dying would remedy this exclusion. This proposal would extend the established precedent in which a person can express their preferences on medical treatment through the procedural mechanism of advance directives and have those preferences enacted, even if they subsequently lose their decision-making capacity. Pope's claim here likewise presumes a concept of moral equivalence: a standard of patient decision-making capacity for medical-assisted dying should be no more rigorous than for execution of an advance directive.

Prognostic Duration and Suffering: The statutes currently legalizing physician prescriptions for hastening death in the United States require a patient to be diagnosed by two physicians of a terminal condition in which there is a reasonable expectation that the patient will die from this condition within the next six months. Pope maintains that this "rigid time frame" excludes "patients with grievous and irremediable conditions that cause suffering intolerable to the individual"[24] (Pope here appropriates language directly from the Canadian law). He proposes that an inclusionary approach would have death be "reasonably predictable" from the disease condition with an open-ended duration rather than restricted by a fallible judgment of a six-month prognostic period. This proposal entails either expanding the concept of terminal illness or expanding the medical indications for access to medical aid in dying beyond terminal illness to encompass chronic illnesses that create intolerable suffering. As the current statutes do not include pain or suffering as a medical indication for a life-ending prescription, the incorporation of suffering shifts the rationale for medical-assisted dying away from a strict reliance on autonomy and towards appeals to beneficence, mercy, and compassion.

Physician Administration: Current state statutes allowing for patients to request a prescription for a life-ending medication all contain provisions for patient self-administration of the medications. Pope contends that this requirement is an obstacle for patients who can't physically self-administer the medication (e.g., some ALS patients), and also places patients who can self-administer at a heightened risk of

---

23. Pope, "Medical Aid in Dying," para. 6.
24. Pope, "Medical Aid in Dying," para. 7.

complications. He proposes revising the statutes to allow for physician administration of medical aid in dying to both increase access for patients and better ensure patient safety. While Pope follows the provisions in the Canadian law almost entirely on these four points of expanded rights, here he retains the requirement of physician participation: he makes no mention of the Canadian permission to allow nurse practitioners to administer the lethal medication or the proposal in the Oregon amendment to allow administration by a designated agent acting under the direction of a physician.

Three significant assumptions underlie Pope's proposal that I wish to call into question. First, Pope assumes that the practice of legalized physician-assisted dying is medically, professionally, and morally unproblematic to such an extent that revisions to expand the scope of patient rights and expanding access will not pose increased risks to patients. For the most part, Pope's analysis draws on the Canadian model of medical aid in dying, for which there is not yet a comprehensive analysis of the empirical data. Studies of euthanasia practices in the Netherlands and Belgium do not, however, provide uniform assurance of a practice that is risk-free for patients, such as misdiagnosis or premature resort to euthanasia in the absence of adequate mental health care.[25]

Second, Pope assumes that the safeguards that he contends have evolved into obstacles were developed entirely with patients as the sole stakeholders. That is, his analysis reflects remarkable libertarian presuppositions: The philosophical and policy assumption is that increased patient autonomy coincides with sound public policy. In fact, the Oregon statute that was appropriated in other state statutes was developed around four priorities: (1) patient rights regarding end-of-life decisions; (2) procedural safeguards for physicians to participate in a patient request without fears of legal prosecution; (3) exemptions for nonparticipating physicians through explicit provisions that stipulate there is no professional duty to participate nor a professional duty of referral; and (4) oversight requirements and procedures to assure public trust that the practice provides professional accountability and can be appropriately regulated.

Pope's critique of the current legal statutes as restrictive or exclusionary relies on a mistaken assumption that patients are the only persons that have interests in the specific details of the policies. His account is oblivious to other stakeholders, including the interests of the profession and individual professionals, as well as the interests of the state and the public in a regulated and accountable practice. Had the statutes had been written with only the concerns of terminally ill patients in mind, they would have been special-interest advocacy proposals rather than efforts to balance the interests of different groups in a reasonable manner. Should the obstacles to access to medical-assisted dying be removed in the manner advocated by Pope, it would be a serious policy mistake to not give due consideration to the impact of expanded medical aid in dying for professionals, professional communities, and for regulatory oversight and public trust.

25. National Academy of Medicine, *Physician-Assisted Death*, 65–72.

Third, Pope's construction of medical aid in dying as encompassing not only physician-prescribed medications to hasten death, but also voluntary euthanasia, and even forms of non-voluntary euthanasia, clearly presumes a conceptual and moral equivalence between the two practices. This is simply a form of moral elision as it begs questions and conclusions in the empirical, professional, and ethical realms for arguments that aren't presented. In this respect, Pope's libertarian analysis converges with the communitarian analysis of Callahan and the legal analysis of Gorsuch that there is not a morally or professionally defensible line that can be drawn between the Oregon model of physician-assisted death and the European model of euthanasia or the Canadian model of medical-assisted dying. I now want to analyze arguments that seek to defend such a line, focusing on three realms of ethical discourse: patient self-determination, physician integrity, and social ethos. Insofar as I critique proposals delineated as medical-assisted dying, I will adopt that nomenclature in my analysis.

The Moral Logic of Patient Rights

The distinction between a right to refuse or terminate treatment and a right to request physician assistance in ending one's life corresponds closely with the conceptual distinction in moral philosophy between negative and positive rights. A negative right is a claim by a moral agent of noninterference against others. The assertion of a negative right provides a realm of moral and legal space within which a person can enact their values and their conception of a meaningful life.

Negative rights tend to be very stringent—that is, there are relatively few moral claims that can justifiably override them. In addition, a negative right is applicable generally against all other persons or institutions (the state, medicine, religious communities, families) who may be in proximity to the moral agent. Negative rights imply a corresponding duty on the part of these persons or institutions to respect the person's choices and not interfere with the enactment of their autonomy, at least insofar as the action does not impose a risk of harm to others.[26] It generally takes minimal physical effort to comply with another person's negative right; essentially, one complies by "staying out of the way" of the choices and actions of the moral agent. A person who disagrees with the exercise of a negative right can rely on methods of persuasion, but insofar as the contemplated action does not present a risk of harm to others, respecting a negative right does not permit paternalistic restrictions on its exercise.

The right to refuse medical treatment is among the most prevalent and significant of negative rights in bioethics and health care decision-making. It stems from a broader negative right to bodily integrity, including what Justice Louis Brandeis called the most comprehensive and valued of any right, "the right to be left alone."[27] In a medical setting, treatments or procedures such as respirators, dialysis machines,

26. Mill, "On Liberty," 955–56.
27. *Olmstead v. United States* 277 U.S. 438 (1928).

pacemakers, feeding tubes, antibiotics, etc., can be understood as invasive procedures that, in the absence of authorization by the moral agent, violate his or her bodily integrity and freedom of self-definition.

A contrasting but complementary set of rights involving a person's claim to *assistance* from another in bringing about a desired end are designated as positive rights. A justified positive right generally is not asserted against all others, but rather against a specified other person with whom the moral agent is in some kind of special relationship. Respect and compliance with the claims of a positive right imply a corresponding positive duty not simply of forbearance from action, but the performance of some action. Positive rights thus tend to have a more limited scope of applicability because they are binding only towards persons within a specified relationship, such as the physician-patient relationship, rather than holding applicability for relationships of strangers, as is the case with negative rights.

I often provide a simple illustration for my students to convey understanding of the difference between a negative and a positive right. We take it for granted as part of the classroom learning environment that they have a negative right against me not to be harmed, either physically or psychologically, in the course of our interactions, and I have a corresponding duty not to harm. The right to not be harmed and duty not to harm is applicable to any social interaction; it has broad scope and stringent application. Moreover, since we are in a specified relationship—that of teacher and student—it can also be said that my students have a positive right for assistance from me with respect to furthering their education and development as critical scholars and citizens, and I likewise have a positive duty to each student to provide the information and educational opportunities that assist them in obtaining their learning goals and aspirations.

My positive responsibility to nourish students' minds and intellectual growth does not mean that I have a broad positive duty, or students have a positive right to my assistance, for their physical nourishment or financial support for their education. The scope of positive rights is bounded by the context of relationship. My interpretation of calling and vocation leads me to understand these commitments as embedded in a covenantal form of relationship and a shared partnership in learning, rather than a contractual and transactional encounter between strangers mediated by rights language. However, rights discourse presents a basis for minimally acceptable conduct and interaction in a culture of strangers.

In general, it is more difficult for a moral culture organized through the values and institutions embedded in liberal political philosophy, with its historical emphasis on freedom from oppression, personal liberty, and equality of opportunity, to generate a robust array of positive rights comparable to the numerous negative rights invoked in political, social, and philosophical discourse. This is attributable in part to the thesis of correlativity—that is, for each right that is affirmed, there is a correlative duty on the part of others, or some others.[28] Some positive rights have broader social applicability in American society, such as the right to education, although the means by which this is exercised are variable—for example, public school, private school, or homeschool. Other positive rights in the social realm are much more controversial, among which is the right to health care. There are also positive rights within health care that are well-accepted and justified because of the special relationship between patient and physician, such as informed consent and rights of privacy and confidentiality.

This brief excursus frames a right to a hastened death through some form of medical-assisted dying as the most contested positive right in medical ethics. Such a claim is morally complex because it can't be honored by "staying out of the way." The statutes legalizing physician-assisted death express a claim by patients for both a negative right of noninterference with regards to respecting his or her choice and a positive right to assistance in facilitating his or her capacity to carry out the choice. The existence of a positive right to medical assistance in dying cannot be derived from a negative right to refuse medical treatment. As a matter of moral logic, negative rights to treatment cessation cannot be the philosophical grounding for the more expansive positive rights to die required in the context of physician-assisted death or medical aid in dying.

The positive rights claim presupposes interpretations not only about the meaning of patient self-determination (the sole focus of Pope and of advocacy organizations) but also about the moral responsibilities of medicine and of the underlying ethos of a society that confers on medicine a status of profession attributable to its distinctive dedication, knowledge, and techniques for healing, curing, and caring. The positive right to die is necessarily about more than the individual patient; its exercise is also a social act insofar as facilitating the desired end of the patient requires the direct participation of others.[29]

Positive Duties of Beneficence

The grounding of a positive right to medical-assisted dying may rely on the distinctive ethos of the medical profession: the core commitments of the profession are not exhausted by refraining from harm, but encompass responsibilities to assist patients through medical care that benefits and promotes patient welfare. The question is whether the general professional duty of beneficence supports a specific positive duty to assist in hastening the death of a patient and a corresponding positive patient right to medical-assisted dying.

Philosopher Margaret Pabst Battin derives from the physician commitment to beneficence ("provide help to those in need") what she designates as a "graduated obligation" on the part of physicians to assist a patient in ending their life according

28. Feinberg, *Social Philosophy*, 59.
29. Callahan, "Reason, Self-Determination," 60.

to the patient's "medical impairment" or "medical need."[30] The physician's obligation increases gradually in strength in proportion to the greater gravity of serious illness or disability afflicting the patient; the most compelling obligation is imposed when patients are "fully disabled or in severe, untreatable, terminal pain."[31]

Battin's argument falls short of providing a robust positive patient right and a correlative duty for physicians for medical-assisted dying. It is not evident at all that terminally ill patients have a medical need for a dying process that can be achieved only through physician prescription or administration of a medication intended to hasten death. There are several last resort methods by which death can be brought about for a terminally ill patient, including the so-called "gold standard" of palliative and hospice care, refusal of medical treatment, voluntary stopping of eating and drinking, and palliative sedation.[32] Indeed, the existence of such alternatives leads scholars like Emanuel to maintain that an expansive positive right to medical-assisted dying is unnecessary: "Patients who are being kept alive by technology and want to end their lives already have a recognized constitutional right to stop any and all medical interventions, from respirators to antibiotics. They do not need physician-assisted suicide or euthanasia."[33]

By framing the patient's request for hastened death as a response to a medical impairment or need, Battin medicalizes the process of dying and perpetuates the presumed necessity for the medical management of death. As delineated in the preceding chapter, part of the plague of bad dying is comprised precisely of the medicalization of dying and death: Hence, we need to ask in what sense is death a medical problem. Excessive use of life-prolonging technology in circumstances of medical futility is a medical problem; inadequate use of pain medications is a medical problem. These can be remedied by appropriate use or cessation of the technology and appropriate medication dosages and palliative care. It is not clear without further argument that a patient's request for medical assistance in dying is similar to these situations such that it grounds both a patient right and imposes a moral and professional duty on the physician. What is clear for Battin is that an argument for an imposed and graduated professional duty of assistance is most compelling in just those circumstances that are not recognized by the state statutes legalizing physician-assisted death. That is, Battin's interpretation of the professional commitment of beneficence concurs with the kinds of claims advanced by Pope and by *The Economist* about expanding patient rights to encompass the full array of hastened death implicit in medical aid in dying. However, by focusing on very difficult and morally anguishing kinds of circumstances as grounds for an imposed professional duty, Battin abandons the principle of patient self-determination for an argument from beneficence, compassion, and mercy.

30. Battin, *Ethical Issues in Suicide*, 219.
31. Battin, *Ethical Issues in Suicide*, 219.
32. Quill, "Physician-Assisted Death," 17–22.
33. Emanuel, "Whose Right to Die," 74.

Daniel Callahan reasons from essentially the same premise as Battin with one important difference: rather than starting from a professional commitment to beneficence, Callahan first affirms an embedded societal duty of solidarity to relieve the suffering of our fellow human beings.[34] The professional duty of beneficence is therefore situated in a quasi-covenantal or moral contractual relationship with society. Society entrusts specific ways of enacting the societal duty of compassionate solidarity to the knowledge and skill of the medical profession. This interpretation similarly shifts the moral ground for medical aid in dying from respect for autonomy to the scope of the ethic of beneficence. The question then arises as to whether a terminally ill patient has a positive right, grounded in the physician's socially bestowed duty, to relief of pain and suffering through a prescribed medication or a lethal injection that hastens death. As Callahan frames the issue: "Ought the general duty of the physician to relieve suffering encompass the right to kill a patient if, in the judgment of the patient, that is desired and seems necessary?"[35] It is not necessary to invoke the polemical language of medical "killing" of patients to appreciate the broader question Callahan raises about the status and scope of professional duties.

Callahan resists medicalizing dying by asserting that the physician's responsibility to relieve pain and suffering is comprised of relieving "only the problem of illness, not the problems of life itself."[36] Medicine lacks the expertise, wisdom, or societal authorization to address mortal problems of the human condition, which may include the patient's or family members' perception of a pointless death. This account likewise rejects Battin's claim that patients have a medical need for relief of existential suffering that may be facilitated through a request for a hastened death. Consequently, the absence of a justifying rationale for expanding the scope of the physician's action to permit medical aid in dying "open[s] the way for a corruption of [the] vocation."[37]

Whether moral analysis starts from the scope of the patient's rights to self-determination or the scope of the physician's responsibility to alleviate pain and suffering, it is difficult to generate moral reasoning that bestows an unqualified positive moral right for patients to a hastened death through medical assistance. Though a patient's right of autonomy is a necessary condition of a moral choice, it is not at all clear that it should be, of itself, a sufficient condition in the manner proposed by legalization advocates. Moreover, a case for a specific professional duty of assistance in hastened death might be more compelling were society and the profession to recognize a patient's positive right to *health care* in the first place; it seems conceptually odd, if not morally perverse, to legitimate a positive right to medical-assisted dying but not recognize a positive right of access to the health care treatments and expertise needed to sustain life or maintain quality of life.

34. Callahan, *Troubled Dream of Life*, 94–95.
35. Callahan, *Troubled Dream of Life*, 95.
36. Callahan, *Troubled Dream of Life*, 102.
37. Callahan, *Troubled Dream of Life*, 102.

The Soul of Medicine

It is not societally, ethically, or professionally compelling to uncouple the issue of the right of a patient to a hastened death from the vocational calling and responsibility of medicine. Patient autonomy is a necessary but not sufficient condition of moral analysis because (a) the precedent-setting negative rights of patient choices to terminate or refuse treatment leave open the issue of whether there is a positive right to die and a positive duty to provide assistance to hasten death, and (b) medicine as a social practice is constituted by a set of values and commitments that comprise its "profession," its ethical integrity and accountability. As Jonas asserted, for scholars "to defend the right to die . . . the real vocation of medicine must be reaffirmed."[38] When patient rights and professional calling are treated as separable questions, or patient rights determine professional responsibility (as is the case in most professional and bioethical literature), medicine becomes a morally neutral profession, and the vocation of physician is morally reduced to nothing more than a skilled technician. The ethics of the profession means that physicians are moral agents, not merely technicians of the body, and that professional responsibility and integrity are necessary features of legalization debates. The values and commitments constitutive of professional integrity are independent of and cannot be reduced to respecting patient self-determination. The central moral mistake in contemporary bioethics, illustrated through the question of the right to medical aid in dying, is to collapse professional responsibility and integrity into patient autonomy.

A distinguished team of physician-ethicists and medical educators (Willard Gaylin, Leon Kass, Edmund Pellegrino, Mark Siegler) composed an editorial commentary in response to a story of a gynecology resident who provided a lethal injection of morphine to an emaciated female patient dying from ovarian cancer. The story presented a clear illustration of voluntary euthanasia and perhaps even nonvoluntary euthanasia, or what now is conceptualized as medical aid in dying. The authors claimed that "the deepest meaning of the medical vocation" had been violated by the resident, and consequently, "the very soul of medicine is on trial."[39] At the moral core (or "soul") of medicine is a principle to not use the entrusted powers for healing, curing, caring, and relieving suffering to engage in direct killing of vulnerable persons.

If the ethics of medicine consisted only of respecting patient autonomy and refraining from killing patients, it's not clear how the professional morality would be at all distinctive from general social morality, let alone distinctive enough to warrant the social trust embedded in the designation "profession." There must be much more to the ethics of medicine than respecting self-determination and *primum non nocere*. The values that the prohibition of medical harm protects include trusting relationships, commitments to healing, and moral identities of comfort and protection of life.

---

38. Jonas, "Right to Die," 36.
39. Gaylin et al., "Doctors Must Not Kill," 2139.

This comprises the moral center of medicine as a social practice for which its members are as accountable for "professing" as much as their accountability for knowledge and technical expertise. The covenantal character of medicine is expressed through commitments to healing, cultivating patient and social trust, principles of responsive beneficence, and responsibilities of non-abandonment of the vulnerable. In the absence of these non-negotiables, medicine can no longer be medicine, but becomes a morally neutral social practice.

Healing Relationship

Philosophical or legalization arguments on the positive right to medical-assisted dying tend to rely on political, economic, or legal assumptions about the relationship between physician and patient that are extrinsic to the ethos of medicine. It is illustrative that Compassion & Choices, the most prominent organization advocating legalization of medical-assisted dying, situates their advocacy within a philosophy of empowerment of *consumers*. The assumption that consumer values should dictate medical practice highlights the technical and transactional nature of an assisted dying relationship even as it diminishes its trusting character and the basic concept of medicine as a moral profession or vocation. This culminates in the paradox observed by William F. May about the relationship embedded in physician actions to hasten death, which "solves the problem of a runaway *technical* medicine by resorting, finally, to *technique*."[40]

It would represent a morally attenuated sense of vocation if medicine had nothing to offer patients when curing disease is not possible. The diseases that afflict terminally ill patients and ultimately bring about their deaths cannot be cured; the diseases experienced by many patients with chronic ailments are not susceptible to cure. Medicine must have complementary objectives to curing and perhaps even a superordinate end or purpose. As developed in preceding chapters, that overarching telos of medicine is summarized by the concept of healing, of making whole what has been fragmented, ruptured, or destroyed. Medicine's claim to be a healing profession and the professional construction of the identity of the physician as a healer manifests an understanding of medical vocation with important relevance for physician responsibilities in end-of-life care.

When medicine cannot save life, when it cannot cure the disease, the professional default to more technology that prolongs biological life is morally inadequate if not immoral. Medical aid in dying, reliant on a technology in its own way, ignores the prospect that medicine can always heal even when cure is impossible, and can remain faithful to its core mission even if there is no prospect for cure. In the mortal responsibility of physicians of presence to the dying,[41] it is a mistake to claim that

40. May, *Testing the Medical Covenant*, 15.
41. Kalanithi, *When Breath Becomes Air*, 114.

when curing (as healing) is not possible, physician responsibility is met by writing a prescription to hasten a patient's death.

The insistent question is whether a physician oriented to a professional identity as a healer compromises professional integrity and the internal ethos of the profession through medical assistance in hastening patient's deaths. Richard McCormick, a pioneering founder of the bioethics field, argued that the question of physician-assisted death can only arise from a convergence of certain cultural and professional trends. Two trends of particular importance were designated by McCormick as the "absolutization of autonomy" and the "independence" of medicine from a moral tradition.[42] A positive right to medical aid in dying will be a coherent moral perspective when patient self-determination is deemed not merely a necessary but a sufficient ethical consideration, and also where medicine's imperatives and integrity lack a narrative and are governed by the instrumental rationality of market efficiency and effectiveness.

Compassion is the virtue and capacity of the witness to suffering to enter into the experience of illness of the patient and bear witness to their ordeal with them. This is the *more* to healing that is not exhausted by curative medicine; compassion is a constituent virtue of the healer. For McCormick, physician participation in assisting terminally ill patients to die manifests a profession that has neglected compassion and the arts that comprise healing for the sake of technical efficiency and human agency. The rationale for medical aid in dying discloses that contemporary medicine is on the cusp of becoming indistinguishable from a business and permeated by its very direct utilitarian morality of instrumental rationality.

My normative claims here are that medicine is not a morally neutral profession, and its commitment to caring and healing, even when curing is not possible, is a distinctive feature of its professional identity and integrity. Physicians as healers have other alternatives to express professional responsibility in their care of dying patients, including witness and presence to terminally ill patients, conversations about patient end-of-life needs and preferences, palliative care and comprehensive pain control, incorporating features of hospice care, and assuming responsibility to bear an embodied witness to the patient's needs for relationship, touch, re-storying, and non-abandonment.

Witnessing Solidarity

The moral witness embodied in the medical vocation encompasses being present to persons who are sick, and to not abandon patients who are terminally ill. The professional vocation to bear witness in solidarity incorporates two interrelated points about human nature rooted in the *imago Dei*. The first claim is that human beings are fundamentally relational and community-oriented beings. We experience our lives

42. McCormick, "Physician Assisted Suicide," 1132–34.

in a web of relationships, with family, friends, colleagues, associates, congregations, professions, and larger communities. Our vulnerability to the vicissitudes of aging, disease, disability, dependency, and dying bursts illusions of independence. A moral community emerges through bearing witness to the presence of the humanity of the other in relationships of interdependency. This claim bears witness against the atomistic individualism of the self presupposed in legalization advocacy.

The second claim is that, in assuming responsibility for caregiving to the ill, medicine expresses an identity-conferring commitment to make common cause with persons who are among society's most vulnerable populations. Terminally ill persons are a very vulnerable population. They experience deprivations of the most fundamental sort: loss of control, loss of a future, loss of story, loss of decision-making authority, loss of bodily integrity, loss of privacy, perhaps loss of home or the familiar, and loss of mobility, ultimately culminating in loss of life. In this context of pervasive loss, medicine has a moral responsibility to assure terminally ill persons that their sickness unto death does not mean isolation or ostracization, and that they have not been abandoned. Though their disease condition may not be amenable to cure, patients can experience a healing and re-storying witness as members of a caring community to the very end.

The witness of solidarity also expresses the shared value of compassion. The etymological meaning of compassion means suffering alongside the afflicted person. The expression of compassion thus requires a relational context; it implies the continual presence of a caring community. The possibility of bearing witness to compassionate caring and healing of terminally ill persons in a setting in which curative medicine is not possible is envisioned and embodied in hospice care. The hospice philosophy of care, which includes commitments to patient self-determination, the highest quality of life while dying, witnessing and alleviating the patient's physical pain and emotional and spiritual suffering, and companionship and non-abandonment of the patient, exemplifies a profound commitment of solidarity with the terminally ill. Hospice is yet another moral community impacted by legalization of physician-assisted death.[43]

I have presented critiques against a positive right to medical-assisted dying through the concepts of healing relationship and solidarity. Taken by themselves, the arguments from relationship, healing, and solidarity cannot sustain an unequivocal or exceptionless prohibition of medical assistance in dying, whether through lethal prescription or euthanasia. However, when these arguments are viewed as complementary and as issuing from what scholars have designated as the "soul" of medicine and its professional integrity, they provide a compelling moral presumption, namely, there should be no positive moral duty or obligation imposed on any specific physician to acquiesce in a patient's request for medical assistance in death. As indicated previously, the various acts legalizing physician assistance in hastening death stipulate that there is no legal duty on any particular physician, health care professional, or

43. Campbell, "Moral Meanings," 223–49.

health care institution to participate in a patient request. That provision witnesses to the proposition that there is more at stake morally in debates regarding the positive right to medical-assisted dying than patient self-determination and welfare, or to put it somewhat differently, the goals and purposes of medicine cannot be reduced without remainder to respect for autonomy or even to curing disease.

Social Witness

The solidarity argument bridges concerns of the professional ethic and the societal ethos. The social impact of legalized physician-assisted death for vulnerable persons is of particular importance in a health care context structured by instrumental rationality and utilitarian commitments to cost effectiveness and rationing of health care services. It is especially problematic and ethically perverse to have inequitable and stratified access to health care everywhere *except* at the end of life, when expanding access to medical aid in dying becomes a priority. The coupling of limited resources for health care with methods of hastening the death of terminally ill persons generates a profound ethical conflict of interest.

This convergence of consumerist health care with initiatives to legalize physician-assisted death presents what May considers to be a profound test to the sustainability of the medical covenant.[44] It would be both terribly ironic and morally tragic were disputes about the ethics of physician-assisted death articulated through discourse on the *right* to die to become intertwined with disputes about rationing end-of-life care, which have sometimes been articulated through the discourse of a *duty* to die.[45] Maintaining a proverbial firewall between costs of treatment and hastened death is a social justice imperative no matter the legal status of medical-assisted dying.

A more encompassing moral critique of the societal commitment to efficiency and the risks this commitment poses to vulnerable persons has been articulated consistently in the past two decades in Roman Catholic moral theology. In this tradition, physician-assisted death and medical-assisted dying are interpreted as a symptom of societal moral decline that places at special risk society's poor and most marginalized persons. This declension narrative contends that actions that are morally wrong have become legitimated by the state through the language of rights. Legal rights can legitimate moral wrongs.

In his 1995 encyclical *Evangelium Vitae* (*The Gospel of Life*), Pope John Paul II drew attention to what he portrayed as the "emergence of a culture which denies solidarity and in many cases takes the form of a veritable 'culture of death.'"[46] This cultural ethos is supported and sustained by "powerful cultural, economic and political currents" that promote excessive concerns with efficiency and instrumental rational-

44. May, *Testing the Medical Covenant*, 13–50.

45. Hardwig, "Duty to Die," 34–42.

46. John Paul II, *Evangelium Vitae*, para. 12.

ity. The papal pronouncement critiqued worldviews of secularism, moral relativism, individualism, and materialism while also objecting to practical manifestations of these worldviews, particularly in social acceptance of legalized rights to abortion, capital punishment, discrimination against persons with disabilities, and practices that exploit the vulnerabilities of persons at the end of their life—that is, persons whose care requires resources that are inefficient from a perspective of technical maximization of efficiency. The argument offered by the Catholic witness views the integrity of the medical profession as inescapably eroded as part of the societal moral decline: "Even certain sectors of the medical profession, which by its calling is directed to the defense and care of human life, are increasingly willing to carry out these acts against the person. In this way, the very nature of the medical profession is distorted and contradicted, and the dignity of those who practice it is degraded."[47]

John Paul II made a clear connection between underlying worldviews, an ethics of instrumentalization and efficiency, and risks to socially marginalized persons: a symptom of the culture of death prevalent in all prosperous societies is "an attitude of excessive preoccupation with efficiency, and which sees the growing number of elderly and disabled people as intolerable and too burdensome. These people are very often isolated by their families and by society, which are organized almost exclusively on the basis of criteria of productive efficiency, according to which a hopelessly impaired life no longer has any value."[48] The social ordering by efficiency, rather than justice, provides an instrumentalized rationale for euthanasia: "euthanasia is sometimes justified by the utilitarian motive of avoiding costs which bring no return and which weigh heavily on society."[49]

Certainly the practices critiqued in Roman Catholic teaching, be it legalized abortion, capital punishment, or euthanasia, have a long history of both practice and philosophical advocacy that predate current preoccupations with industrialized efficiency. Moreover, while the utilitarian rationales cited in *Evangelium Vitae* are present in some justificatory arguments, they are really a secondary legitimation to the primary rights-based arguments for medical-assisted dying. With these caveats in mind, a person need not concur with the background theological teaching to recognize the validity of questioning the cultural context within which the medical vocation comes to incorporate medical-assisted dying as comprising best practices in care for dying persons. It is the coupling of practice with an ideology of consumerism and efficiency that manifests the cultural problem medical-assisted dying both creates and reflects. The ethics of medical-assisted death, however much it is correctly concerned with personal self-determination and individual autonomy, cannot be reduced morally to a private self-regarding action. The issue itself is situated within a particular cultural context, influenced by prevalent worldviews, medical and nonmedical narratives,

47. John Paul II, *Evangelium Vitae*, para. 4.
48. John Paul II, *Evangelium Vitae*, para. 64.
49. John Paul II, *Evangelium Vitae*, para. 51.

ideologies, and mythologies, and has impacts on families, professions and moral communities like hospice, and the broader commitments of society to protect vulnerable persons.

Conclusion

Although legalized physician-assisted death is still relatively rare in the United States, the focus of much current professional, bioethical, and policy debate on the right to die has anticipated legalizing voluntary and nonvoluntary euthanasia, as well as making intolerable suffering a medical indication for medical-assisted death. I have sought to challenge the thesis of moral equivalence that underlies the expansion of a positive right to die and the corresponding legitimation of various practices in medicine on several grounds. Within the moral logic of rights, a positive right to assistance from a physician cannot be derived from a negative right to noninterference. It is misleading furthermore to characterize a right to assistance as entirely a question of a private action: all rights-claims presume some moral community and relationships, and the most significant communities with respect to medical-assisted death are the medical profession and hospice programs. Furthermore, a more compelling case for a positive right to medical aid in dying could be made were society to first recognize a positive right to a basic minimum of health care services. It is instructive in this regard that the countries seen as exemplary by legalization advocates such as Belgium, Canada, and the Netherlands all have universal access health care systems.

My interpretation of medicine as a calling and a covenantal relationship oriented by the end of healing entails that medicine is not a morally neutral profession, nor should its practitioners be reduced by patients, the profession, or society, to the status of skilled technicians: medical practice is shaped by defining commitments of integrity of relationships, healing, and solidarity with vulnerable persons. Insofar as individual rights are historically articulated as claims of the person for freedom from tyranny and political oppression, the social and political context of the right to die bears careful scrutiny. Moral assessment requires differentiating between the discourse and the exercise of rights in health care from cost-effectiveness movements and the ethics of instrumental rationality such that patients' exercise of their rights is not a manifestation of economic oppression or deprivation. Ultimately, arguments advocating legalized medical aid in dying for terminally ill patients, for chronically ill patients experiencing protracted pain and suffering, or for patients who have lost decision-making capability, all bear a substantive burden of proof. They must not only rely on claims of patient self-determination as morally decisive, but must show that they can meet justificatory standards of authorization, cause, proportionality, intention, discrimination, and last resort.[50]

50. Campbell, "Aid in Dying," 128–34.

PART FOUR

The Public Witness

10

Bioethical Cultures

Critiques of Pure Religion

The landscape of contemporary bioethics is largely devoid of a religious presence. The pedagogical cultures of bioethics rely on textbooks and other authoritative sources in which ethical reflections from a religious tradition or theological perspective are almost entirely absent. The occasional exception to this pedagogical profile is the inclusion of a statement from a religious perspective portrayed as a representative expression of a conservative position, such as a Vatican document about reproductive choices or euthanasia. This selective style of presentation means that many students who take very popular courses in bioethics are educated to understand that religious traditions are either not interested in or have no relevance to the issues that comprise the terrain of bioethics. Religious discourse may also be portrayed as an obstacle to bioethical inquiry, a conversation stopper. Philosophical argument by contrast provides a way to "sidestep religion" and "the deadlock and futility characteristic of religious disagreement."[1] Most undergraduate bioethics courses are under the purview of programs in philosophy, which tend to structure religious ways of thinking about ethics through an intellectualized construction of divine command theories.

The professionalized discourse of bioethics no less displays a peripheral presence of religion.[2] At a recent annual meeting of the field's professional scholars, just over 1 percent of the presentations contained some content that reflected issues with direct relevance to religious understandings of health and disease. The professional associations continue to affirm the important role of pastoral care in diverse clinical settings, including ethical consultations, especially in end-of-life decision-making. However,

1. Ridley, *Beginning Bioethics*, 6–7.
2. Eckenwiler and Cohn, *Ethics of Bioethics.*

this pastoral role is constructed around matters of clarity in communication and does not reflect an engagement by bioethics scholars and by scholars in religious studies with the serious intellectual questions and issues of the field. Academic journals perpetuate this culture of a bioethics without religion.

The public policy realm of bioethics discourse occasionally manifests attentiveness to the views of religious traditions or scholars from religious communities, with the caveat that arguments offered in the public square of discourse need to be accessible to all persons regardless of literacy about religion. Alternatively, as illustrated by the policy appropriation of my own scholarship on two occasions, religion may be assimilated under the concept of "culture" or interpreted through an overlay of the principles and paradigms of liberal political philosophy (see chapter 1). These interpretative maneuvers reflect the trend articulated by law professor Stephen Carter nearly two decades ago to trivialize religion and dismiss its pertinence to matters of the public good.[3]

These three examples surely do not constitute the entirety of the bioethics field. In the cultures of institutional bioethics comprised of deliberations of hospital ethics committees about problematic cases or institutional policy formulation, religious contexts, issues, and beliefs continue to be encountered. However, often in institutional bioethics cultures, matters of religion are constructed as a "problem" for conversation participants, especially when religious considerations lead to requests for continuation of technological treatment deemed medically futile. Furthermore, institutions or professional health care associations encounter religion as a problem when accommodation must be made for conscientious objections or refusals of health care professionals regarding the provision of legal and otherwise accessible healthcare services.[4]

This chapter explores the rationales for this limited religious presence in the pedagogical, professional, and policy cultures of bioethics. It is important to acknowledge that there are a variety of forums and realms of discourse in which bioethics is practiced that are suffused with religious values, including religious-based health care institutions and hospitals or pastoral care and chaplaincy programs integrated within clinical ethics discourse. My focus will instead primarily be on the three cultures of bioethics delineated in these examples. My own educational learning of the questions important to bioethics was indelibly shaped through discussion with important figures and analysis of central texts that assumed that, in conversation with medicine, law, philosophy, and the anthropology, sociology, and politics of medicine, religion was part of the bioethics landscape.

3. Carter, *Culture of Disbelief*, 23–43.
4. Campbell, "Meaningful Resistance," 1–29.

Pioneers in Religious Bioethics

I discussed in chapter 2 the various narratives and stories of origins of bioethics. However differently these origin stories are constructed, a common feature is the role of different religious perspectives, communities and traditions, and thinkers. It is thereby a bit problematic to witness how contemporary bioethics tends to construct religion as an intellectual monolith. Historically, this orienting diversity of religion is often represented through the conflicting positions of two pioneering scholars, Joseph Fletcher and Paul Ramsey.

An early proponent of autonomy and choices as expressed through the moral discourse of rights, Joseph Fletcher's work illustrates the broader bioethics narrative of patient empowerment. As exemplified in a groundbreaking book, *Morals and Medicine*, Fletcher saw in various biomedical technologies, such as assisted reproductive methods, human genetics, organ transplantation, and life-extending technologies, a way to liberate moral choices from the normativity of the natural as well as what he considered to be the freedom-oppressing nature of legalistic morality and religious authoritarianism.[5] Fletcher's embraced the expanding scope of medical technologies due to the prospect for expanding human choices. His approach to medical morality expressed well a secularized separation from moral traditions, especially religious traditions and their historically embedded (and perhaps anachronistic) rules or principles, and their displacement by the primacy of individual moral choices. In this respect, Fletcher was an anticipatory prophet of the commitment to respect for self-determination that eventually became ascendant in bioethics generally.

Fletcher's elevation of individual choice was reflected in his critiques of religious-based morality, which he maintained were characterized by a legalistic fixation on rules and by the supplanting of persons with principles. These features created a prefabricated moral system in which moral choices effectively had already been made by the moral wisdom of predecessors and tradition. This prefabricated morality was inattentive to the situatedness of moral choice, and thus was woefully inadequate for the new moral horizons opened up by medical technologies. Fletcher's construction of religious morality as legalistic, principle-based, and prefabricated allowed virtually no place for individual freedom and autonomy. A decade after *Morals and Medicine*, Fletcher published his more well-known and influential *Situation Ethics*, which popularized a "new morality," in contrast to the "old" principle and rule-based morality of religion and medicine. *Situation Ethics* likewise celebrated the empowerment of the individual now emancipated from restrictions of religious law, community, and tradition.[6]

Fletcher's ethics of self-determination was complemented by a moral decision-making method that he appropriated from the classical hedonistic utilitarians, Jeremy

5. Fletcher, *Morals and Medicine*, 3–33.

6. Fletcher, *Situation Ethics*, 17–56.

Bentham and John Stuart Mill. Mill had articulated a position in his own writings that the substance of Christian morality, such as the golden-rule ethic, was the "ideal perfection" of the greatest happiness principle of utilitarianism.[7] Fletcher developed this point even further, affirming moral equivalence between the Christian concept of neighbor-love, or *agape*, and the utilitarian imperative to maximize happiness (or minimize suffering) for the greatest number; utilitarian ethics was the secular version of Christian ethical teaching. While Fletcher's incorporation of *agape* could be understood as retaining a minimal form of a religious ethic, his thesis of moral equivalence effectively rendered religious ethics unnecessary and superfluous in moral decision-making. There is no need to draw on an otherwise discredited account of religious morality when a philosophical method accessible to all persons (indeed, on Fletcher's view, a method already used by most persons) can generate the same conclusions. Fletcher's method of utilitarian-style maximization as informed by *agape* is subsequently made over in the image of the secular bioethics principle of beneficence.

For these reasons, Joseph Fletcher is not a terribly compelling exemplar of religious thinking in bioethics as much as a secular moralist engaged in a sharp critique of authoritarian morality and its applications and restrictions in the context of moral choices in medicine. Notably, Stephen Toulmin portrayed Fletcher primarily as a pioneer in reviving the ethics of casuistry that Toulmin maintained contributed to the life-saving character of medical praxis for the discipline of philosophy.[8] Fletcher was a sharp critic of historical religious ethics whose arguments and methods displayed that, despite some historical reliance of morality on religious communities, in a new era organized by scientific, engineering, and mechanistic assumptions and technologies, there is no necessary or logical dependence of ethics upon religion; indeed, religion can be a regressive obstruction against scientific knowledge, medical developments, and moral progress. Fletcher preceded and anticipated an era in which moral choices pervade medicine, and in which much of the moral discourse is framed by versions of an ethics of self-determination and individual rights and an ethics of caring and beneficence (the thin moral residue of *agape*) without any recourse to religious-based argumentation. The thesis of moral equivalence of *agape* and utility makes for an entirely secularized ethics.

While Fletcher modernized and medicalized the historical Protestant commitment to Christian freedom, the conservative counterpoint to his autonomy-expanding embrace of innovative technologies was articulated in the positions of Christian ethicist Paul Ramsey. Ramsey made substantial contributions to interpretations of Christian ethics and the theory of just war before turning his attention to some of the very same technologies of reproductive choice, genetic controls, and life extension that so captured Fletcher's imagination and ethics.[9] Theologically, Ramsey presented an un-

7. Mill, "Utilitarianism," 34.
8. Toulmin, "How Medicine Saved Ethics," 740.
9. Smith, "On Paul Ramsey," 7–29.

sparing critique of modernist ideologies of progressivism and human perfectionism, especially as they were manifested in science and medical technology. This informed a far more probing analysis of the moral anthropologies and existential situatedness of contemporary medicine than Fletcher developed and led Ramsey to find in some aspects of contemporary medicine a misguided inquiry to "relieve the human condition of the human condition."[10]

Ramsey claimed that the optimistic proposals of the progressivist science of reproduction and genetic manipulation assumed "operating, unspoken premises" that risked conflation of human nature and aspirations with divine responsibility. Such premises supplanted ethical concepts with constructs drawn from engineering and design conducive to refashioning humanity biologically and environmentally in the image of human beings. A moral orientation of boundless human freedom (as illustrated by Fletcher) pushed inevitably towards human subjugation of nature and mastery of mortality and the human condition. In a world that no longer knows God, Ramsey maintained, human beings encounter no inherent limits, biological or moral, to their aspirations of mastery over the infinitely malleable and contingent, including human nature: "Where there is no God, no destiny towards which men move and which moves in them, then self-modifying freedom must be the man-God."[11]

Despite the areligious and increasingly amoral character of modern scientific medicine, Ramsey strikingly discerned in the literatures, languages, and metaphors of the biological and medical sciences a profoundly religious and eschatological impulse. He portrayed the anticipatory genetic and medicalized manipulations of human reproduction increasingly as "not the findings . . . of an exact science as such, but a religious view of where and how ultimate human significance is to be found. It is a proposal concerning mankind's final hope."[12] The modernist project envisioned through the biological sciences of unlimited self-modification pushes beyond the moral and professional boundaries embedded in the goals and purposes of medicine and ultimately approaches the existential boundary of human nature and the divine. For Ramsey, popular discourse over the "prohibition against 'playing God'" necessitated resisting human hubris and the overreaching aspirations of mastery of mortality to "learn something about the *context* of decision and action that is properly human."[13] The wisdom of learning what is properly human meant that "men should not play God before they have learned to be men and . . . when they learn to be men they will not play God."[14]

Ramsey understood medicine as a school for learning the moral wisdom of being human. In contrast to Fletcher's *agape*-informed freedom of the individual self,

---

10. Ramsey, "Ethics and Chronic Illness."
11. Ramsey, *Fabricated Man*, 93.
12. Ramsey, *Fabricated Man*, 144.
13. Ramsey, *Fabricated Man*, 143.
14. Ramsey, *Fabricated Man*, 143.

Ramsey contended that love was embedded in various rules and principles that mediate human relationships in general, including the special form those relationships assume in medicine. The concept of covenantal loyalty played a mediating and bridging role for Ramsey between theological convictions and medical ethics. The moral character of relationships between physician and patient or researcher and participant was expressed through "the Biblical norm of *fidelity to covenant*";[15] this covenantal context extended beyond the clinical relationship to broader communities as well, such as the "covenant between the living and the dying, [and] the covenant between the well and the ill."[16] In these various covenantal relations, Ramsey identified the central ethical question to consist in asking, "What is the meaning of the *faithfulness* of one human being to another in every one of these relations?"[17]

With covenantal fidelity rather than boundless self-defining freedom as a moral foundation for medical ethics, Ramsey acknowledged the moral propriety of "playing God" in specific contexts, such as decisions about allocation of scarce medical resources. Instead of relying on the inescapable fallibility of human judgments regarding the social worth of other persons, or of procedures designed (in an engineering rather than aesthetic sense) to achieve greater social utility and instrumental rationality, covenantal faithfulness is manifested in commitments to the equal worth of persons and indiscriminate care, as well as processes of randomization to assure equal opportunity. Moral decision-makers can then "'play God' in the correct way: he makes his sun rise upon the good and the evil and sends rain upon the just and the unjust alike."[18]

Joseph Fletcher's affirmation of freedom, rights, and technological control were repeatedly countered by Paul Ramsey's relentless restraint, rules, and critiques of scientific and medical aspirations that pushed towards mastery of mortality. Although the moral genealogies are not as direct as this comparison, contemporary bioethics bears much more the markings of Fletcher's emphasis on autonomy and utility and of his relegation of religion to a peripheral and dispensable presence. When the kinds of methods, questions of meaning and of ultimate ends, and critiques of medical progress that Ramsey articulated reemerged in the early twenty-first century through the voices of Leon Kass, Gilbert Meilaender, Michael Sandel, and other contributors to the President's Council on Bioethics, the objections within the bioethics community were strident and initiated a form of culture war within bioethics.[19] The kinds of theoretical questions that could be asked and the form of prophetic voice in bioethics that Ramsey embodied no longer seemed conducive of dialogue.

This framing provides a point of departure for examining the specific bioethical cultures of pedagogy, professionalism, and policy-making. I have found for nearly

---

15. Ramsey, *Patient as Person*, xii.

16. Ramsey, *Patient as Person*, xii.

17. Ramsey, *Patient as Person*, xii.

18. Ramsey, *Patient as Person*, 256.

19. Charo, "Endarkenment," 95–107.

three decades that there is one primary phrase about bioethics in popular culture that resonates with my students, that of "playing God." If students know nothing else about "bioethics" upon enrolling in class, they know it has something to do with "playing God." They take this phrasing to imply a critique of decisions and decision-makers who engage in consequential decisions about creating and ending human life while under the constraints of human finitude and fallibility. Bioethics seems to represent decisions without wisdom. This suggests a more limited scope for responsible human moral choice that is actually rather close to what Ramsey had in mind but very different than the expanding realm of freedom coupled with technological control that Fletcher affirmed and that is so resonant with the ethos of the contemporary age. The concept of "playing God" provides one way into the pedagogical culture of bioethics.

Pedagogy: "Playing God" and Getting Two Words In

Does religion have a place in the bioethics classroom? Is the public space of a classroom setting open to the bioethical positions affirmed by various religious communities and traditions? Or is the classroom also assimilated into the naked public square? Discussions of the presence and presentation of religious perspectives in the bioethics classroom should hinge ultimately on the purposes and goals of ethics education. The general goals of ethics education certainly seem to not only invite but require discourse about religious understandings and framings of bioethical issues. These goals, formulated in research projects at the Hastings Center, include encouraging moral perception, engaging and enlivening moral imagination, cultivating consciousness of personal moral responsibility, exercising moral deliberation methods and processes, and developing attentiveness to moral ambiguity and the need for tolerance of diverse moral opinions.[20] These are not exclusively matters for philosophical, legal, or scientific pedagogy, but are broad-based objectives grounded in a humanistic study of ethics and medicine, with humanistic approaches understood to be interdisciplinary in nature, including the critical study of religion, rather than exclusive and disciplinary-based.

Some further directions for bioethics education, particularly pertaining to citizenship and processes of democratic deliberation, have more recently been articulated by the Presidential Commission for the Study of Bioethical Issues under the Obama administration. In a very thoughtful report, the Commission encouraged bioethics education as part of what it called "ethics education across the lifespan."[21] It further underscored a need for bioethics pedagogy to make use of empirical studies on "how best to cultivate moral sensibilities and normative reasoning skills into the institutional and individual practices of scientists and health care professionals."[22] My one

20. Callahan, "Goals," 61–80.
21. Presidential Commission, *Bioethics for Every Generation*, 51–71.
22. Lee et al., "Teaching Bioethics," 10–11.

reservation is that the Commission did not seem to think it important to consider how religious values might be integrated into bioethics education or the broader civic educational objective of cultivating skills of citizenship and democratic deliberation.

The increasing professionalization of the field has gradually dissipated the interdisciplinary nature of bioethics education; courses in bioethics in a philosophy classroom, and the accompanying texts or resource books, are rigorously disciplinary. It is certainly possible for such a pedagogical setting to achieve many of the conventional goals for ethics education, but not all, and not without some diminishment of what bioethics is about, and who bioethics is for. K. Danner Clouser, the first philosopher to teach ethics in a medical school setting (Pennsylvania State-Hershey), portrayed the medical ethics taught in the medical school setting prior to the emergence of philosophical methods as "a mixture of religion, whimsy, exhortation, legal precedent, various traditions, philosophies of life, miscellaneous, moral rules and epithets uttered by wise or witty physicians."[23] Whatever comprised the content of the traditional medical ethics, it was lacking in the systematic methods, consistency, and organizing questions that philosophy brings to the world of biomedicine. However, Clouser's description begs the question I originally asked: If religion is considered by philosophers and other bioethics educators as morally on a par with "whimsy," "exhortation," or pithy statements of mentors as far as authoritative sources for ethical guidance, is there a place for a religious presence in the bioethics classroom?

Virtually all the recent bioethics teaching anthologies exclude religious thought or include a single essay as a foil for philosophical or policy-oriented articles on an issue that implicates the value of the sanctity of human life. Addressing religious considerations seems to guarantee pedagogical futility. Bioethics educators do best, it has been argued, to "sidestep religion" in order to engage ethical deliberation and argument, for engaging in a religious approach to ethical issues is "certain to produce a breakdown in communication and then a standoff," a circumstance readily demonstrated by numerous historical examples.[24] One text introduces students to bioethics in its opening chapter through one such exemplary standoff, the 2005 case of Terry Schiavo, to illustrate how a prevailing secular-constructed bioethics is challenged by conservative religious perspectives in particular.[25] The bioethics classroom in short seems to replicate the polarization of the culture wars. Whether bioethics discourse relying only on philosophical methods, or narrative pedagogy, or legal or medical casuistry, can do much better in avoiding dialogic breakdown is seldom examined in these interpretations.

As bioethics has evolved from an interdisciplinary inquiry to a more professionalized study that privileges traditions of reasoning reliant on secular concepts and constructs drawn from philosophy, law, and policy, it stands to reason that a dominant

23. Clouser, "Bioethics and Philosophy," S10.

24. Ridley, *Beginning Bioethics*, 6–7.

25. Barry, *Bioethics in Cultural Context*, 1–11, 68.

secular construction will be reflected in the teaching resources for pedagogical bio-ethics. This is symbolic of a narrowing of the pedagogical cultures of bioethics, not an opening. Even as the field reflects increasing inclusionary wisdom from different cultures, such as minority traditions or disability perspectives, it is exclusionary, indifferent, or hostile towards religious traditions in a manner that does not serve students' educational needs or the professional and civic purposes of teaching ethics well.

Having associated religion with whimsy and exhortation as a source for bioethics reflection, secular pedagogical bioethics is structured on the pretense that religion and religious convictions are largely ethically irrelevant in the otherwise diverse and welcoming public space of the academic classroom. This approach invariably gives a misleading impression to students about the nature of ethical inquiry and discourse, which first consists in asking the right questions. It also overlooks the pervasive pluralism of methods, norms, and positions in bioethics. Students who are educated that religious thought generates impasses in communication are not challenged to find modes of common ground that can be inclusive of religious views that inescapably emerge in controversies outside the classroom. When students are inculcated to interpret bioethics as a window on the culture wars, they seldom critically evaluate stereotypes of various religious, professional, and philosophical traditions.

Conversely, students with religious convictions may come to see bioethics as primarily about procedures for reaching consensus, but otherwise substantively shallow and spiritually vacuous. It is as if bioethics has no soul, no enlivening and animating presence. Within the predominantly secular construction of bioethics, it can require considerable courage for a student to appeal to a religious value in a classroom setting. Not only does the student have to confront the conventional power dynamics of the classroom, but the pedagogical culture itself is oriented to delegitimate religious values as obstacles to rational consensus. Sometimes a particular issue compels the expression of a religious claim, most frequently when the value of the sanctity of life is contested in moral arguments about reproductive issues, medical-assisted death, or euthanasia. However, this constricted scope of classroom conversation (it cannot be called dialogue) also ill serves students, for it seems to replicate the conclusions of an argument the student wasn't even aware had occurred. The invisibility of religious discourse in the classroom reflects the arguments that in a pluralistic culture, religion is best kept out of public discourse, that religious positions are only and invariably a source of moral conflict (very seldom does a pedagogical reading portray religious values as contributing to moral resolution), and that religious-based arguments almost inevitably support a form of vitalism in ethics.

It might seem that religious discourse in one respect is spoken fluently in pedagogical bioethics, for language that comes readily to almost all students is that of "playing God." This phrasing is not used with a great deal of substantive meaning and reflection; it typically functions as a kind of all-encompassing shorthand description for what is occurring in a very complex situation requiring a life-or-death decision, or in circumstances when concepts of human nature are contested, such as the issues of genetic manipulation that so concerned Ramsey. The phrase "playing God" signifies that, for some persons, a moral limit of grave magnitude is threatened, although precisely what the limit is and why it should be retained or rescinded is often not clear. As Allen Verhey has observed, the phrase "playing God" generally "invokes a perspective," but this perspective requires critical exposition.[26] A discursive appeal to "playing God" can be a rich pedagogical moment—indeed, the proverbial "teaching moment"—but if the occasion is not seized or disregarded because a religious idea has entered the conversation, the moral point will be diluted and vacuous. The phrase will become a conversation-stopper, rather than opening what it can do, which is to invite deeper conversation when ethics cannot so easily be detached from meaning and ultimate values.

I have often thought that one of the most under-recognized philosophers of the twentieth century was Bill Watterson, author and illustrator of the "Calvin and Hobbes" comic strip. In one particular strip, he wonderfully and comically illustrates some of the issues embedded in the phrase "playing God." The comic heroes are off on one of their numerous sledding adventures, and on this occasion, Calvin declares his aspirations to "be a scientist" and to a reshaping of the world according to personal whimsy. Unfortunately, the aspiring scientist has his head turned backwards to Hobbes and isn't aware of the sled's direction and its impending collision with a tree. As the backseat rider, Hobbes is looking ahead and can of course see the tree, but in his position, he is powerless to change the direction of the sled, or to even utter a warning. Just after Calvin asserts that his goal is to create new life forms, a perennial life form, the tree, sends the intrepid explorers careening into the air. Hobbes finds it an opportune moment to ask Calvin, "So, you want to play God?"; though having completely lost control of the sled, Calvin doesn't miss a beat and confidently predicts he'll not only play God, he'll one-up God by patenting his new creations.

Watterson is poking fun at both scientific aspirations that are "up in the air" and have no basis in empirical or natural realities as well as the reactionary criticisms often directed against modern science, biotechnology, and its genetic applications that often search for an argument and articulate but a vacuous phrase. In the ironies of his characters' adventures and conversation, he captures important features of popular conceptions of this resonant phrase. "Playing God" may refer to:

1. A bold human attempt to use scientific expertise and technique to *reshape or master the contingencies* of the world and nature. For some persons, such as Ramsey, such boldness is really a form of rashness that reflects a form of disrespect or irreverence towards the natural world and of the giftedness of human experience in the world.

26. Verhey, "'Playing God,'" 347–64.

2. A *moral myopia or blindness*, a failure of moral imagination, and an absence of the corrective vision of ethics. This myopia may be attributable to the myth of perpetual progressivism embedded in western science, even though the myth provides no knowledge about which direction a particular scientific proposal or biotechnology is headed or its most probable end. The progressivist vision or imaginative capacity is closed off to the potential outcomes, particularly negative outcomes, such as losing control of the process.

3. A neglect of the ways *natural barriers* to the scientific pretensions to mastery of nature, contingency, finitude, and fallibility can be resistant to desired or anticipated manipulation. As Calvin ultimately learns, the tree will not move and gravity cannot be defied.

4. Knowingly initiating actions (sledding) on *a slippery slope* in the confidence of control as pace of progress accelerates.

5. Transforming the natural or the giftedness of experience into a human commodity for patenting, transfer, sale, or other disposition.

I don't mean to imply here that the phrase "playing God" is so meaningless as to now be useful only for caricature and comic relief; to the contrary, deeply substantive issues are intimated in Watterson's portrayal, which is why it works so well and is so applicable in the classroom context. My analysis suggests that five substantive claims of critical import in bioethics discourse are embedded in a four-panel cartoon phrasing of "playing God" (my discussion in chapter 2 delineates some additional meanings). At the same time, this brief excursion into the pedagogy of cartoons also is illustrative of why an appeal to this concept can be so frustrating and even annoying in a classroom context, let alone a professional or policy setting. The issue isn't so much wariness of venturing into the religious or sacral realm as that the phrase is multivalent. It should nonetheless be evident that some contextualization of the metaphor of "playing God" as a resonant phrase in popular culture about the nature of bioethics can achieve some of the basic objectives of bioethics education, such as enlivening moral perception and engaging the moral imagination, assuming (or evading) moral responsibility, and foregrounding the inescapability of moral anguish and distress in circumstances of moral ambiguity.

The discursive dissonance prompted by an appeal to "playing God" can invite sustained discussion on both the notions of "play" and of "God," reflection that is necessary to give content to the interpretive force the phrase is presumed to have. The background context of "God" typically presupposes an idea of a transcendent authority and judge whose cosmological position is purportedly threatened when human beings come up against boundary-limiting decisions in circumstances of extremity or aspiration. While this conception of the divine or sacred authority is present in several religious understandings of the West, it is hardly exhaustive of the ways that the divine being is understood to be in relation with human beings, including a covenantal relation. Similarly, the metaphor of "play" seems to presume human arrogance in decision-making when the stakes are high and life is on the line. But "play" is an extraordinarily rich concept, invoking notions of aesthetic creativity, imagination, cooperation and even rules, all aspects of the *imago Dei*.

The concept of playing God can present more than a restrictive, negative, or skeptical perspective on bioethical questions. Certainly, one common function of the phrase is to signify a *limitation or boundary*. The claim of limitation is not necessarily directed towards a restriction or prohibition of technology per se as much as it aims to heighten awareness of limitations inherent to human nature, including our finitude, our fallibility, our pride and our arrogance, which can lead to overreaching. The limitation function is a reminder that, like Calvin in the comic strip, we sometimes don't have a good idea of where we are going or where we land.

A second kind of function embedded in the phrase is that of *procedural accountability*. Even if God is not (on some theological views) accountable to human beings for the exercise of power or decisions, our own finitude and fallibility mean that transparency, oversight, and accountability are essential for proceeding with biomedical research and clinical applications. Contemporary bioethics has no place for isolated physicians or researchers conducting inquiries into the creation of life or the constitution of life forms without collegial review and processes of public accountability.

A third function is what I would call *invitation to imitation*. While religion is frequently perceived as an obstacle to scientific inquiry and progress, it is striking how frequently the religious traditions most prominent in the broader culture use language of "co-creatorship" or "partnership" with the divine to provide a distinctive set of motivations for collaboration with scientific inquiries, medical research, and applications of medical technology. This perhaps surfaces most frequently in Jewish reflection on the meaning of *tikkun olam* for bioethics—that is, that the world is divinely designed to be in need of repair and improvement by the human community, a mandate that can be fulfilled at least in part through scientific and biomedical developments. I have previously discussed how the biblical concept of the *imago Dei* warrants the fundamental value of human creativity, including the creation of technologies, to alleviate and cure disease and promote human wellness. Even Ramsey developed an imitation interpretation of playing God, though restricted to the context of deliberations about resource allocation.

My claim is simply that insofar as this metaphor is familiar to many students as part of the broader culture, it provides a realm of engagement in bioethics education, and really cannot be understood or explicated without giving some space to religion and religious modes of interpretation in the bioethics classroom. The pedagogical question is whether it evokes silence or a deeper exploration in the teachable moment. The culture of pedagogical bioethics is centered on a social practice, that of teaching, which inevitability pushes back from the resolution of concrete problems to reflection on how the problems were generated in the first place. These are issues for bioethics discourse precisely because of the meanings persons attach to their lives, relationships, and values. This method of "backing up" into reflection is characteristic not simply of this two-word evocative phrase, but also much of the scholarship of religious bioethics. When bioethics textbooks thus present the enterprise of bioethical inquiry as removed from religious discourse and engaged in principally if not exclusively by philosophers, legal scholars, professional societies, and policy-making bodies, they neglect what bestows to bioethics its spirit and soul, a witness to the human experience of vulnerability and the shared quest for meaning.

Professional Bioethics: Compromise and Jurisdictions

The impediments to conversation and dialogue by or about religion in bioethics is indicative of a professional field and discourse finding its way toward its own acquiescence with what philosopher Richard Rorty referred to as "the Jeffersonian compromise" that the intellectual Enlightenment made with religion.[27] For Rorty, this compromise was comprised of three interrelated features:

Privatized Religion. Religious conviction needs to be privatized. This social situatedness was deemed acceptable for religious communities because it was accompanied by guarantees of religious liberty enshrined in foundational documents. The privatization of religion was likewise acceptable to political elites in order to ensure the viability of a liberal, democratic, pluralistic society unthreatened by wars of religion or surrogate wars of culture.

Civic Discourse. The social corollary of privatizing religion is that the public square would be free from religious discourse. This would provide social space for the lifeblood of a democratic system, civic and civil discourse regarding the common good. Such a differentiation was necessary for the vibrancy of the civil society and the integrity of religion, a Jeffersonian and Madisonian insight that de Tocqueville would validate a generation later. Rorty is clearly not terribly interested in religious integrity, but he does have a great stake in pluralistic public and political discourse for which some religious mixture could be corrosive insofar as "in political discussion with those outside the relevant religious community, [religion] is a conversation stopper."[28]

Restructuring. An extension of this corollary of civic discourse is that it will be in what Rorty refers to as "bad taste" to interpose religion into discussions of public policy. The claim of "taste" suggests concerns not of moral violation, but rather of aesthetic preference. This aesthetic consideration entails that arguments or positions rooted in religious worldviews need "restructuring" into secular terms. For Rorty, restructuring involves "dropping reference to the source of the premises of the arguments,"[29] such as

27. Rorty, *Philosophy and Social Hope*, 169.
28. Rorty, *Philosophy and Social Hope*, 171.
29. Rorty, *Philosophy and Social Hope*, 173.

appeals to Scripture, religious authority, or tradition. In the context of public policy, the source of moral appeals, be they religious, professional, or secular, should not matter: "the only test of a political proposal is its ability to gain assent from people who retain radically diverse ideas about the point and meaning of human life, about the path to private perfection."[30]

Rorty contests the objection that privatizing religion to the lives of individual believers and to their corporeal communal structures diminishes religion; what he portrays as "the path to private perfection" can be comprised of religious convictions and community as well as nonreligious pursuits, such as writing poetry. What it clearly does imply is that religious traditions will have an implicit boundary imposed should they want to say something of significance about the moral meaning of professional life, such as in medicine, or about the goods and purposes of health care, or broader questions about the nature of the good society. Religious communities are not restricted from addressing such issues to audiences outside the particular religious community, but they do so as a community of politically-concerned citizens rather than as a religious tradition. In Rorty's perspective, acceptance of the Jeffersonian compromise is for the faith traditions "a reasonable price to pay for religious liberty."[31]

Rorty's primary investment in the compromise is clearly securing a domain in civic life and in public policy that is immune from religious influence; this position perpetuates the assumption of the liberal philosophical tradition that the primary moral relationship is between the individual and the state entity. The central concern for the examined life in this tradition is directed to justifying, legitimating, and enacting those moral and political rights the individual can assert against state authority to protect their liberties, respecting their private paths to meaning and happiness. However, the separationist compromise strikingly neglects to address the issues of religious presence within intermediate associations and communities, including professions like medicine, and especially for my present purposes, the value and validity of religious discourse or influence in various cultures of bioethics, including professional academia.

Philosopher Vincent Barry has extended Rorty's critique of religions as conversation stoppers in political and public life and the need for a compromise into both the pedagogical and professional cultures of bioethics. In his narrative of the emergence of bioethics, Barry maintains that, as bioethics assumed a greater public profile through incorporation into higher education, professional associations, and in federal commissions, it adopted its own form of a "Jeffersonian compromise." The bioethics equivalent of the Jeffersonian compromise is essentially instantiated or ratified through *The Belmont Report* and its trinity of ethical principles, respect for persons, beneficence, and justice. These principles provided a foundation for a common morality and discourse into which religious language and arguments "would get translated into

30. Rorty, *Philosophy and Social Hope*, 173.

31. Rorty, *Philosophy and Social Hope*, 173.

secular terms."[32] Barry's narrative seems to reflect another retrospective myth of the origins of bioethics. It's unclear to me that this bioethics compromise was intentional and formalized, in the way that the political compromise was articulated by Jefferson and Madison, but perhaps was a more informal, evolving, and implicit assumption of professional scholars. Hence, while Jonathan Moreno refers to the fragmentation of the "great bioethics compromise" as part of the culture wars of the early twenty-first century,[33] it isn't at all clear that Moreno's account of the compromise contains the same content as does Barry's account. It may be that the bioethics equivalent of the political compromise contains its own mythic projections and assumptions. Assuming Barry's gloss on Rorty to have some validity (and Rorty acknowledged that the political compromise was under "continual renegotiation"),[34] I am still not convinced that the religious communities of moral discourse received anything in the bioethics compromise comparable to the preservation of religious liberty that motivated the political compromise. Barry indeed acknowledges that while the bioethics version of the compromise maintained "religious and philosophical neutrality," it also "had the effect of marginalizing religious questions, analysis, and insight about many bioethical issues."[35]

Why Bioethics Should Take Religion Seriously

Even in an academic culture that prides itself in openness to diverse perspectives of all kinds, incorporating insights from, or even attentiveness to, religious traditions can be vigorously challenged. Why, after all, take religious ethical perspectives on medicine seriously? I want to discuss three kinds of critiques within the bioethics professional literature. One critique, principally articulated by philosophical bioethicists, is that religious argumentation borrows intellectual legitimacy and credibility from questions it purports to answer. Traditions of religious bioethics can provide interpretative frameworks for addressing deep substantive questions or questions of ultimacy, as well as methods for answers to practical questions, such as moral choices presented by life beginnings and life endings. Such discourse may be illuminating and of value for the tradition's adherents, or for comparative studies in religiosity, but commands little broader interest or audience. The core issue in the philosophical critique is that the questions religious communities and scholarly discussion are attentive to may not be perceived as terribly significant or relevant for medicine or bioethics discourse, while the answers for practical questions, such as pertain to life beginnings or life endings, are inextricably tied to substantive metaphysical assumptions that are largely

32. Barry, *Bioethics in Cultural Context*, 67.

33. Moreno, "Great Bioethics Compromise," 14–15.

34. Rorty, "Religion in the Public Square," 141.

35. Barry, *Bioethics in Cultural Context*, 67.

inaccessible, perhaps even incomprehensible, to the general educated public or to policymakers that bioethics claims as its audience.

There is undoubtedly some validity to this criticism. Discussions of the ethics of contraceptives, or in my own tradition, perennial discourse about a health code that imposes requirements of abstinence from tobacco, alcohol, coffee, and tea, may seem trivial to persons outside the specific religious community. Even in posing or addressing shared human questions of ultimacy and meaning—inquiry into our origins, our nature and identity as persons, the point to pain and suffering, the meaning of mortality, our destiny—religious thought can be tentative, exclusive, and exasperating. Yet, features embedded in the professional culture of bioethics witness to the inescapability of attending to constitutive questions of human being and well-being as part of the agenda of bioethics. Embedded in the ethics of debates about birth control are meaning-rich understandings of human relationships, responsibility, sexuality, and embodiment. And, even if contraceptive ethics doesn't prompt vigorous bioethics dialogue, federal mandates for insurance for contraceptives are certainly not seen as insignificant bioethical matters. As a further illustration, procedures and priorities in organ transplantation are not only matters of feasible policy and practical philosophy, but invoke deep matters of meaning about community, sharing, the ethics of gift, stewardship, and embodiment. More normatively, I would claim that philosophical and civic discourse in advocacy of a dignified death is impoverished because it has not engaged questions about the meaning of dying well and of mortality (chapters 8 and 9) that are really distinct from the issue of choice and self-determination. Religious traditions bear witness to questions to which the professional cultures ought to be attentive, questions that are evaded at the cost of intellectual integrity and the moral meaning of a profession of healing.

A second critique of religion in the academic professional culture of bioethics is that the intellectual credibility of religious argumentation is primarily attributable to the limits of scientific discovery. While Einstein proposed that art, science, and religion had a common origin in awe and wonder at the mysterious,[36] as scientific understanding advances with new discoveries about the origins of human life and the procreative process, the influence of genetics in disease prevalence, the cellular and genetic changes that accompany aging and diseases of dementia, and the prospects of genome editing, religious interpretations of health and disease seem increasingly diminished in relevance. Religious understandings that once provided an explanatory paradigm retreat to a "god of the gaps" posture, filling in holes where science has not yet exerted its progressive methods, empirical knowledge, and cultural authority. As Verhey articulated the point, "the God of the Gaps is only invoked . . . where doctors are powerless,"[37] and, as just indicated, medicine rarely claims an area over which it has little power or control except in the contexts of suffering, dying, and mortality.

36. Einstein, "Strange is Our Situation," 204.
37. Verhey, "Playing God," 353.

Insofar as the limits to human knowledge and technologies are provisional and temporary, technological advances imply an unveiling of those areas of human and biological life where the mysterious ruled and human powerlessness prevailed. The expansion of human knowledge and manipulation of the genetic constituents of life involves a corresponding diminishment of the realm of the mysterious and the routinization of awe into the ordinary and mundane. "God" may be invoked in circumstances where doctors are powerless to cure disease or to alleviate suffering, but for everything else, biomedical science, reason, and technology are considered sufficient. Indeed, given the scope and power of medicine to intervene in genetics, in life beginnings, and in life endings, to say that, for example, the dying course of a terminally ill person is "in the hands of God" is to imply the near-blasphemous claim that God's will is conditioned by the state of current technologies.

While this critique reflects deeper cultural chasms between religion and science in the society, it is an overgeneralization and sometimes misrepresentation to portray religious discourse in bioethics as in an invariable adversarial relationship with scientific methods and developments. There are religious motivations for the quest for knowledge and understanding undertaken by science. Such a context is presumed by Francis Collins, the current National Institutes of Health (NIH) director who previously oversaw the federal human genome research program: "For the scientist who is also a Christian, science is a form of worship. It is an uncovering of the incredible, awesome beauty of God's creation."[38] This sentiment is echoed by the Abrahamic traditions in general: scientific inquiry is not a threat, but a witness to the wondrous complexity and gift of creation. It is a careless oversimplification to see scholars in religious bioethics as engaged in a rearguard effort to save space for the sacred in a secular world.

This is not to deny that there are some significant differences in interpretations of scientific knowledge that issue in controversies in bioethics. On certain issues, some religious traditions embody what Carter portrays as a "community of resistance."[39] However, moral resistance is typically manifested not in challenges to the epistemic credibility of scientific data as much as to the meaning imputed to research results and their potential applications. It is important to be clear that the philosophical and bioethical critique of "religion," and the controversies enmeshed in the bioethics culture wars, is really directed at conservative, Christian, evangelical communities and the influence of the evangelical movement in politics generally. Not coincidentally, these seem to be the religious communities who resist both the Jeffersonian compromise and its corollary compromise in bioethics.

Without developing the arguments in detail here, the bioethical and policy controversy over both research and funding on embryonic stem cells is an evident ongoing example of contested interpretations. I contend that the resistance and opposition

38. Collins, "Human Genome Project," 101.

39. Carter, *Culture of Disbelief*, 40.

expressed by some religious traditions and scholars in conservative traditions, resistance that is not universally shared within religious bioethics, is largely an objection to scientific reductionism. That is, given that embryonic stem cells are derived from very primitive biological forms of human life, this doesn't mean that the early embryo is solely the moral equivalent of other forms of cellular life subject to scientific study. The early embryo symbolizes the beginnings of human life, even if it does not yet possess the biological characteristics that warrant the conferral of full moral standing bestowed on more developed forms of human life. My position is that it is morally necessary to recognize the prospect for significant knowledge and treatments that stem cell research may generate and refrain from impeding this research beyond conventional regulatory oversight. At the same time, I have expressed the importance for cultivating a sentiment, however vestigial, of the awe in the presence of mystery that Einstein maintained was necessary for any scientific researcher. The attitude of awe supports protections and legitimates moral restraints as expressed in the current regulatory provisions. A diminished sensibility of awe invites scientific reductionism and a view of the human embryo as merely cellular material.[40] The warrants for regulatory restraints do not reflect an adversarial paradigm of science with religion, but instead presume a common commitment that scientific research is a basic human good, the application of which requires careful professional and moral assessment.

A third philosophical critique of religious argumentation in bioethics is that it borrows selectively from authoritative sources such as formative texts, narratives, or practices. Some issues in bioethics generate this particular propensity more than others; it is prevalent, for example, in the views of some religious communities on abortion or on faith healing of children. While this critique raises interesting questions of hermeneutical interpretation and authority, it sets the standard of consistency and coherence in moral reasoning untenably high for even philosophical bioethics to meet. Very few bioethicists would dismiss the wealth of philosophical and ethical insight from a figure such as Aristotle, as well as most of his successors in the Western philosophical tradition, on the basis of gendered biases about the nature and reasoning capacities of women that we would reject now. Similarly, the indispensable contributions a figure like Kant has made to philosophical and moral reasoning in contemporary bioethics should not be discarded simply because Kant took an absolutist view on the subject of prohibiting lying and deception or found tooth transplantation a violation of perfect duties to one's self.

The kind of argumentation I have presented about "bearing witness" is clearly one interpretation of a particularly resonant religious metaphor, but it cannot be claimed to represent the whole of the moral wisdom of the biblical, Christian, or even LDS religious traditions. I have made choices and selections according to criteria of coherence, comprehensiveness, and experience. A vibrant moral tradition necessarily engages in interpretation, selection, and application of relevant historical materials

40. Campbell, "Awe Diminished," 44–46.

and the wisdom of moral tradition; philosopher Michael Walzer designates this as the "interpretative" path in moral philosophy.[41] The process of retrieval and the interpretative path of ethics and moral reasoning applies not simply to religious bioethicists, but to scholars in any field and culture of bioethics.

The professional culture of bioethics has perennially been the beneficiary of searching and compelling critiques of sociologists; in the pioneering days, two women, Renee Fox and Judith Swazey, brought to the largely male-dominated bioethics world distinctive insights about the cultural assumptions and methodological limits of bioethical methods that drew on modes of analytical philosophy. The legacy of sociological critique has recently been undertaken by John Evans, who has brought critical sociological scrutiny to bear in *The History and Future of Bioethics*. Evans identifies in the course of his discussion a further consideration relevant to displacement of religious discourse in bioethics, that of the "professionalization" of bioethics.[42]

Evans frames his account of bioethics and its emerging professionalization through the legal and political metaphor of "jurisdiction." In the jurisdictional or territorial narrative, bioethics presents a challenge to the jurisdictions of medicine and science over healing and understandings of disease in four particular areas: health care consultations, research, public policy, and culture. Needless to say, this narrative of jurisdiction domain builds an inherently adversarial element into the professions and a competitive, conflictual character into bioethics in general. Within this narrative, it makes little sense to understand bioethics, as many of its pioneers did, as an interdisciplinary method of scholarly inquiry. The jurisdiction metaphor instead suggests continual conflicts over who gets to define the questions and control the practical agenda of bioethics. These conflicts can expand beyond the legal to the extralegal, as implied by other metaphors Evans employs of a more militaristic nature. For example, in the bioethics realm relevant to religious discourse, Evans's interpretation intimates the intellectual equivalent of warfare: Scientists issue a "call to arms" against theologians, while theologians wage a "battle" to "defend" their own jurisdiction (matters pertaining to life's meaning). The theological community relies on various "allies," but ultimately the scientific community is successful in "winning the war."[43] This account implies that bioethics has really been marked by an ongoing culture war, separate from although related to, the broader culture war in the society. The bioethics war simply emerges more openly and publicly in the early twenty-first century in the United States. Although Evans does not self-consciously reference his own language, it clearly seems that he understands debates in bioethics, or conflicts between jurisdictions, through the metaphorical construct of argument as warfare.[44]

41. Walzer, *Interpretation and Social Criticism*, 17–30.

42. Evans, *History and Future of Bioethics*, 33–72.

43. Evans, *History and Future of Bioethics*, 28–38.

44. Lakoff and Johnson, *Metaphors We Live By*, 3–6.

Evans claims the jurisdiction of theologians is comprised of articulating "a sense of meaning and source of ethics for human society,"[45] but this oversight of meaning and social ethics is continually challenged from scientific interpretations, and eventually from the professionalization of bioethics. Rather than retreat from the jurisdictional conflict, Evans contends that leading theologians (with Paul Ramsey as the exemplar) developed what he calls "condensed translations" of various theological concepts into secular ends. His "translation" metaphor bears similarities to Rorty's concept of "re-structuring": the content of a theological claim is condensed into publically accessible terminology (the ethical principles of respect, beneficence, and justice) such that the concept "crosses over communities and traditions," although the totality of the content does not.[46] Hence, the resort to the method of a condensed translation by theologians effectively writes the recipe for the demise of a religious presence in bioethics.

What on Evans's account ultimately brings about the theological "retreat" from bioethics is the emergence of the professionalization of bioethics, which is marked by the development and utilization of "methods in a system of abstract knowledge" that seek to reflect and represent widespread, if not universal, claims about the values held by the public or by non-professional elites.[47] The professionalization of bioethics coincides in the jurisdiction narrative with the formulation of a common-morality ethics of principlism. As the scope of application for a system of principles of non-maleficence, beneficence, justice, and respect for persons expanded from its original context in *The Belmont Report* of protecting human subjects in biomedical research to an all-encompassing foundation for decisions in medical relationships, institutional ethics committees, and public policy, the jurisdictional domain of theologians and the presence of religion in bioethics increasingly diminished. The condensed translations of theological concepts are supplanted in bioethics by the four principles of the embedded common morality. Consequently, though "theology had defended its jurisdiction from scientists, [it] had subsequently lost the jurisdictional challenge to the bioethics profession"[48] and to its ethics of a common, rather than a particularistic, communal, or professional, morality.

The jurisdictional narrative converges with what I referred to as the "declension" narrative in chapter 2. While on the whole insightful, the narrative engages in some very problematic oversimplifications. On Evans's understanding, theologians are engaged with bioethics, but not religion or religious traditions. There is some legitimate warrant for making the jurisdictional conflict about theology as a professional discipline rather than religion as an embodied practice of moral communities, but such a rigid distinction does not always hold up. Furthermore, Evans claims that, with the ascendance of the bioethics profession and common morality principlism,

45. Evans, *History and Future of Bioethics*, 5.

46. Evans, *History and Future of Bioethics*, 17.

47. Evans, *History and Future of Bioethics*, xxi.

48. Evans, *History and Future of Bioethics*, 66.

"theologians (and others) lost interest" in the various debates, "abandoning attempts at jurisdiction."[49] However the declension narrative and a diminished religious presence of bioethics may be characterized, I don't think it stems from "losing interest" in the issues of bioethics on the part of theologians or scholars of religion. Unlike philosophers, or lawyers, or even physicians, religious thinkers and theologians participate also in the moral discourse of actual embodied communities in their faith traditions. Within these living moral communities, questions about relationships with medicine and physicians, the moral status of human life and stem cells, infertility treatments, research into the genetic and environmental etiologies of diseases, access to health care, and dying well are a matter of faithfully living out commitments and covenants, not intellectual abstractions or policy recommendations divorced from actual experience.

A striking result of this jurisdictional narrative of Evans is that there is really no intrinsic jurisdictional domain for professional discourse, let alone interprofessional discourse; there is no prospect for a coming together for a common, collaborative inquiry, but simply discussions and debates that reflect power and territorialism. The professions that come to be interested in medical ethics seem to inevitably have expansionist and imperialistic interests. Theologians and their "allies" are of necessity seeking to "defend its jurisdiction over ethics from science/medicine" as a response to "elite scientists [who] were attempting a jurisdictional expansion into the jurisdiction held by theology."[50] There are narrative implications not only for the professional culture of bioethics, but also the pedagogical cultures. What is neglected in the story of ongoing jurisdictional conflicts is precisely who has the jurisdiction for ethics education, teaching, and the communication of knowledge. Precisely those questions regarding pedagogical bioethics I delineated previously seem to be of no interest in the jurisdictional narrative, and yet that seems to me one shared domain intrinsic to the responsibilities of academic professionals in diverse communities or disciplines.

Just as pedagogy seems almost irrelevant in the narrative of competitive jurisdictions, so also medicine seems to be of purely instrumental value and to not possess its own professional integrity and ethic. The purposes of medicine are for Evans established by the principles of the common morality, constructed not by members of the medical and healing professions, but by members of the bioethics profession. These principles are themselves manifestations of public values, not values inherent to the medical profession. A central difficulty, then, with both the jurisdictional narrative of the professionalization of bioethics and its exemplification in a common morality of principles is that neither can really account for inherent values embedded in and witnessed by particularistic moralities, be they those of religious communities, or those historically carried by the medical profession. In other words, the jurisdictional and professionalization narratives reinforce the neglect of the ethics of intermediate communities characteristic of liberal political philosophy. As indicated previously, it is

49. Evans, *History and Future of Bioethics*, 65–66.
50. Evans, *History and Future of Bioethics*, 5.

within these intermediate communities that the morality of most persons is enacted. The jurisdictional interpretation of bioethics has explanatory power with respect to the construction of a system of abstract knowledge and an ethics amenable to the goals of public policy, but it is less clear that it is attentive to intrinsic issues of bioethics that emerge in the discourses of the classroom, the professions, or intermediate moral communities.

Ironically, however, the jurisdictional narrative illuminates what can be at stake in a bioethics without religion. The jurisdictional domain of theology and religion for Evans has to do not simply with ethics, but with ethics situated within a framework of human and social meaning. Once the professionalization of bioethics and its common morality principlist methods takes over the task of ethics that had historically been the province of theology, it is not clear on the jurisdiction narrative just which community assumes responsibility for bearing witness to broader meanings regarding human life and mortality. I have long claimed that the issue of meaning is a historical commitment and contribution of religious faith traditions.[51] If the question is raised as to what substantive difference does it make for bioethics or medicine if there is a diminished or silenced religious presence, the response in part is why we should be content with the portrait Evans leaves us with of a bioethics culture and medical culture that is agnostic about meaning on the most important issues of our lives.

Public Policy and Purely Religious Claims

I now turn to examining illustrations of the limited policy presence of religious perspectives, focusing particular attention on two examples: the controversy over human cloning taken up by the National Bioethics Advisory Commission (NBAC) in 1997, and a policy analysis on the science, ethics, and policy issues on mitochondrial replacement treatment issued in 2016 by the Institutes of Medicine. The policy deliberation process in both of these instances was informed by testimony, presentations, and written analysis prepared by scholars in religious studies and theology from diverse traditions, as well as discourse regarding scientific, philosophical, and policy questions. Religious understandings were more fully integrated into the policy conversation than seems to be the case in professional discourse. The policy deliberation culture nevertheless imposes a standard or threshold of public reasoning to which religious discourse and religious traditions need to conform. The public reasoning standard means that ethical concepts or norms must be intelligible and accessible to a public that is necessarily broader than the religious community, tradition, or narratives within which the concepts were historically formed and given meaning. One consequence of the public reasoning standard is that policy conclusions, as distinct

---

51. Campbell, "Religion and Moral Meaning," 4–10.

from policy deliberation, can appear as though religious reasoning and reasons have been excluded or not considered.

The culture of policy bioethics is framed not only by the orienting principles of beneficence, respect for persons, justice, and social utility, but also situated within a general consensus about the characteristics of the underlying political ethos as liberal and pluralistic. Legal philosopher Kent Greenawalt provides a thoughtful exposition of what he calls the "premises" or assumptions of liberal democracy, which include (a) democratic governance; (b) extensive personal liberty; (c) a secular, or nonreligious, justification for government and the state; (d) governmental non-sponsorship of religion; (e) laws that are supported by secular objectives, or that promote some good "that is comprehensible in nonreligious terms"; and (f) commitments to rationalism and individualism.[52] Once these assumptions are instantiated, then moral pluralism seems to necessarily follow—that is, a liberal and pluralistic society will, within these constraints, be agnostic about the human good or the good society, and will leave these more philosophical and religious questions to be addressed through the realms of personal liberty and voluntary community associations, including religious communities and their particularistic discourses. It also follows that public expression of particularistic goods, be it from religious or other intermediate communities, can become what Rorty refers to as "conversation stoppers."

While these principles and premises of liberal pluralism preclude religious justifications for policy or law, in general and with respect to health care and bioethics specifically, I contend that they permit and sometimes even require the involvement of religious argumentation in policy deliberation. Principles of liberty, equality, and the common good, as well as the foundational commitment to democratic governance, secure space in the culture of policy bioethics for the ethical discourse of religious traditions. As theologian Lisa Sowle Cahill articulates the point, "public bioethics discourse (or public policy discourse) is actually a meeting ground of the diverse moral traditions that make up our society."[53]

Regardless of whether or not such a meeting ground is necessitated by the nature of the issue, religious argumentation in policy bioethics must be conveyed in a constricted moral discourse of standards shaped largely by secular moral categories. One such standard is what I refer to as *informed citizen comprehension*; it is implicit in Greenawalt's view that public justification requires framing an argument so it is comprehensible in nonreligious terms. This standard is likewise embedded in Rorty's concept of "restructuring" religious concepts and what Evans contends are "condensed translations" of religious concepts in the bioethics policy culture. The difficulty with such a standard for public discourse is that it effectively precludes the voicing of distinctive religious interpretations or moral norms; a religious concept needs to be articulated in language that is not only accessible but capable of being understood by

52. Greenawalt, *Religious Convictions*, 14–26.
53. Cahill, "Can Theology Have a Role," 11.

the informed citizen.[54] This is not an unreasonable requirement given that the audience in the policy setting is not one's religiously-literate peers in the academy, nor a confessional community, but the general public—that is, what I am referring to as "informed citizens." However, if the policy discourse is entirely vitiated of distinctive religious language, symbols, or imagery, it can seem that whatever religious residue is retained serves merely to underwrite conclusions the policy deliberation has already arrived at through nonreligious reasoning.

If the influence of religious ethical thinking is unnecessary for generating moral rationales for policy conclusions, and if it is equally dispensable in formulating ethical questions that should be addressed (as implied by other bioethics policy analyses),[55] that seems to leave only the confined process of policy deliberation amenable to religious or theological thinking. It in this respect that the attentiveness to religious thought exhibited by both the NBAC—in addressing the ethics of human reproductive and therapeutic cloning—and the Institute of Medicine committee—in its consideration of the ethics of mitochondrial replacement treatment—are instructive.

The Cloning Controversy

The National Bioethics Advisory Commission (NBAC) undertook its examination of the science and ethics of human cloning in the spring of 1997 at the request of President Bill Clinton.[56] The consideration given by NBAC to religious views, including hearing public testimony from scholars of various Christian, Jewish, and Islamic traditions, as well as devoting a chapter in its public report to an overview of religious themes presented by human cloning (a chapter that drew on an invited background paper I had prepared),[57] was challenged by some scientists and bioethics scholars. Biologist Richard Lewontin in particular gave voice to an interpretation of religion and of theological reflection that, if valid, would certainly warrant understanding a religious presence in even the policy discourse of bioethics as contrary to the purposes of a deliberative public policy process. Lewontin argued that theological reflection in general attempts to "abolish hard ethical problems" and evade "painful tensions."[58] In contrast to moral philosophy, which has more credibility as a serious intellectual endeavor, Lewontin asserted: "What religious revelation does is to provide the certainty that in all situations there is an unambiguously right thing to do, as given by Divine Law, and leaves only the question of how to know God's will."[59]

54. Campbell, "Religious Ethics," 271–76.

55. President's Commission, *Splicing Life*, 51–80.

56. National Bioethics Advisory Commission, *Cloning Human Beings*.

57. Campbell, "Religious Perspectives on Human Cloning," D1–D64.

58. Lewontin, "Confusion over Cloning," 22.

59. Lewontin, "Confusion over Cloning," 22.

The critique from bioethics scholars pushed in an entirely different direction, contending that, far from religious traditions providing a clear and unambiguous right position, the account of religious views in the NBAC report "mechanically array competing perspectives on the appropriateness of human cloning, which appear to cancel each other out."[60] The authors failed to see how their interpretation should actually work to dispel the bioethics illusion that religious ethical traditions comprise an intellectual monolith. The primary objection was not about religious pluralism, however, but that inclusion of religious viewpoints on human cloning violated the core principles of a liberal democratic society. Echoing the premises presented by Greenawalt and the basic terms of Rorty's "Jeffersonian compromise," the bioethics critique claimed that the NBAC report presented no argument for considering religion "in a political system governed by a core commitment to the separation of church and state and marked by pervasive pluralism. It fails to clarify why or how religious views and voices could or should shape public policy with respect to cloning."[61]

Several members of the Commission were compelled to respond to Lewontin's critique, addressing their perception of his mischaracterization of the NBAC policy outcome on human cloning and defending the integrity of the policy process, including the reliance on the witness of religious scholars.[62] Furthermore, the policy arguments for attentiveness to the ethical traditions of religious thought about human cloning, the omission of which had so irked the bioethics scholars, were succinctly summarized in a separate analyis by James F. Childress, one of the NBAC commissioners and a pioneer in formulating the intellectual infrastructure of bioethical principles. Childress presented a central premise of the relation of public policy and religion embedded in NBAC's own process: "public policy in the United States cannot be based on considerations that are purely religious in nature."[63] There are two aspects of this premise that bear examination. First, the claim of Childress is that religious considerations cannot be the foundation or justification for public policy. This does not, however, preclude the articulation of religious stories or claims in the deliberative process that precedes a policy conclusion, which is what NBAC exemplified. A further question that arises from this statement of the basic bioethics premise for public policy is just what would constitute a "purely" religious consideration. Presumably, a direct appeal to a moral injunction contained in a scriptural text, or a more general understanding that civic laws are subject to veto by biblical morality, would comprise purely religious matters and are thus proscribed. However, restricting purely religious claims in public policy justifications would not seem to rule out mixed moral considerations supported by nonreligious as well as religious-based appeals.

60. Miller et al., "Dealing with Dolly," 266.
61. Miller et al., "Dealing with Dolly," 265.
62. Shapiro et al., "Confusion over Cloning," para. 46.
63. Childress, "Challenges of Public Ethics," 11.

The possibility of a mixed moral consideration is explicitly addressed by Childress in two of the five rationales he presents in explication of the religious presence in the NBAC policy deliberations. The background construct that underlies these two rationales for inclusion of religious discourse is the notion of an "overlapping consensus" developed in the writings of John Rawls, in which a democratic pluralist society presupposes a significant core of common moral commitments.[64] Citing examples of appeals in religious moral discourse to "nature," "basic human values," or "human dignity," Childress observes that "religious traditions often present moral arguments that rest on premises that are not merely or exclusively religious in nature."[65] The modifiers here are carefully chosen and important: Insofar as a moral position or premise is not "exclusively" religious, it doesn't seem to violate the policy premise of avoiding a "purely" religious consideration as a basis for policy. Appeals in religious discourse to the normativity of the natural, or the essential imperatives of basic human values, can be understood as "accessible to citizens of different or no faith commitments" rather than emerging exclusively from the commitments of any particular faith tradition.[66] The conceptual presupposition is that religious traditions of ethics can in certain instantiations reflect and represent an embedded common or shared morality of the public in general. *This* common morality can be a legitimate source and basis for policy recommendations.

A similar assessment is relevant to Childress's subsequent observation that NBAC sought out a religious witness in its deliberations to assess "the extent to which religious traditions—and secular traditions—overlap on moral positions on human cloning to create children."[67] A position that "overlaps" with that of another tradition cannot be said to be "purely" or distinctively unique to one moral community. The claim presupposes a shared morality at least at some level.

A substantive account of the values that comprise this consensus would require searching analysis, interpretation, and exposition of concepts such as "nature" or "human dignity," and it is likely that at some point a religious account will present distinctive content relative to a scientific interpretation of the plasticity and malleability of the natural or the human. Concurrence of positions at a very general level of analysis would not preclude the emergence of substantive differences in specific instances or applications. However, even if there is agreement at a fairly high theoretical level regarding the importance of respecting nature or procreative dignity for a salient bioethical issue like human cloning, the question still persists as to why the religious interpretation is actually necessary for policy deliberation when a nonreligious account can provide the same background of moral intelligibility for an ethical concept.

64. Rawls, *Political Liberalism*, 134–49.
65. Childress, "Challenges of Public Ethics," 11.
66. Childress, "Challenges of Public Ethics," 11.
67. Childress, "Challenges of Public Ethics," 11.

The argument for a religious presence in policy deliberation and the NBAC rejoinder to Lewontin's critique cannot reside entirely on ascertaining shared moral premises or overlapping positions. As important as determining the degree of coherence between religious and secular or nonreligious claims may be, perhaps the more significant policy consideration consists of assessing both dissent from common morality and especially the intensity of such dissent. Childress acknowledges that the feasibility, effectiveness, and benefits of a social policy are influenced by "the nature, extent, and depth of opposition to those policies by various religious and secular communities."[68]

I don't dispute the genuineness with which the NBAC sought to both incorporate and impose standards of public accountability for religious traditions in their policy deliberations. The difficulties with this mindful attentiveness should nonetheless be evident. The analysis of the resonance of religious reflection around criteria of consensus or dissent implies that the ethics of religious traditions either are irrelevant for deliberative purposes, because their positions have sufficient substantive overlap or generalized accessibility such that they can be derived from the shared morality, or their distinctive content will be expressed in a position of "opposition." It does not seem possible in this construction for religious traditions to manifest support or participation in a way that is recognizably of a religious nature. This policy construction then sets up traditions of religious ethics precisely for two kinds of problematic, if popular, misrepresentations: (1) As illustrated in the Lewontin caricature, religion avoids the hard ethical questions and always seeks certainty and the "unambiguously right thing to do";[69] or, (2) distinctive religious content that diverges from the overlapping consensus will be understood as necessarily in an adversarial and oppositional relationship with the proposed biomedical research inquiry or clinical application. Any claim that religions might offer distinctive support for such research or application is diluted as part of the consensual overlap.

The convergence of these philosophical, cultural, and political constructions of religion for policy is precisely what was displayed in the concluding policy recommendations made by NBAC on human cloning. The guiding policy premise means there should not be any expectation of a policy recommendation rooted in an "exclusively" religious value or religious argument. However, the recommendations eviscerate even the mention of the term "religion" altogether; instead, the term "culture" is invoked as a surrogate for moral considerations about cloning besides those of science, philosophical ethics, and the law. The recommendations stress the importance of improving the scientific literacy of citizens, including citizen awareness of the scientific impact on ethical, social, and cultural concerns about human cloning. This is an important endeavor to be sure, but the recommendations make no mention of improving the ethical literacy of citizens, or any intertwining of reproductive and genetic science and

68. Childress, "Challenges of Public Ethics," 11.
69. Lewontin, "Confusion over Cloning," 22.

medicine with religious values. They do not identify any specific learning forums for science literacy programs despite the fact that a great deal of continuing civic education is convened not only in public meeting spaces, like community libraries, but also in houses of worship. The assimilation of religion into a broad pluralistic "culture" seems to undermine the purposes of seeking out religious understandings and values on cloning (or on other issues that emerge from new reproductive or genetic technologies). It also is oblivious to the substantially problematic relationship of religion *to* culture.[70]

Policy and Religion on Mitochondrial Genetics

The scientific and biomedical context for mitochondrial replacement treatment (MRT) in 2016 was different than for the issue of human cloning: While the cloning discussion invoked substantial hype, media speculation, and philosophical conjecture, transmission of mitochondrial genetic disease is a real and immediate issue for many couples and inhibits them from having a genetically-related child. This immediacy meant there was no need for a broad canvassing of the philosophical and religious landscape on MRT or an exploration of different scenarios under which it might be permissible. No less significant, the MRT discussion occurs following the bioethics culture wars that the human cloning discussion preceded. There is thus a more narrow and constricted moral context for policy consensus. Significantly, the chapter in the Institutes of Medicine (IOM) report that makes a brief allusion to a religious context for MRT, "Whether Ethical and Social Considerations Preclude MRT," is structured by a policy presumption in favor of proceeding with MRT embedded in its title.

Very little in the IOM report could be considered "purely" or "exclusively" religious; religious content is essentially reduced to the two-word phrasing, "playing God," which the IOM committee assessed to be "too vague and indeterminate to guide such judgments without additional premises and arguments."[71] Unfortunately, the committee neglected to present an exposition of those arguments. The committee determined that engaging a framework that would give intelligibility to the phrase as it pertains to MRT "was not an appropriate or useful grounding for the committee's analysis."[72] This assertion begs the question of why religious accounts, which are certainly much broader regarding creative methods of reproduction than "playing God," are not only inappropriate, but not even helpful as "grounding" for an analysis.

The language of "grounding" resonates with the NBAC concern to avoid having a purely religious perspective be the "basis" for public policy. Both the NBAC and IOM accounts of moral foundations for public policy entail that arguments that appeal to purely religious premises will fail to meet the conditions for public reasoning of

70. Niebuhr, *Christ and Culture*, 1–44.

71. Institute of Medicine, *Mitochondrial Replacement Treatment*, 91.

72. Institute of Medicine, *Mitochondrial Replacement Treatment*, 91.

accessibility and intelligibility. This threshold test for public reasoning doesn't affirm neutrality between religious and secular arguments, but clearly endorses nonreligious discourse as both necessary and sufficient as a basis for policy-making. Although as suggested in the discussion of the pedagogical culture of bioethics, the meaning and scope of "playing God" can be specified more substantively, there is little question that on its own, the phrase is indeed too "vague" to be useful grounding for policy. The IOM report, however, is making a different kind of claim, less about moral substance and more about public deliberation: invoking an appeal to an admittedly imprecise phrase is a way to evade moral accountability. In this respect, religious views (though they are not considered in any meaningful fashion in this report) may well be seen to limit public debate and inhibit public policy.

Prophetic Resistance

My two illustrations suggest different approaches to the issue of religious discourse in policy bioethics. The NBAC narrative reflects policy engagement with and incorporation of traditions of religious ethics. The IOM narrative, by contrast, finds religious discourse to be an obstacle to sound policy. These differences reflect in part the nature of the issue under discussion. Although religious thinkers, including Fletcher and Ramsey, had addressed human reproductive cloning speculatively along with some biological scientists three decades prior to NBAC, developing policy pertaining to reproductive cloning was really a case of "first impression." By contrast, the primary issues raised by MRT, such as inheritable genetic modifications, have been the subject of practical deliberation at least since the advent of the completion of the human genome project. The different approaches of incorporation or exclusion are also reflective of the societal ethos with respect to religion and the culture wars in bioethics. Religious views and values have been politicized (or political ideologies have sought backing in religious forms) and proven to be particularly polarizing for the culture, and this is no less true for various pedagogical, professional, and policy cultures of bioethics.

The culture of policy bioethics often seems to replicate the assumption of professional bioethics that religion is necessarily an adversary or obstacle to scientific advancement. While I concede that my experience at the federal policy level is limited, on the two occasions I have been invited to submit summations or interpretations of religious thought, I have been specifically requested to focus on the objections that religious communities or traditions might have to new advances in biotechnology, whether human cloning or research use of human body tissues. This focus is understandable if the question is determining the political feasibility of an otherwise ethically sound policy. While I have stressed the importance of differentiating the policy process from policy conclusions, religious perspectives seem appropriated only insofar as they are part of a mixed or overlapping consensus, in which case they are not necessary, or they are recognized for the frequency and intensity of their dissent from the consensus. The structure of the policy process thereby contributes to a caricature of religion as a regressive, tradition-bound perspective inimically opposed to scientific advances—that is, the policy structure echoes the narrative presented by Fletcher about the necessity of emancipation from religious morality.

Given this construction of the policy questions, it may seem not all that surprising that religious views are so readily dismissed in the policy and professional bioethical cultures. This construction of religion as necessarily oppositional to scientific inquiry and advances fits within the broad narrative of perpetual scientific progress, but this myth overlooks occasions when religious views can provide distinctive support or distinctive motivations for scientific research and advances in health care applications. If the bioethical policy question were ever to shift to address health care inequalities and universal access to health care, religious support would be substantial. The professional and public policy cultures of bioethics need to reflect fair-mindedness and the spirit of philosophical charity towards religious views rather than perpetuating caricatures.

It is nonetheless important to retain the distinction between deliberation in the policy process and justification for the policy outcome. Religious traditions of bioethics can have an indispensable role of witnessing to values and ideals in the former context, even if they have a diminished or negligible role in the latter. Religious discourse in policy bioethics is characterized by symbolic or expressive rationality, expressed as a concern about why this matter is important, that a genuine pluralism should recognize as a necessary complement to the "What should we do?" emphasis embedded in the policy tradition of instrumental rationality. The discourse of symbolic rationality focuses less on realizing goals, and is directed instead to expressing values, virtues, attitudes, and symbols that witness to moral considerations that have intrinsic value or are not reducible to policy concerns of efficiency, effectiveness, and feasibility.

The rootedness of religious ethics in traditions of communal experience and history means that the relevant principle of ethics for these traditions may be less autonomy or utility and more so the principle of universalizability, of treating similar cases similarly. Patterns of analogical reasoning and moral imagination, and appeals to symbols and metaphors, can bring the moral wisdom of sacred texts or formative narratives to bear in the reasoning process. A first (though not last) question for ethics in religious communities is to examine whether a proposed area for biomedical research and clinical application reflects similarities with some experience, story, or covenant in texts, rituals, or community practices. Creation narratives are particularly generative of ways of interpreting contemporary innovations, and sometimes may be interpreted as anticipating scientific developments rather than offering dispensable anachronistic attitudes. Policy deliberations about innovative medical interventions are more pluralistic and constructive when attentive to reliance on creative imagination, analogy, metaphor, and symbolic rationality.

Although beyond the purview of policy bioethics, strictly speaking, religious traditions of ethics can bear witness against the cultural addiction to embrace the new, or the relentless quest for the "next big thing." The scientific ideology of ongoing progress generates what may be categorized as an idolatry of the innovative. This does not imply restrictions on the freedom of scientific inquiry, but it can suggest different ways to understand progress other than linear, and as necessarily connected with technological innovation. A further moral concern is that investment of resources towards the next innovation that may benefit persons in the future may divert resources critically needed for caring of persons in the present. In such instances, the benefits may be speculative while the deprivations are both immediate and tangible. Since the vast majority of citizens experience (and die from) chronic illness, substantial resource commitments to prospective curative or enhancement measures can represent a distortion of moral priorities. Social and community responsibilities to future generations should not mean neglect of the present needs of vulnerable persons.

The moral credibility of traditions of religious ethics is bound up with a commitment to resist the cultural tendency to ethical polarization and divisiveness without dialogue. Pluralism does not mean that sound moral and policy judgments cannot be articulated, nor does it mean subscribing to a subjectivist ethics, but it does come with a responsibility and moral accountability for infusing civility in contexts of controversy. That is where the core goals of pedagogical bioethics can illuminate and interact with the responsibilities in policy bioethics. Religious traditions have a shared stake in ensuring that the public square retains its public-ness. A method that is feasible, even in the context of many bioethics issues that have potency for polarization such as gene editing or physician-assisted death, is to begin ethical discourse with areas of agreement and points of common ground rather than delineation of differences and points of adversarial contention.[73] This does not deny the emergence of differences and disagreements over the scope, interpretation, and implications of ethical commitments in a pluralistic society, but the philosophical and religious traditions that inform bioethics entail shared respect for different interpretations and positions so long as they are rooted in ethical values and arguments, not political or legal posturing, caricature, or personalization. The virtues of philosophical charity and intellectual humility are essential elements for the diverse discourses of bioethics.

73. McCormick, "Abortion," 26–30.

11

The Sacred Rights of Conscience

The hospital ethics committee had been convened to consider an ethical question presented by a cardiologist at the hospital. The physician had been treating an elderly male patient, who had undergone a second hospitalization following a spell of recurrent vomiting. The patient experienced ongoing nausea, diarrhea, and consequent dehydration following his initial discharge from the hospital. The physician indicated that the patient's medical history included some diminishment of kidney function, as well as a heart ailment that required insertion of a pacemaker; however, neither of these chronic conditions were deemed factors leading to his current hospitalization. During the current hospital stay, medical staff noted that the patient had on file an advance directive indicating no resuscitation, intubation, or feeding tubes should any of those interventions be required to keep him alive.

The patient's condition gradually stabilized and improved, and he was close to being discharged again. However, the day prior to his anticipated discharge, the patient made a request that startled and created moral distress for the attending physician and the caregiving team: the patient requested that his pacemaker be "turned off" so that he could be allowed to die. A palliative care physician called for a consultation on the case confirmed this request. A psychiatric evaluation assessed the patient as having capacity to make health care decisions.

The patient's family, consisting of his son and daughter, supported their father's request. They had communicated to the treating team that their father lived in a mobile home adjacent to his son, and was largely dependent on the son for assistance in his daily needs. In the meeting with the ethics committee, the son acknowledged that his father did not have a diagnosable terminal illness, but questioned whether upon discharge from the hospital his father would be able to live without the around-the-clock care provided by an assisted living facility, especially given his recent recurrent hospitalizations. The son also commented that his father had been a man who took pride in his independence and autonomy, and he anticipated that he would not do well in an assisted living setting, but would experience severely diminished quality of life.

The patient's request for his pacemaker to be turned off posed medical and professional conflicts for the professional staff that they sought moral clarity on from their meeting with the hospital ethics committee. The staff concurred that the patient was decisionally-capable, and they agreed among themselves that the patient was not terminal, even if he wanted his life to end. They acknowledged that were the man to experience an acute recurrence of heart or kidney failure, they would respect the provisions of his advance directive to refuse additional medical interventions such as resuscitation or tube feedings. The pacemaker was different, however; discontinuing the pacemaker would mean stopping an intervention that had provided medical support to the patient for over five years.

Upon communication of the patient's request, the physician and patient engaged in a conversation, during which the physician informed the patient that were the electrical current to the pacemaker stopped, there was no guarantee that the outcome would be death. The physician indicated three different outcomes as possible: (1) the patient might continue to live in his current condition because his heart function was sufficiently independent of pacemaker support; (2) the patient would continue to live, but be physically and cognitively incapacitated because of low ventricular rhythm; or, (3) the patient's heart would stop, and death would occur from cardiac arrest. However, the physicians did not know prospectively what would happen. The patient indicated that incapacitation would be a worse outcome for him than the other alternatives, but even with these uncertainties, the patient persisted with his request, with the support of his children.

The attending physician informed the committee that he was unsure about the ethics of the patient's request, but that he, personally, would need to remove himself from further participation in the patient's care should the patient's request be deemed acceptable and autonomous. The physician stated that his continued participation would mean his actions could be the direct cause of the patient's death, and that was contrary to his understanding of his medical commitments: his medical responsibility, he affirmed, was to help save the lives of his patients, not bring about their deaths. The physician acknowledged that not everyone at the hospital or amongst his professional colleagues would agree with him; he was willing to transfer care for the patient to another qualified physician who would accommodate the patient's request.

The members of the hospital ethics committee had initially assumed they were going to be engaged in another ongoing deliberation about the ethics of stopping medical treatment, based on concerns about futility, efficacy, or familial pressures. However, as the narrative unfolded, the committee found themselves confronting a conscientious refusal of a physician to participate in a patient's decision because participation was deemed to compromise the physician's personal sense of integrity. It was a different kind of conscientious refusal insofar as the physician was not declining to provide a medical service requested by the patient, but rather was refusing to stop a treatment the patient now no longer wanted.

The physician's refusal was not based on a shared professional ethic, per se; he recognized that not everyone would agree with his views, especially a physician to whom care of the patient might be transferred. He held a commitment that physicians (or other professional staff) should not abandon their patients, and this was an overriding consideration in his willingness to transfer care of the patient to another physician. However, on this matter and for this patient, he could not bring himself to acquiesce in the patient's request without a sense of profound moral compromise: "I could no longer be the physician I am." The physician in this circumstance did not use the language of conscience explicitly, but rather invoked his personal values and integrity as the form of expressing his conscience and conscientiousness.

The health care professions are experiencing an increasing prevalence in the frequency and the scope of conscience-based refusals by physicians, nurses, and pharmacists to either decline to offer what are legally available medical services or, as illustrated in this situation, refuse to remove treatments deemed medically efficacious. The scope of these refusals remains largely in the purview of decisions pertaining to preventing life, such as refusals to provide emergency contraception, or perform an abortion or a sterilization; or creating life, such as refusals to provide certain fertility services, such as IVF treatments, or offering sex selection for nonmedical reasons; or, circumstances of hastening death, such as cessation of life-support technology, stopping medical nutrition and hydration, provision of palliative sedation, or declining to participate in a patient's request for medical aid in dying. This is to say, circumstances of conscientious refusals involve momentous and integrity-defining considerations for both the patient and the physician.

The emergence of conscience-based objections and conscientious refusals to offer or provide services in health care, or decline to stop treatment, reflects features of the bioethics culture wars, as well as a form of backlash by some professionals against the perceived secularization of medicine and bioethics. This is not to say that all conscientious refusals in medicine are comprised of religious objections as such, although many are. Insofar as the medical relationship has become informed by market models of consumer sovereignty and empowerment, and some accounts of professional bioethics have seemed to endorse reducing the ethics of medicine to the choice of the rational, informed patient as consumer, some health care professionals have felt compelled to opt out of providing certain services or procedures or of discontinuing certain procedures. This chapter aims to explore the moral terrain of conscientious refusals and claims of conscience in disputes over the compatibility of professional life and personal integrity.

Concepts of Conscience

If James Madison had had his way, claims of conscience would have received the same level of protection as other foundational rights such as freedom of religion, speech, press, assembly, or petition for redress of grievances. In his speech introducing a formal bill of rights to the US Constitution, Madison's "first" first amendment read: "The civil rights of none shall be abridged on account of religious belief or worship, nor shall any national religion be established, nor shall the full and equal rights of conscience be in any manner, or on any pretext infringed."[1] Most of the deliberative records we have from the Congressional debates focus on the meaning of "national religion"; the protection of the rights of conscience from infringement was retained in various iterations of what became the First Amendment in both the House and the Senate until a motion passed in the Senate to strike the clause entirely. Historians are unclear why the proposal was so modified. However, writing nearly a quarter of a century later as President, Madison still saw the rights of conscience to be embedded in constitutional protections. The Constitution, Madison affirmed, guaranteed "to each individual security, not only of his person and his property, but of those sacred rights of conscience so essential to his present happiness and so dear to his future hopes."[2]

Madison's efforts sought to secure conscience from infringement by a feared tyrannical government and hostile religious persecution; he was not addressing the matter of infringement of conscience by state governments, let alone what may be involved in the practice of medicine (which had yet to be organized under the American Medical Association). My claim here is simply to indicate that the discourse of conscience is not merely a byproduct of twenty-first-century controversies in medical ethics. It has a rich history in religion, in philosophy, and in political discourse, and pointed to some human good or capacity that, at least for Madison, was both sacred and could not be entirely protected by ensuring civil or political-based rights. The adjective "sacred" did not mean that protecting conscience was a matter only for believers, or a back-door way of protecting religious expression, but rather referred to a human capacity that should not be infringed by government, legal institutions, or organized religion; the phrase "rights of conscience" was invoked because of its applicability to all human beings, regardless of religious belief or (of special concern in the age of Madison) of no belief.

However, the current discourse of conscience does seem to make conscience the close conceptual equivalent of religiosity; conscience language and conscientious refusals are flash points in debates over social tolerance for religious appeals and presence in public and professional life, even when such tolerance can be inimical to the welfare and interests of patients who health professionals are committed to serve. Legal scholar Alta Charo has made this point succinctly in her concern about

1. Madison, "Speech in the First Congress," 420.
2. Madison, "Proclamation," 458–59.

the basis and scope of legal protections of conscience, or "conscience clauses," in the provision of medical care. She maintains: "the surge in legislative activity surrounding conscience clauses represents the latest struggle with regard to religion in America. Should the public square be a place for the unfettered expression of religious beliefs, even when such expression creates an oppressive atmosphere for minority groups? Or should it be a place for religious expression only if and when that does not in any way impinge on minority beliefs and practices?"[3] There is no straightforward answer to these questions, for in the context of medicine, claims about who comprises the "minority" and who is subject to "oppression" are advanced by professionals and patients alike. However, Charo contends: "health care professionals can claim the right of conscience as necessary to the nondiscriminatory practice of their religion, even as frustrated patients view conscience clauses as legalizing discrimination against them when they practice their own religion."[4]

Several important conceptual and ethical questions are embedded in claims about conscience and conscientious refusals in health care. It is first important to be clear about the importance of conscience in the moral life. A second important issue is whether, when a conflict of conscience arises in health care, some integrity-preserving compromise can be sought for individual professionals, particular patients, and the profession as a whole. The outlines of an integrity-preserving compromise: (a) guaranteeing continuity of care and non-abandonment to particular patients; (b) respecting conscientious refusals of health care professionals; and (c) coordinated responsibility of the profession to provide necessary care and accommodate conscience were embedded in my initial story. However, on some accounts, conscience should also be subject to what philosopher Richard Rorty calls the "Jeffersonian compromise"[5] and thereby excluded from professional life; compelling arguments are made by both professional caregivers and bioethicists against any accommodation for claims of conscience made by health care professionals in medical care. Some commentators about medical professionalism have argued that perhaps aspiring health care professionals should make a determination to choose to follow the professional standard of care or code of conduct or choose a different profession. These two primary questions, the moral meaning of conscience, and the professional significance of conscientious objection, provide the framework for my analysis. My exposition relies on the moral and conceptual frameworks developed by philosophers Martin Benjamin[6] and Mark Wicclair.[7]

3. Charo, "Celestial Fire of Conscience," 2472.

4. Charo, "Celestial Fire of Conscience," 2473.

5. Rorty, *Philosophy and Social Hope*, 169.

6. Benjamin, *Philosophy & This Actual World*, 100–148.

7. Wicclair, *Conscientious Objection in Health Care*, 12–86.

Conscience and Moral Integrity

In the early months of his presidency, President Barack Obama was invited to give a commencement address to graduates at Notre Dame University. The invitation provoked controversy because of Notre Dame's historical affiliation as a Roman Catholic institution, including its commitments to the sanctity of human life from conception onward, whereas President Obama was a long-standing advocate of a woman's right to choose regarding the termination of her pregnancy. In a speech that reflected his own commitments of personal integrity, Obama challenged his audience to seek out common ground in the otherwise polarized social controversy over abortion rights. As part of this challenge, Obama asserted: "Let's honor the conscience of those who disagree with abortion, and draft a sensible conscience clause, and make sure that all of our health care policies are grounded not only in sound science, but also in clear ethics, as well as respect for the equality of women."[8] Though the Obama Administration later passed legislation in the form of the Affordable Care Act that prompted claims of conscientious exemption, I first want to explore the meanings of the concept of conscience presupposed in Obama's assertion of the necessity to "honor conscience."

What is it about conscience that requires respect, honor, and at times, legal protections? Different conceptions of conscience contribute to controversies about whether a claim of conscience warrants respect from others, within professions, and as a matter of law. A common understanding of conscience embedded in various historical religious traditions is that conscience refers to an internal moral sense that enables a moral agent to differentiate between right and wrong action. A concept of conscience as an internal faculty for moral discernment is reflected in LDS Scripture: "it is given unto [persons] to judge that you may know good from evil; and the way to judge is as plain, that you may know with a perfect knowledge as the daylight is from the dark night . . . [T]he Spirit of Christ is given to every man, that he may know good from evil."[9] In this understanding, conscience is a universal phenomenon; a capacity for moral discernment is a gift inherent in all human beings. Furthermore, conscience is quite literally a matter of "in-sight," that is, a capability internal to a person that involves looking inward to identity-constituting and identity-conferring values to make discriminating judgments about right and wrong conduct. Conscience is not the sole source or primary authority for moral decision-making. It can be complemented by other sources of moral understanding, including parental, social, and religious moral teaching, as well as particular professional moralities; a moral agent engaging in conscientious self-reflection can nonetheless use the capacity of moral discernment embedded in conscience to assess the validity of these diverse sources of ethical values.

A second interpretation of conscience is that it is the echo and voice of various norms and mores that have been internalized in the course of a person's social

8. Obama, "Commencement Address," para. 23.
9. Moroni 7:15–18.

experience. Conscience does not refer to an inherent and universalized faculty, but instead is a social construction. In this interpretation, a person's conscience is primarily a product of how a person is raised, and the content of conscience will necessarily differ from person to person; there is no generalizable capacity, let alone a standard, for moral judgment. Conscience is not recognized to involve a capacity of moral discernment and discrimination independent of socialization. The view of conscience as socially constructed seems to underlie the perspectives of many critics of conscientious objection in medicine; an appeal to conscience cannot be relied on as a sound source of personal ethics insofar as conscience was inevitably shaped and tainted by various forms of bias and prejudice experienced in the socialization process.

A third interpretation understands the phenomenon of conscience as consisting of self-reflection on personal integrity and wholeness. In this interpretation, a person who appeals to conscience in objecting to the performance of some action is expressing a claim that concerns the impact of the action on their self-identity as a moral person. An action contrary to conscience constitutes a violation of personal moral integrity and commonly will be accompanied by "pangs of conscience" or moral residue, including regret, guilt, and self-recrimination. Insofar as a person may deem that fulfilling the responsibilities of their professional vocation could require them to perform actions that violate their conscience, a restriction on conscience-based actions threatens personal moral integrity. Protection of conscience is clearly a matter of substantial ethical and existential importance. The appeal to personal integrity presented by the cardiac physician as related in the opening narrative reflects this third account of the moral status of conscience.

The perspective of conscience on which I will rely in ethical analysis of conscience and conscientious objection in medicine and health care integrates elements of the first interpretation of conscience as a capacity for moral discernment and the third account of conscience as self-reflection on personal integrity. For these purposes, I leave aside questions about the metaphysical origins or social constructionist interpretations of conscience. Whatever else conscience may comprise, at its core, a claim of conscience represents (1) a basic human capacity for moral discernment and discriminating judgments regarding moral actions. This means that an appeal to conscience presupposes a prior determination of a proposed course of action as right and obligatory, permitted but nonobligatory, or wrong and prohibited. Furthermore, the concept of conscience also refers to (2) a reflective assessment of personal integrity and wholeness in contemplating an anticipation action. This prospective contemplation includes anticipation by the moral agent that, in performing the action in question, he or she will experience the peace of a "clear" conscience or the "pangs" of a remorseful, guilty, or wounded conscience. This anticipatory assessment is often referred to in religious discourse as the activity of a "legislative" conscience as distinct from a "judicial" conscience that emerges in retrospective assessments of past conduct.

The exercise of compulsion, coercion, or obligation by persons or institutions with authority (religious, political, professional, etc.) to prescribe the performance of an action contrary to personal conscience will thereby be experienced as profoundly threatening and disrupting to the integrity of the moral self and the inviolability of the person's moral identity. If the claims of conscience are routinely ignored by the agent or violated by externally imposed power or compulsion, the presence of conscience in the moral life can be substantially diminished. A person past the capacity of feeling of peace or pangs is a person whose conscience is lost. It follows that there is a moral presumption requiring respect for a person's claim of conscience. As philosopher Martin Benjamin writes, "appeals to conscience must always be taken seriously and should, if consistent with other equally important claims and values, prevail."[10]

Benjamin's account of an ethics of integrity provides a compelling illustration of why it is important to honor and, where possible, respect a person's claim of conscience even when it may issue in a conscientious objection to a legally permitted practice.[11] Ethical decision-making involves a highly fluid and dynamic interrelationship and interaction between particular moral judgments in concrete situations, ethical principles and norms or rules that provide moral justification for the judgment, and background theories and beliefs, including religious convictions about nature and human nature, understandings of knowledge and epistemic certainty, and interpretations of the world and the divine nature. (Many of my background convictions for medicine and medical ethics were articulated in chapter 3.) Benjamin claims that moral agents seek coherence or "fit" between these three aspects of ethical decision-making, as well as between moral commitments that reflect and preserve our wholeness or integrity as moral selves. Ethical talk and moral action requires critical self-reflection over the whole of a person's life, not merely discrete actions, in order to experience clarity and congruence between moral choices and "one's basic identity-conferring, moral, religious, and philosophical convictions."[12]

Our experience of integrity or its absence is profoundly influenced by ways of life that are ordered and organized according to shared moral commitments in moral communities as well as by personal ethical values, and by worldviews that correspond with the various background beliefs and pre-moral assessments regarding human nature and destiny, the world, God, and other matters of ultimate concern. Benjamin formulates a "way of life" to consist in "a set of patterns of living, admired ideal types of men and women, ways of structuring marriage, family relationships, governance, educational and religious practices and so on."[13] When these patterns of living are carried out in the context of professional conduct, I have maintained, we are able to refer to those patterns as reflections of the person's "calling" or "vocation." A worldview

---

10. Benjamin, "Conscience," 691.

11. Benjamin, *Philosophy & This Actual World*, 135–47.

12. Benjamin, "Conscience," 690.

13. Benjamin, *Philosophy & This Actual World*, 129.

within which such life patterns are situated refers to "a complex, often unarticulated (and perhaps not fully articulable) set of deeply held and highly cherished beliefs about the nature and organization of the universe and one's place in it."[14]

Benjamin understands these elements of ethical decision-making to likewise be dynamically interrelated. A way of life organized, for example, according to an ethos of gift and a pattern of covenantal relationship will presuppose and embody a view about the world and human nature, such as persons as inherently relational beings who find meaning in community. A worldview of the ultimate powers as creative, nurturing, and transforming will structure the way of life around patterns of creativity, caring, and change in relationship, while a worldview that finds in nature or the cosmos indifference or hostility, abuse, and cruelty, will sanction more attentiveness to individualistic quests or patterns for preservation and protection that mediate all relationships with strangers through rights-claims.

One of the central challenges of an agent's personal moral experience is to achieve balance, wholeness, and a fit between ways of life, including particular judgments and ethical norms, and worldviews, including background beliefs and pre-moral convictions. It is a long-life process carried out over time and in relational encounters, and helps form and constitute personal moral integrity. Although it is very unlikely that there will be a convergence and harmony between persons of the interrelationships of ways of life—including their ethical structure—and worldviews—including their background beliefs—various intermediate communities such as family, friendships, and religious communities may provide approximations of convergence and unity of increasing complexity. It is also possible not only in moral communities but also in professions and in relationships of moral strangers to find consensus or agreement about central ethical principles or norms, even in the midst of substantive disagreement about particular moral judgments or decisions and incompatibility or irreconcilability of background worldviews. This at least is the claim made by bioethics scholars who affirm a variation of a common morality ethic.[15] The common morality thesis reasoning of ethical reasoning claims to evade not only the issues raised by moral relativism, moral nihilism, and ethical skepticism, but also those of particularistic moralities, including religious and professional ethics.

An exposition of the broader interrelation of ways of life and worldviews with ethical principles and particular concrete moral judgments bears great significance for issues of conscience and conscientious objection. A person who makes an appeal to conscience in civic life or as part of their professional responsibility is claiming that performing an action will threaten their integrity and personal wholeness because the action (a) challenges or runs contrary to the ethic embedded in their way of life and likely also is (b) incompatible with their understanding of the world as well as their

---

14. Benjamin, *Philosophy & This Actual World*, 129.

15. Beauchamp and Childress, *Principles of Biomedical Ethics*, 2–5; Veatch, *Hippocratic, Religious, and Secular*, 149–58.

place and meaning in the world. A claim of conscience is not then an insignificant or easy-to-set-aside matter; acting contrary to conscience constitutes betrayal of not only ethical standards but also of commitments to ways of being through which a person situates their moral self within the world. Ultimately, actions contrary to conscience reflect self-betrayal rather than staying true to one's self. The retention of integrity and the protection of conscience thereby is a matter of bearing witness to what matters most in the moral self.

Principles of Accommodation

Implicit in the appeal to honor conscience, and in providing structures of professional and legal protection for claims of conscience, is a social and professional context of ethical pluralism. Ethical pluralism presents a contrast to theories of ethical or moral harmony in which any and all moral decisions or conflicts are in principle resolvable by appeal to a basic or superordinate ethical imperative. By contrast, a context of ethical pluralism means moral agents will experience conflicts between various important ethical principles and values or conflicts between particular moral judgments that are not readily reconcilable. Numerous elements in moral decision-making, including human finitude, fallibility, and different organizing worldviews (not to mention the significance of religious convictions and adherence to professional ethics) contribute to a pluralistic context for ethics in society and in the professions.[16] As noted, my own position is that there is broader agreement on questions of ethical principles in medicine, and to some extent in society, such as minimalistic considerations of respecting liberty and refraining from harm, than there may be about particularized moral judgments. This reflects in part the influence of the pre-moral judgments and interpretations that bear on moral perception and moral vision and the embodied limits of human finiteness and fallibility.

Moral conflicts that emerge in foundational principles and commitments, such as between respecting life and liberty of choice, or between liberty and equality, often reflect matters of prioritizing and tension in particular situations of moral conflict. It is important to recognize that even in deep, apparently intractable moral conflicts, such as over abortion rights and corresponding claims by some professionals for conscientious exemption from provision of such contested services, it is rarely the case that a moral argument reflects a complete discarding of an otherwise central moral principle for professional ethics or ethical relationships in civic life. Contested interpretations emerge in religious tradition over the relation of the norms of love and justice. Both principles or values are always relevant for moral agents, but disputes arise, for example, over whether love and justice are in conflict, are morally equivalent, are in a hierarchical/preferential relationship, or manifest a context-bound relationship

---

16. Beauchamp and Childress, *Principles of Biomedical Ethics*, 24.

(justice is the form that love takes in broad civic and political interactions), or display a transformational relationship. These tensions may manifest particularly in situations of concrete judgments.[17] The general presumption of respecting and honoring conscience must thereby be situated within a background context of moral, civil, and professional pluralism. Moral agents in a pluralistic ethical and professional world can experience conflicts between ethical principles or requirements applicable to everyday moral life or professional life and those values and moral commitments that are constitutive of that person's moral integrity—that is, those values that comprise the moral conscience of a person.

Historically, the most common context for the assertion of claims of conscience and conscientious objection has involved refusal by persons with religious convictions (or their secular equivalent) to participate in military service and warfare. A person whose moral self is shaped by a commitment to an absolute moral principle not to kill other human beings can experience a conflict with principles of civic responsibility and fairness that require citizens to support the requirements of the state for defense and security, including the taking of human life in armed conflict, if necessary. There is a robust and sustained ethical and legal precedent in these circumstances in which the state attempts to accommodate claims of conscience and personal integrity regarding nonviolence or refraining from killing in ways that do not pose a threat to security or civic responsibility. What philosopher Martha Nussbaum designates as the "principle of accommodation" is an embedded cultural protection of conscience through exemptions from otherwise generally applicable requirements to participate in military service for persons who voice a conscientious objection to such requirements.[18]

The accommodation principle that sanctions exemptions from military service on grounds of conscience does not create "duty-free" citizens or "free-riding" citizens who receive the benefits of defense and security while not assuming any of the burdens. These exemptions have instead commonly entailed provisions for the conscientious objector to perform alternative forms of civic service that contribute to the greater social welfare, such as service in hospital or medical settings. Such persons enact what the pragmatist philosopher William James referred to as "the moral equivalent of war."[19]

The practical application of the principle of accommodation for conscience through alternative forms of civic service in the historical context of conscientious objections to military service, which in part reflects principles of equality and fairness in contributing to the common good, has made it possible to achieve what Benjamin considers an integrity-preserving compromise.[20] That is, pluralistic ethical claims and principles that initially appear to generate an irreconcilable conflict between the

17. Outka, *Agape*, 75–92.
18. Nussbaum, *Liberty of Conscience*, 22–26.
19. James, "Moral Equivalent of War," 4–14.
20. Benjamin, *Philosophy & This Actual World*, 140–42.

citizen and the state can be honored through an accommodation that preserves the moral integrity of the conscientious objector and the legitimacy of the state interest in promoting civic participation and security. The question is whether such an integrity-preserving compromise is possible in the context of conscientious refusals by professionals in medicine, which then can be institutionalized and given legal recognition.

The necessary moral structure that provides the basis for such a compromise in the health care setting requires commitments to: (a) ensuring continuity of care for patients, (b) protecting the moral integrity of the professional, and (c) advancing fairness and accountability as part of professional responsibility. Strikingly, Benjamin grounds the prospect for accommodation and an integrity-preserving compromise in medicine in a shared professional commitment to healing and wholeness: "The values underlying appeals to conscience in the health care system are similar to the underlying values of medical and nursing care—preserve or restore wholeness."[21] Insofar as the patient, the professional, and the profession itself express a common interest in the "fundamental commitment to preserving and restoring personal wholeness or integrity," it should be possible to achieve "some sort of workable compromise or accommodation" when a physician or other health care professional appeals to conscience.[22]

Two other conceptual and normative presuppositions for accommodating claims of conscience also are present in the medical context. An acknowledgement of professional pluralism on certain matters of ethical concern corresponds with the normative commitment to the principle of respect for self-determination. A patient's request for services that are legally accessible can nonetheless infringe or violate deeply-held personal, philosophical, or religious-based commitments of a health care professional. The occasions of a claim of conscience have primarily emerged in addressing the availability of legal medical services and interventions concerning the creation, prevention, or termination of human life. They may also emerge from specific genetic-related contexts of decision-making such as pre-implantation genetic screening or sex selection methods. In ethical decisions regarding circumstances of the boundaries of human life and death, some conscientious professionals can experience a claim of conscience. Should the professional undertake the course of action stipulated by the principle of respect for patient self-determination, they contend they would have to cross the identity- and integrity-constituting line of their conscience. In examining the prospects for an integrity-preserving compromise in these contested contexts, I first consider arguments made by medical professionals and by bioethicists that medicine should be a conscience-free zone of professional practice.

21 Benjamin, "Conscience," 691.
22 Benjamin, "Conscience," 691.

Medicine as "Conscience-Free"

In the most comprehensive ethical analysis of the question, philosopher Mark Wicclair differentiates three types of approaches to conscience-based refusals in health care. Wicclair's argument builds off of the precedent of political discourse about conscientious refusal or objection to certain civic duties. A first approach, which Wicclair ultimately defends, is the idea of an integrity-preserving compromise for professional, profession, and patient that provides both limited justification for conscientious refusals and also builds in certain ethical constraints on the exercise of conscience. I first explore the two perspectives that Wicclair rejects because they either do not place constraints on or do not permit justification of appeals to conscience.

Wicclair designates one approach to the issue of conscientious refusal as "conscience absolutism."[23] This position affirms that it is within the sole purview of health care professionals to refuse to provide any service that may violate their conscience. Safeguarding conscience and preserving the personal moral integrity of the professional are considered to be sufficient justifications for conscientious refusal. Conscience absolutism imposes no strong ethical constraints on the actual exercise of a right of conscience.

Conscience absolutism not only encompasses refusals of professionally accepted and legally available services or interventions, but also supports professional refusal of referrals to other providers who could meet the needs of a patient, and even refusals to disclose information about alternative options a patient may have, such as for different contraceptive methods or for prescriptions to hasten the end of life. Conscience absolutism considers professional referrals or information disclosure about objectionable legal services to involve a compromising degree of moral complicity in the patient's action or access to the service, even if it is not as extensive or as direct as providing the service. The absolutist interpretation of the stringency and scope of conscience presumes the moral sovereignty of the conscience of a health care professional and fails to provide any grounds for a compromise to ensure the patient is not abandoned and their health care needs are met. The absolutist position affirms that a health care professional should be exempt from any conscience-infringing or complicity-inducing practice.

The polar approach to conscience absolutism is designated by Wicclair as "the incompatibility thesis."[24] This position affirms that the conventional professional practice regarding a patient request for a legally accessible service is normative; there is no space whatsoever for a professional to refuse to provide a legally available medical procedure or service, let alone evade referrals to other practitioners or withhold information necessary to the informed decision of a patient. The question of ethical constraints on conscience does not arise as it does for both the compromise and abso-

23. Wicclair, *Conscientious Objection in Health Care*, 34–44.
24. Wicclair, *Conscientious Objection in Health Care*, 33.

lutist positions because there is no justification of a claim of conscience independent of professional responsibility in the first instance. The only qualification to the thesis of incompatibility between professional norms and personal convictions arises in circumstances where the professional doesn't have the requisite knowledge or technical competence to provide the procedure or information. In such a situation, the professional could and should refuse on grounds of lack of qualification and the duty to avoiding harming patients, but this is a foundational principle intrinsic to medical professionalism, not a claim that emerges from personal conscience. This distinction is exemplified in the originating narrative for this chapter in which the particular physician did not appeal to lack of professional competence as grounds for refusal, but rather to personal convictions about his sense of medical vocation.

The incompatibility thesis is coupled with a thesis of generalization: if the procedure can be done ethically by any professional with the requisite professional competence, it can be performed ethically by every professional with such competence. A procedure that can be done technically should be at least offered ethically; it would be unprofessional, if not also unethical and paternalistic, to refuse to provide the intervention when requested by a patient with decision-making capacity. The incompatibility thesis holds that a refusal of a patient request for a legally available service is an act of defiance that places the physician outside the boundaries of professional identity and integrity; indeed, refusals based on a conscience claim can mean the person may have a responsibility to pursue a different professional path. The incompatibility thesis thus creates what can be understood as a conscience-free zone in medicine, nursing, and health care. I will analyze the arguments regarding the incompatibility thesis insofar as the position has been advocated vigorously by prominent medical professionals and prominent bioethicists, and I have encountered variations on it in professional discourse much more frequently than an absolutist position.

The arguments over professional responsibility in physician-assisted dying and medical aid in dying can provide a focused illustration. The statutory provisions in law permitting a physician's prescription upon the request of a terminally ill patient to end the patient's life also affirm there is no legal duty of participation required of any health care provider or institution in a patient request. Moreover, providers or institutions that refuse to participate are also under no obligation to refer the requesting patient to another physician or institution. The burden of responsibility for identifying a participating physician falls to the patient and his or her advocates. In short, the legal statutes allow for physicians and pharmacists to opt out of providing a life-ending medication or providing referrals. Since there is no legal or professional duty of participation, the statutes do not frame professional nonparticipation as a matter of an exemption based on an appeal to conscience. However, the nonparticipation provisions are commonly interpreted in bioethical and professional discourse as protection for conscientious refusals to requests to participate in hastening death. The nonparticipation provision appears to have effectively the same function as a conscience clause. This illustration is a reasonably close approximation of what Wicclair has in mind by the concept of conscience absolutism.

A physician's refusal to participate in prescribing the medication can create a significant burden of access for a patient, although in all circumstances that I am aware of in the Oregon context, the access issue was ultimately alleviated through referral to a hospice program. While 0.6 percent of licensed Oregon physicians have participated in writing a prescription to hasten death under the law,[25] there is no published data on the frequency of physician refusals or the nature of the burdens imposed by such refusals for terminally ill patients. Nonetheless, some physicians and some advocates of patient rights have recently argued that physician or pharmacist adherence to the statutory provisions is not as professionally discretionary as otherwise may appear. The claim is that the law provides a kind of minimalist morality: the responsibility of a professional with the requisite training requires a commitment to best practices that is more elevated than legal compliance. This is a version of the incompatibility thesis in that a professional ethic cannot be reduced to the law. Physicians make a commitment of fidelity to medicine and its inherent moral responsibilities, which confers moral primacy on respect for patient choice and commitments to patient welfare displayed through physician beneficence.

Furthermore, arguments reflecting the incompatibility thesis hold that the moral commitments of medicine do not allow for a selective professional morality: once a person has set out on the career path to become a physician (or pharmacist), they must be "all in" morally. If an aspiring professional is considering becoming an oncologist, and could be practicing in a jurisdiction in which they may receive requests from their patients for a medication to end life to which they have a conscientious objection, they should select another medical specialization for practice in which claims of personal conscience will not emerge. Benjamin has likewise advanced a similar critique with a more general scope: "An individual whose moral or religious convictions are incompatible with a common, essential type of health care has no business deliberately seeking a position in which such care is a routine expectation."[26]

It is certainly difficult at this point in the practice of physician-assistance in dying in which some 0.2 percent of patients die through a prescribed medication to end life[27] to consider physician prescriptions to hasten death a "common" or "routine" form of medical treatment (or "health care," to put a more polemical point on it). Furthermore, Benjamin makes a moral distinction between a person who inadvertently finds themselves in a situation where their conscience may conflict with a patient expectation of a professional—for example, a physician who entered oncology prior to the passage of laws on physician-assisted dying—and a physician who deliberately enters a specialization with the purpose of obstructing a legally available service. The Oregon

25. Hedberg and New, "Oregon's Death with Dignity Act," 581.

26. Benjamin, "Conscience," 691.

27. Hedberg and New, "Oregon's Death with Dignity Act," 582.

legal statute that assures professional communities and the public of the voluntary nature of professional participation, but again is not framed as an explicit conscience clause, is understood as providing a legal option. The question posed by the incompatibility thesis is whether this is an option that should be selected by an ethically responsible professional.

The difficulty presented in these illustrations of the incompatibility thesis is that the moral agency of the physician as a physician (or pharmacist as pharmacist) is displaced. The decisive moral decision for a health care professional is understood to occur prior to their entry into the profession. Once that decision is made and ratified through schooling, residency, and practice setting, the moral commitments of the profession, including the virtue of conscientiousness in medical practice, eclipse personal reservations or questions of conscience. The incompatibility thesis implies that physicians are merely the technical extension of the patient's will; this reflects, as discussed in previous chapters, the technician and provider model of the physician's vocation and the consumer or market model of medicine.

My own assessment is that what is really driving these arguments for an incompatibility claim is not the legal provision allowing nonparticipation. Physician-assisted death legislation is less than a generation old in almost all jurisdictions, and there is hardly a settled consensus on the question from a professional, societal, or religious set of perspectives.[28] Instead, the principal contentious issue is the statutory provision that exempts physicians or pharmacists from a duty of referring patients who request physician-assisted death. An implicit professional expectation is that referral is a professional responsibility and the trade-off for the preservation of conscience and personal integrity. That is, it seems mistaken to claim that there is a moral equivalence in the degree of complicity involved in referring a patient to another physician as there is in participating directly in the objectionable action. In its discussion of professional claims of conscience, the AMA Code of Medical Ethics maintains: "In general, physicians should refer a patient to another physician or institution to provide treatment the physician declines to offer."[29] While I have talked to many physicians in Oregon who have exercised their right not to participate in a patient's request for a prescription to hasten death, all of these physicians have indicated that they are willing to refer a patient to another physician who will provide the prescription.

If referrals in the physician-assisted death statutes were a matter not just of professional discretion but legal responsibility, I think arguments questioning the moral and professional legitimacy of nonparticipation of professionals in requests for a prescription to hasten death would diminish. A consequence of the current scope of the nonparticipation provision that includes non-referrals is that it impedes not only patient self-determination but also access to a legal medical service or procedure. The need to delineate precisely the scope of decisions about conscientious refusal

28. National Academy of Medicine, *Physician-Assisted Death*, 7–52.
29. American Medical Association, "Physician Exercise of Conscience," para. 11.

ultimately becomes a feature of the approach of the integrity-preserving compromise to be discussed subsequently.

With this context of physician-assisted death and claims of conscience in mind, I wish to consider two arguments in the professional literature that exemplify advocacy of the incompatibility thesis. Julian Savulescu is a prominent British philosopher and bioethicist who finds claims of conscience morally suspect: indeed, appeals to conscience may perhaps mask evidence of moral corruption and professional dereliction of responsibility. On Savulescu's construction, conscience claims represent a reemergence of the old ethics of paternalism that threatens the primacy of patient self-determination and autonomy. However, Savulescu raises the moral stakes involved in conscientious objection from assessments of actions to moral character. Appeals to conscience in medicine really comprise a form of moral evasion and an excuse for vice, particularly the vice of injustice as reflected in discriminatory refusals to provide access to legal health services, especially in the context of reproductive health care. Alternatively, he argues that a claim that conscience will not allow a particular professional to provide a legal health care procedure is simply a bad-faith manipulation by the professional to avoid enacting their professional duty.[30]

Professional moral evasion rooted in claims of conscience is thus a matter of critical significance, so much so that Savulescu makes the willingness to discard personal values that may potentially conflict with professional responsibilities a threshold test of professionalism. Echoing the critique of Benjamin, Savulescu contends that "if persons are not prepared to offer legally permitted, efficient, and beneficial care to a patient because it conflicts with their values, they should not be a doctor."[31] Savulescu exemplifies the understanding that the health care professions should be conscience-free zones of professional ethics: "A doctor's conscience has little place in the delivery of modern medical care."[32]

Professional, ethical, and even legal ramifications must follow from this position. Structures and regulations at professional and organizational levels should be implemented to assure that medicine becomes and remains a conscience-free realm of professional life. This seems to hold the further implication that part of professional licensure should include the development of medical conscience review boards not, as some have suggested, to assess the genuineness of the conscience claim and its strength in the moral life of the conscientious objector, but instead to preclude in advance any prospect of circumstances of conflict between personal values and professional responsibilities. Certainly, there is no warrant on this argument for instantiating conscience clauses in legal statutes or professional standards of care, and entirely strong professional and policy reasons for rescinding such clauses.

---

30. Savulescu, "Conscientious Objection in Medicine," 294.

31. Savulescu, "Conscientious Objection in Medicine," 294.

32. Savulescu, "Conscientious Objection in Medicine," 294.

In the setting of reproductive health issues, especially patient requests for contraception or abortion, Christian Fiala and Joyce Arthur raise the professional stakes of conscientious objection even further. Fiala and Arthur reject the proposal that conscience claims relating to military service provide any kind of precedent and legitimation for conscience claims in medicine. Rather than affirming a need to respect conscience and establish conscience clauses, the authors believe that conscientious objection in medicine is best understood as "dishonorable disobedience."[33] Conscientious refusals violate the core tenet of *primum non nocere* by imposing a form of harm on patients seeking legal services from an authorized medical provider. This means that conscientious objection represents an "ethical breach that should be handled in the same way as any other professional negligence or malpractice, or a mental incapacity to perform one's duties."[34] It clearly follows from this interpretation of the incompatibility thesis, as well as that of Savulescu, that persons of conscience need to seek out other professional opportunities.

These arguments clearly reflect the incompatibility thesis that there is no legitimate conscience claim in the provision of medical care and that medicine should be a conscience-free practice. An embedded presupposition in the claim that medical responsibility and conscience are incompatible is that medicine is a career, not a calling or vocation. An appeal to conscience is invariably unprofessional and immoral and misconstrues the essential technical nature and responsibility of the profession. For Savulescu, some circumstances of conscientious objection are not only unethical but also should be illegal, a position about as far removed from developing and honoring a conscience clause as is possible. Savulescu contends that a legal prohibition of conscientious objection is applicable in circumstances of professional evasion of a "grave duty"—that is, a denial of a procedure that is potentially health-transforming or life-threatening, such as refusal to perform an abortion or to prescribe emergency contraception following a sexual assault. These cases of medical emergency and moral necessity are an important constraint on conscience absolutism; is it possible to craft an integrity-preserving compromise should patients be in a circumstance of last resort?

It is important to clarify the nature of the paternalism that Savulescu maintains underlies conscientious objection in medicine. In most circumstances in bioethics, paternalism represents a restriction on the decision-making authority of patients by an authority such as a physician or the state. A determination of whether or not the paternalistic restrictions or interventions are justifiable commonly depends on whether the patient is assessed to be decisionally-capable or instead "suffers from some defect, encumbrance or limitation in decision-making or acting."[35] Paternalistic restrictions regarding the decisions of patients whose autonomy is compromised and

33. Fiala and Arthur, "Dishonourable Disobedience," 18.
34. Fiala and Arthur, "Dishonourable Disobedience," 20.
35. Childress, *Who Should Decide*, 17.

whose decision-making reflects impaired judgment is often characterized as limited or restricted paternalism and can be morally justified by the principles of beneficence and patient welfare. By contrast, paternalistic interventions regarding an autonomous and decisionally capable patient represent extended or extreme paternalism and are difficult to justify morally because "it overrides a person's wishes, choices, or actions because they are risky for that person."[36]

Like Savulescu, James F. Childress questions whether conscientious objection in medicine is simply a form of paternalism with a new conceptual nomenclature. Childress identifies four main rationales for physician nonacquiescence in a patient's request, including protection of third parties from harm, considerations of justice and fairness, moralism (a judgment that a person's actions are immoral by another person with different values), and paternalism. He contends that "conscientious objection is only the bottom line of an extended argument," and that "in practically all cases, conscientious objection can be restated in terms of the four major reasons for not acquiescing in a patient's wishes and choices."[37] That is, an appeal to conscience is not an independent moral claim, but is rather socially constructed and derivative of other moral principles. Childress concurs that conscience discourse can reflect concerns of a moral agent about the potential for loss of personal integrity and wholeness, but conscience is most often doing the work of another moral principle in medical contexts, such as justice or preventing harm, and thus can be held to standards of public and professional accountability rather than simply personal accountability. A physician who refuses to provide a legally available service for an autonomous patient with decision-making capacity is not only engaging in extreme or extended paternalism, but also "hard" paternalism—that is, "impos[ing] values that are alien to the patient."[38] At the very least, then, a claim of conscience by a health care professional should be the beginning of moral exploration, not the end of discussion, as is the position of conscience absolutism.

The bioethics arguments presented by Savulescu and, to a certain extent, by Childress are echoed by a recent argument within professional medicine by Ronit Stahl and Ezekiel Emanuel.[39] The premise of this argument is that the ethic of physicians is entirely encompassed by professional roles and codes, to which physicians subscribe or profess upon entering the profession. The argument of Stahl and Emanuel likewise hinges on the voluntary choice of a person to determine to enter the medical, nursing, or healing professions or to select another career path; it is, in short, a voluntaristic argument.

Stahl and Emanuel concur in the critique of the proposed parallel between military and medical conscientious objector. The voluntary nature of the choice to

36. Childress, *Who Should Decide*, 17.

37. Childress, *Who Should Decide*, 15.

38. Childress, *Who Should Decide*, 18.

39. Stahl and Emanuel, "Physicians, Not Conscripts," 1380–85.

pursue medicine as a career (not, as previously, a vocation) differentiates the situation of a person who may raise a conscientious objection in the context of medicine from the involuntary nature and context of coercion faced by a person conscripted into military service. Medical professionals are "physicians, not conscripts." Since the choice to pursue medicine is presumptively autonomous in that it reflects criteria of sufficient information about the nature of medical practice, as well as voluntariness to undertake such a practice, rather than the involuntary nature of conscription, once a person says "yes" to medicine, physicians necessarily forgo any subsequent "no" to their participation in a specific procedure, intervention, or service that is otherwise legally available and accessible. They contend that the accommodations made by the state and the military in the context of conscientious objection to participation in war, including the possibility for alternative forms of civic service, are intelligible only against the backdrop of state paternalistic coercion. Since no one is coerced into pursuing a career in the medical profession, claims of conscience lose this resonant structure of moral intelligibility.[40]

Both the bioethics and the professional arguments that seek to establish medicine as a conscience-free zone are problematic on several grounds. These exemplifications of the incompatibility thesis of conscience and medical professionalism endorse a social contract model for medicine between physicians and their profession, in which all expectations and responsibilities are delineated in advance. There is a diminished sensibility to the interpretations I have defended regarding medicine as a calling and vocation; certainly, the assumption that medicine articulates a monolithic professional morality contrasts sharply with the more fluid and open-ended relationship characteristic of a covenantal ethic. Furthermore, the image of physician as value-free technician or functionary is embedded in the argument that claims of conscience are to be circumscribed, and crises of conscience as well as conscientious objections are inimical to the profession of a medical ethic.

The incompatibility thesis embedded in these arguments presumes a remarkably static conception of medicine and medical practice. Contemporary medicine is certainly marked by developments in medical technologies as well as by changes in the legality of certain procedures that have expanded the options for patient choices and requests of practitioners. As a couple of rather obvious illustrations of a more dynamic practice than the voluntaristic argument accommodates, the possibility for couples to request preimplantation diagnosis for not only genetic screening but also sex selection purposes is a development only of the most recent generation. The prospect of gender reassignment surgery is now an alternative choice for some persons to make a request of medical professionals in a way very different than previous eras. This illustration reveals how very elastic the conceptions of "health" and "disease" and medicine are. The opportunity for patients with a terminal illness to request a lethal medication from their attending physician to end their life is likewise a comparatively

---

40. Stahl and Emanuel, "Physicians, Not Conscripts," 1380–81.

recent innovation in the structure of choices at the end-of-life. Hence, it can be coherently claimed that medical professionals have voluntarily abandoned their personal values and claims of conscience upon entering the conscience-free zone of medicine only on the presumption that medical practice in the next decade will be precisely the same as it has been in prior decades. As one critique of Stahl and Emanuel puts it, the voluntaristic position presumes that "*all* 'standardized' interventions of a particular specialty are *essential* to the practice of that specialty."[41] The voluntaristic claims seem simply a mistaken account of the nature of medicine in the twenty-first century.

The voluntaristic position also reflects a truncated view about the ends and purposes of medicine. The core claim of each of the voluntaristic authors about what medicine is for is to promote the well-being of patients. This leaves the concept of "well-being" up for negotiation in the interaction between specific physician and particular patient. However, given the present circumstance of a market model of medicine, within which is embedded the professional roles of physicians as technicians and providers responsive to requests of consumers, as well as the background societal ethos of respect for self-determination, it is not at all clear how the content of patient well-being is largely not going to be shaped by the requests of patients exercising their rights of autonomy. The concept of the incompatibility thesis makes patient autonomy into a moral trump.

A physician who assumes a professional role as a value-free technician in relation to patient requests for a specific intervention or legally available service effectively concedes that the medical ethos is determined primarily by respect for patient autonomy. Medicine is not distinctively shaped by ends and goals of caring or curing, let alone healing; rather, the moral substance of conceptions of "health," "disease," "well-being," or "pain" becomes the exclusive province of patient preference. This seems a rather problematic, if not entirely inconsistent, position for someone like Emanuel to advocate, given his long-standing objection to legalized physician-assisted dying. That restriction, however much it has given way in the past two decades, only makes sense if there is an ethic to medicine distinct from respecting patient autonomy.

The case for medicine as conscience-free implies a compartmentalization of the moral self. In the private realm of life, the voluntaristic arguments must permit conscience to have unrestrained governance, but upon assuming the mantle of professional responsibility, a person's conscience is not permitted to have any claim on moral beliefs or conduct. As indicated, this presumes a very problematic view of conscience—primarily, the second conception of conscience as a matter of internalized social mores, which may include bias, prejudice, and discrimination of varying types. By contrast, the kind of perspective on conscience I have affirmed is that conscience manifests reflection on a person's wholeness and integrity. In that respect, the argumentation that claims of conscience in medicine are unprofessional and should be delegitimated institutionally and perhaps legally enforce a moral separation of the

41. Stark and Stark, "Physicians without Chests," para. 6.

person as professional. This objection is acknowledged by Fiala and Arthur in their account of conscientious objection as dishonorable disobedience. Having advocated professional screening so that medicine succeeds in eliminating conscientious objection, the conscience-free professionals that do remain in practice can "adopt an attitude of 'professional distance' in order to separate their personal beliefs from their work duties."[42] The advocacy of professional distance entails a commitment to provide necessary health care with which the professional disagrees on moral or religious grounds.

The voluntaristic argument against allowing, let alone respecting or making provisions for, claims of conscience seems then to work against a physician's wholeness and integrity, expressed not only in private life, but through a profession that is a calling and vocation, and not simply a self-driven career. There is legitimacy in the concern articulated by Stark and Stark: "Driving out conscience in favor of blind devotion to professional standards will create a class of providers who have neglected to cultivate virtue and have ceded their humanity."[43] A sign of the moral health of a professional and of the profession as a whole is the experience of a degree of moral anguish about the performance of certain responsibilities, even if, and perhaps especially when, the moral anguish does not culminate in a conscientious objection. The alternative—an aspiration that medical professionals never experience moral anguish in the course of their practice, and that medicine is a conscience-free profession—presumes the prevalence of a technician model of professional life.

Conscience and Integrity-Preserving Compromises

Neither the incompatibility thesis nor the position of conscience absolutism provides a prospect for finding common ground on the question of respecting conscientious objection in medicine. The incompatibility thesis, as delineated in the previous examples, makes a conscience-free zone a matter of professional identity, even at the loss of personal integrity; or alternatively, requires a person of conscience to withdraw from the profession, and rejects legal protections for conscience-based objections. The perspective of conscience absolutism affirms personal integrity with respect to refusing patient requests for procedures, referrals, and information, thereby leaving patients potentially abandoned and imposes on other members of the profession to assume the responsibility of meeting patient needs. The question is whether there is some way through this apparent impasse of a conflict between personal conscience and professional integrity.

Though Benjamin tends in some instances to affirm the primacy of professional responsibility over personal integrity, his exploration of the concept of a compromise that preserves integrity strikes a balance of accommodation of conscience and

42. Fiala and Arthur, "Dishonourable Disobedience," 20.
43. Stark and Stark, "Physicians without Chests," para. 22.

fulfillment of professional responsibility, and offers a middle path between the absolutist claims of incompatibility or conscience absolutism.[44] The possibility of a compromise that preserves rather than betrays integrity first requires the establishment of various characteristics or circumstances of compromise:

(a) Existence of *factual or metaphysical uncertainty* about the issue in question. If the issue can be resolved on factual or empirical grounds, then a claim of conscientious objection loses its moral standing. For example, in the initial years of the introduction of emergency contraception, there was empirical uncertainty over whether some forms of Plan B acted to prevent conception or rather to prevent implantation of a fertilized egg. The latter possibility led to conscientious objections on the part of some pharmacists. Subsequent research has now indicated that emergency contraception acts primarily as a contraceptive.[45]

(b) The existence of *moral complexity*—that is, that there are compelling values in conflict. In most of the occasions for conscientious objection in medicine previously delineated, moral complexity is framed through conflicting values of respect for self-determination; professionalism, fairness, and beneficence; preservation of the sanctity of human life; and personal integrity. Neither the incompatibility thesis nor conscience absolutism sees the alternative view as reasonable. That is, both views reject the minimum condition of moral complexity.

(c) The importance of preserving a *continuing, cooperative relationship*. This circumstance is clearly at stake in conscientious objection in medicine. The physician who expresses a claim of conscience is placing a cooperative relationship with their patient in jeopardy, while the voluntaristic arguments embedded in the incompatibility thesis threaten to end the relationship between the professional and their profession or specialization.

(d) The necessity of an *impending, non-deferrable decision*. In most of the circumstances of conscientious objection, at least those pertaining to the beginnings of life, there is an urgency to the decision such that the patient who requests emergency contraception or a sterilization procedure can avoid a pregnancy, or a woman who requests an abortion procedure can avoid a potentially health- or life-threatening pregnancy. Those decisions cannot be deferred without some risk to the well-being of the woman. The nondeferrable nature of a decision is less compelling in circumstances of requesting assistance with a pregnancy or with sex selection.

(e) The prospect of *limited resources*. The issue of limited resources, including not only medical resources but availability of qualified professionals, arises especially in the context of reproductive medicine services in which available alternatives

44. Benjamin, *Philosophy & This Actual World*, 134–47.
45. American College of Obstetrics and Gynecology, "Limits of Conscientious Objection," 1206.

to a requested service may limit the scope of conscientious objection. The existence of resource-deprived or medically-underserved areas, such as rural areas of a state, may make it more difficult to support a conscientious objection to a requested health care procedure in the absence of alternative providers.

If these five circumstances—factual uncertainty, moral perplexity, continuing relationship, impending decision, and resource scarcity—occur and are realized in a specific situation of controversy, Benjamin contends that it may nonetheless be possible and morally preferable to construct a middle ground between the alternatives of conscience absolutism or a conscience-free profession. The question of a compromise aims to resolve the issue of whether a professional can legitimately refuse to provide a medical service about which they experience a claim of conscience "on terms that pay equal respect to the contending reasonable positions and that stand a chance of public acceptability."[46]

The ultimate objective is comprised of formulating a compromise on conscientious objection that preserves integrity, which would encompass (1) respecting the conscience claim of the professional, (2) fulfilling the request of a patient for a legitimate legal service, and (3) designating responsibilities assumed by the profession as a whole, even if not by every member of the profession. A moral agent's quest to preserve integrity means "pursu[ing] that course of action that seems on balance to follow the preponderance of [the agent's] central and most highly cherished and defensible values and principles."[47] Benjamin stipulates that among these values must be a commitment to a "democratic temperament,"[48] which should incline persons or organizations to share decision-making power with others who are directly affected by the decision.

Although Wicclair's analysis of conscientious objection in medicine does not make the preservation of integrity a central feature, he nonetheless develops the burden of his normative argument towards defending a middle ground between conscience absolutism and the incompatibility thesis. The incompatibility thesis contends that there is no moral justification for conscientious objection because the totality of professional life is encompassed in professionally articulated responsibilities. The position of conscience absolutism justifies and permits the exercise of conscience as always sovereign and does not concede that professional responsibilities to care for patient welfare can place constraints on conscience. Both of these positions are defended as absolutist in nature. By contrast, the shared ground model advanced by Wicclair maintains that there is both justification for conscience-based refusals as part of professional life (thus differing from the incompatibility thesis) and also justifiable limitations on the exercise of conscience because of the presumptive relevance

---

46. Benjamin, *Philosophy & This Actual World*, 141.

47. Benjamin, *Philosophy & This Actual World*, 141.

48. Benjamin, *Philosophy & This Actual World*, 131–34.

of professional responsibilities to patients (thus differing from conscience absolutism). This means that core professional obligations impose ethical constraints and conditions on the exercise of the core moral beliefs of the person as a professional. Justifiable conscientious refusals will always be "context-dependent"[49] rather than a matter of absolute prohibition or absolute legitimation, taking into consideration the seriousness of the patient's condition, the urgency of their need for a service, and the availability of alternative means of access.[50]

A moral structure of justification and limitation characterizes the distinctiveness of a compromise model that preserves integrity. This structure is not present in the alternative models insofar as they manifest an unwillingness to reflect moral complexity. The moral structure of justification and limitation is instructively illustrated in an opinion on conscientious refusals in reproductive medicine issued by the Committee on Ethics of the American College of Gynecology and Obstetrics (ACOG).[51] The committee opinion acknowledges the prevalence of conscientious refusal in reproductive medicine due to "deep divisions regarding the moral acceptability of pregnancy termination and contraception" and emphasizes the importance of seeking to "maximize accommodation of an individual's religious or moral beliefs" in the setting of providing reproductive health care.[52] However, the limits on conscientious refusals alluded to in the document title are generated from core professional obligations and values assumed on entering the profession of medicine. These include commitments to deliver health care in a way "that is respectful of patient autonomy, timely and effective, evidence-based, and nondiscriminatory."[53]

In developing its own guidelines, the ACOG Committee manifests a compromise or non-absolutist model by clearly acknowledging the presumptive legitimacy of claims of conscience, of professional responsibilities to patients, and of professional norms that mediate the relationship between physician or practitioner and patient. The committee opinion reflects clear acknowledgement of moral complexity and, to some extent, acknowledgment of factual uncertainty. However, the ACOG committee maintains that sound scientific research supports the claim that disputed forms of emergency contraception are indeed contraceptive rather than contra-gestational agents. In that respect, conscientious objections based on erroneous interpretations of the science would not be allowed. The ACOG Committee approach is also context-dependent; the document explicitly asserts that, in some circumstances, conscientious refusal cannot be justified because it contravenes core professional norms and manifests abandonment of a patient or disrespect of their request. The circumstances of restraints on conscientious refusal include (1) a high potential for imposition of the

49. Wicclair, *Conscientious Objection in Health Care*, 87.

50. Wicclair, *Conscientious Objection in Health Care*, 141.

51. American College of Obstetrics and Gynecology, "Limits of Conscientious Objection," 1203–8.

52. American College of Obstetrics and Gynecology, "Limits of Conscientious Objection," 1203–4.

53. American College of Obstetrics and Gynecology, "Limits of Conscientious Objection," 1205.

professional's beliefs on the patient due to refusals to provide medication (emergency contraception), reproductive health procedures (abortion, sterilization), or withholding information critical to decision-making (including referral information); and (2) the rationale for the refusal "contradicts the body of scientific evidence," such as the dispute over the pharmacological mechanism of Plan B medication.[54]

In other circumstances, the ACOG Committee is cautious but open to the permissibility of conscientious refusal provided that the paramount professional responsibility of care and well-being of the patient is fulfilled by a responsible and qualified member of the profession. This requires that the refusing professional provide an advance notice of their objections to patients, present a timely referral to another provider, and otherwise refrain from impeding access to safe and legally available services, or from perpetuating patterns of injustice or discrimination, such as in rural health care settings. The paramount commitment to the patient's welfare also means that, in emergency circumstances where timely referral is not possible without serious risk to the patient's health—that is, those circumstances that reflect Benjamin's category of an "impending" and "non-deferrable" decision—"providers have an obligation to provide medically indicated and requested care regardless of the provider's personal moral objections."[55] The position works out a limited justification of conscientious refusal within the constraints imposed by professional ethics, including respect for autonomy, beneficence, non-maleficence, and justice. The burden of the justification falls on the professional making an appeal to conscience rather than on the patient; the burden of responsible practice likewise falls on the professional to initiate collaboration with other members of the profession.

A structure of justification for conscientious refusal can also be framed through the moral logic of prima facie duties. The paramount duty of promoting patient welfare is the presumptive ethical responsibility of the health care professional. Overriding this commitment in order to preserve the personal moral integrity of the professional imposes a substantial burden of justification, including the following criteria:

1. *Justifiable purpose*: The underlying objective of a conscientious objection by a health care professional is to preserve personal moral integrity and protect conscience. This means that the request that initiates the prospect of a refusal must clearly infringe on a core moral or religious conviction of the professional that has been affirmed for a sustained period of time. This also means that the objective cannot be to obstruct access to a legal medical service that the professional finds morally objectionable.

2. *Reasonable prospect of effectiveness*: The conscientious refusal of the professional should be an effective and efficient means to achieve the aim of preserving moral integrity. The conscientious refusal will protect the professional from

---

54. American College of Obstetrics and Gynecology, "Limits of Conscientious Objection," 1206.
55. American College of Obstetrics and Gynecology, "Limits of Conscientious Objection," 1207.

experiencing remorse and self-recrimination had they instead participated in the patient's request, and will also not diminish moral integrity through a sense that the professional failed in their moral responsibility to the patient or abandoned the patient.

3. *Necessity*: This consideration entails that the only way for the professional to maintain their integrity is to engage in a conscience-based refusal of the patient's request. As some conscientious refusals may be rooted in different interpretations of scientific evidence, ensuring scientific competency on the relevant issue is necessary. Other options to avoid a conflict should be undertaken, including advance notification to patients about possible conflicts, candid conversations with specific patients that disclose sufficient information about the patient's range of choices and treatments that facilitate informed decision-making, and recourse to institutional intermediaries, including providing advance notice to supervisors or an explanation to an ethics committee. Affirming that justifiable conscientious refusal is context-dependent means it is a last resort: a sincere effort to seek other alternatives to fulfill the physician's commitment to the patient, to relational continuity, and to preserve the physician's moral integrity is morally required.

4. *Proportionate benefit*: The benefits for the professional of preserving their moral integrity should be greater than any burdens imposed on the patient or on the profession as a whole (as borne by the refuser's colleagues). Ultimately, the burdens of access to care experienced by the patient or burdens of additional care assumed by colleagues or other providers to whom the patient may be referred should be minimal not substantial.

5. *Conscientious intentionality*: Conscientiousness involves remaining true to a person's own moral commitments and undertaking actions to avoid personal moral complicity in a perceived moral wrong. A conscientious commitment to the patient's good requires providing an explanation to patients about why the physician cannot participate in the patient's request and retain their integrity, while at the same time foregoing recourse to "professional authority to argue or advocate [the] position."[56]

6. *Least imposition*: Preserving the integrity of the health care professional should impose the minimal amount of burden or imposition to the patient and also the minimal amount of infringement to other values. As Wicclair contends, it is important to differentiate between "permitting x to refrain from acting against x's conscience [and] enabling x to prevent y from performing legal actions that are contrary to x's (but not y's) ethical or religious beliefs."[57] This consideration can

---

56. American College of Obstetrics and Gynecology, "Limits of Conscientious Objection," 1207.

57. Wicclair, *Conscientious Objection in Health Care*, 113.

typically be satisfied through a referral process to a colleague or professional who is willing to facilitate the patient's request.

The conventional recourse to the referral process as an ethical compromise through the conflict of conscience for all parties implies that there is a sufficient number of health care professionals who are willing to assume some additional burdens of caregiving so that a colleague can preserve their moral integrity. Wicclair contends that such a practice is "virtuous and laudable,"[58] which seems to place accepting care for a patient from a conscience-based referral in the realm of supererogation rather than as part of the professional responsibility of collegiality. The ethical principle of fairness should provide an important framework to ensure that any particular participating professional isn't assuming a disproportionate or excessive burden of conscience-based caregiving.

A justifiable conscientious refusal in medicine should meet these moral criteria and also be limited by the constraints of central professional norms, including non-abandonment of the patient. This proposal bears witness to the moral status of conscience in medical decision-making and avoids transforming medicine into a conscience-free profession. It is morally important for medical professionals and for the profession as a whole to take measures to preserve integrity and also limit the occasions for conscientious objection in medical care in order to best serve the needs of patients.

58. Wicclair, *Conscientious Objection in Health Care*, 127.

Bibliography

79th Oregon Legislative Assembly. "Senate Bill 893." https://olis.leg.state.or.us/liz/2017R1/Downloads/MeasureDocument/SB893.

ABIM Foundation, et al. "Medical Professionalism in the New Millennium: A Physician's Charter." *Annals of Internal Medicine* 136 (2002) 243–46.

Alexander, Shana. "They Decide Who Lives, Who Dies." *Life* 53 (1962) 102–25.

Allen, Joseph L. *Love and Conflict: A Covenantal Model of Christian Ethics.* Nashville: Abingdon, 1984.

American College of Obstetrics and Gynecology, Ethics Committee. "The Limits of Conscientious Objection in Reproductive Medicine." *Obstetrics and Gynecology* 110 (2007) 1203–8.

American Medical Association, Code of Medical Ethics. "Opinion 1.1.7: Physician Exercise of Conscience." https://www.ama-assn.org/delivering-care/ethics/physician-exercise-conscience.

American Pharmacists Association. "Code of Ethics for Pharmacists." https://www.pharmacist.com/code-ethics.

Aristotle. *Nicomachean Ethics.* Translated by Martin Ostwald. New York: Macmillan, 1986.

Austin, Michael. *Re-reading Job: Understanding the Ancient World's Greatest Poem.* Salt Lake City: Kofford, 2014.

Bainton, Roland. *Christian Attitudes Toward War and Peace.* Nashville: Abingdon, 1980.

Barnard, David. "The Physician as Priest, Revisited." *Journal of Religion and Health* 24 (1985) 272–86.

Barry, Vincent. *Bioethics in a Cultural Context.* Boston: Wadsworth, 2012.

Battin, Margaret P. *Ethical Issues in Suicide.* New York: Simon & Schuster, 1995.

Beauchamp, Tom L. "Origins and Evolution of the Belmont Report." In *Belmont Revisited: Ethical Principles for Research with Human Subjects,* edited by James F. Childress et al., 12–26. Washington, DC: Georgetown University Press, 2005.

Beauchamp, Tom L., and James F. Childress. *Principles of Biomedical Ethics.* 7th ed. New York: Oxford University Press, 2013.

Beecher, Henry K. "Ethics and Clinical Research." *New England Journal of Medicine* 274 (1966) 1354–60.

Benjamin, Martin. "Conscience." In *Bioethics,* edited by Bruce Jennings, 688–93. 4th ed. New York: Macmillan, 2014.

———. *Philosophy & This Actual World: An Introduction to Practical Philosophical Inquiry.* New York: Rowman & Littlefield, 2003.

Bernardin, Joseph Cardinal. "Renewing the Covenant with Patients and Society." In *The Seamless Garment: Writings on the Consistent Ethic of Life*, edited by Thomas A. Nairn, 267–74. Maryknoll, NY: Orbis, 2008.

Bouma, Hessel, III, et al. *Christian Faith, Health and Medical Practice.* Grand Rapids: Eerdmans, 1989.

Bowler, Kate. *Blessed: A History of the Prosperity Gospel.* New York: Oxford University Press, 2013.

Buber, Martin. *I and Thou.* Translated by Ronald Gregor Smith. 2nd ed. New York: Scribner, 1958.

Byock, Ira. *Dying Well: Peace and Possibilities at the End of Life.* New York: Riverhead, 1997.

———. "Physician-Assisted Suicide Won't Atone for Medicine's 'Original Sin.'" *Stat News*, January 31, 2018. https://www.statnews.com/2018/01/31/physician-assisted-suicide-medicine/.

Cahill, Lisa Sowle. "Can Theology Have a Role in 'Public' Bioethics Discourse?" *Hastings Center Report* 20 (1990) 10–14.

Callahan, Daniel. "Bioethics and the Culture Wars." *Cambridge Quarterly of Health Care Ethics* 14 (2005) 424–31.

———. "Bioethics as a Discipline." *Hastings Center Report* 1 (1973) 66–73.

———. "Goals in the Teaching of Ethics." In *Ethics Teaching in Higher Education*, edited by Daniel Callahan and Sisela Bok, 61–80. Boston: Springer, 1980.

———. "Reason, Self-Determination, and Physician-Assisted Suicide." In *The Case Against Assisted Suicide: For the Right to End-of-Life Care*, edited by Kathleen Foley and Herbert Hendin, 52–68. Baltimore: Johns Hopkins University Press, 2002.

———. "Religion and the Secularization of Bioethics." *Hastings Center Report* 20 (1990) 2–4.

———. *The Troubled Dream of Life: Living with Mortality.* New York: Simon & Schuster, 1993.

———. "Why America Accepted Bioethics." *Hastings Center Report* 23 (1993) S8–9.

Camenisch, Paul. "Gift and Gratitude in Ethics." *Journal of Religious Ethics* 9 (1981) 1–34.

Campbell, Alistair. *Health as Liberation: Medicine, Theology, and the Quest for Justice.* Cleveland: Pilgrim, 1995.

Campbell, Courtney S. "Aid in Dying and Taking Human Life." *Journal of Medical Ethics* 18 (1992) 128–34.

———. "Awe Diminished." *Hastings Center Report* 25 (1995) 44–46.

———. "Meaningful Resistance: Religion and Biotechnology." In *Claiming Power Over Life: Religion and Biotechnology Policy*, edited by Mark J. Hanson, 1–29. Washington, DC: Georgetown University Press, 2001.

———. "Metaphors We Ration By: An Interpretation of Practical Moral Reasoning." *Soundings* 96 (2013) 254–79.

———. "Moral Meanings of Physician-Assisted Death for Hospice Ethics." In *Hospice Ethics: Policy and Practice in Palliative Care*, edited by Timothy W. Kirk and Bruce Jennings, 223–49. New York: Oxford University Press, 2014.

———. "Mormonism, Bioethics in." In *Bioethics*, edited by Bruce Jennings, 2124–31. 4th ed. New York: Macmillan, 2014.

———. "Religion and Moral Meaning in Bioethics." In *Hastings Center Report* 20 (1990) 4–10.

———. "Religious Ethics and Active Euthanasia in a Pluralistic Society." *Kennedy Institute of Ethics Journal* 2 (1992) 253–77.

———. "Religious Perspectives on Human Cloning." In *Cloning Human Beings: Report and Recommendations of the National Bioethics Advisory Commission*, 2:D1–64. Rockville, MD: Government Printing Office, 1997.

———. "Ten Years of Death with Dignity." *The New Atlantis* 22 (2008) 33–46.

———. "What More in the Name of God?: Theologies and Theodicies of Faith Healing." *Kennedy Institute of Ethics Journal* 20 (2010) 1–25.

Camus, Albert. *The Plague*. Translated by Stuart Gilbert. New York: Vintage, 1991.

Carter, Stephen L. *The Culture of Disbelief: How American Law and Politics Trivialize Religious Devotion*. New York: Basic, 1993.

Cassell, Eric J. *The Nature of Healing: The Modern Practice of Medicine*. New York: Oxford University Press, 2013.

———. *The Nature of Suffering and the Goals of Medicine*. 2nd ed. New York: Oxford University Press, 2004.

———. "Pain and Suffering." In *Bioethics*, edited by Bruce Jennings, 2283–91. 4th ed. New York: Macmillan, 2014.

Catholic Bishops' Joint Bioethics Committee. "Catholic Social Teaching and the Allocation of Healthcare." In *On Moral Medicine: Theological Perspectives in Medical Ethics*, edited by M. Therese Lysaught and Joseph J. Kotva Jr., 130–38. 3rd ed. Grand Rapids: Eerdmans, 2012.

Chapman, Audrey R., et al. *Stem Cell Research and Applications: Monitoring the Frontiers of Biomedical Research*. Washington, DC: American Academy for the Advancement of Science, 1999.

Charo, R. Alta. "The Celestial Fire of Conscience: Refusing to Deliver Medical Care." *New England Journal of Medicine* 352 (2005) 2471–74.

———. "The Endarkenment." In *The Ethics of Bioethics: Mapping the Moral Landscape,* edited by Lisa A. Eckenwiler and Felicia Cohn, 95–107. Baltimore: Johns Hopkins University Press, 2007.

Childress, James F. "The Challenges of Public Ethics: Reflections on NBAC's Report." *Hastings Center Report* 27 (1997) 9–11.

———. *Practical Reasoning in Bioethics*. Bloomington, IN: Indiana University Press, 1997.

———. "Religion, Theology, and Bioethics." In *The Nature and Prospect of Bioethics: Interdisciplinary Perspectives*, edited by Franklin G. Miller et al., 43–69. Totowa, NJ: Humana Press, 2003.

———. *Who Should Decide? Paternalism in Health Care*. New York: Oxford University Press, 1982.

Churchill, Larry. *Rationing Health Care in America: Perceptions and Principles of Justice*. Notre Dame, IN: University of Notre Dame Press, 1987.

The Clinton Foundation. "Health Care is Local." https://www.clintonfoundation.org/main/clinton-foundation-blog.html/2013/07/17/healthcare-is-local.

Clouser, K. Danner. "Bioethics and Philosophy." *Hastings Center Report* 23 (1993) S10–11.

Cole, Thomas R., et al. *Medical Humanities: An Introduction*. New York: Cambridge University Press, 2015.

Collins, Francis. "The Human Genome Project." In *Life at Risk: The Crises in Medical Ethics,* edited by Richard D. Land and Louis A. Moore, 100–113. Nashville: B. & H., 1995.

Cruess, Sylvia R., and Richard L. Cruess. "Professionalism and the Social Contract." In *Healing as Vocation: A Medical Professionalism Primer*, edited by Kayhan Parsi and Myles N. Sheehan, 9–21. New York: Rowman & Littlefield, 2006.

de Tocqueville, Alexis. *Democracy in America*. Edited by J. P. Mayer. New York: Doubleday, 1969.

Dik, Bryan J., and Ryan D. Duffy. "Calling and Vocation at Work: Definitions and Prospects for Research and Practice." *The Counseling Psychologist* 37 (2009) 424–50.

Eckenwiler, Lisa A., and Felicia Cohn, eds. *The Ethics of Bioethics: Mapping the Moral Landscape*. Baltimore: Johns Hopkins University Press, 2007.

Editorial Board. "Aid-in-Dying Movement Advances." *The New York Times*, October 10, 2016. https://www.nytimes.com/2016/10/10/opinion/aid-in-dying-movement-advances.html.

Einstein, Albert. "Strange Is Our Situation Here upon Earth." In *The World Treasury of Modern Religious Thought*, edited by Jaroslav Pelikan, 202–5. Boston: Little, Brown, 1991.

Emanuel, Ezekiel J. "Whose Right to Die?" *The Atlantic*, March 1997. http://www.theatlantic.com/magazine/archive/1997/03/whose-right-to-die/304641/.

———. "Why I Hope to Die at 75." *The Atlantic*, October 2014. https://www.theatlantic.com/magazine/archive/2014/10/why-i-hope-to-die-at-75/379329/.

Emanuel, Ezekiel J., and Linda L. Emanuel. "Four Models of the Physician-Patient Relationship." *Journal of the American Medical Association* 267 (1992) 2221–25.

Evans, John H. *The History and Future of Bioethics: A Sociological View*. New York: Oxford University Press, 2012.

Fadiman, Anne. *The Spirit Catches You and You Fall Down*. New York: Farrar, Straus and Giroux, 1997.

Feinberg, Joel. *Social Philosophy*. Englewood Cliffs, NJ: Prentice-Hall, 1973.

Fiala, Christian, and Joyce H. Arthur. "'Dishonourable Disobedience'—Why Refusal to Treat in Reproductive Healthcare Is Not Conscientious Objection." *Women: Psychosomatic Gynecology and Obstetrics* 1 (2014) 12–23.

Filene, Peter G. *In the Arms of Others: A Cultural History of the Right-to-Die in America*. Chicago: Dee, 1998.

"Final Certainty." *The Economist* 415 (June 27, 2015) 16–20. http://www.economist.com/news/briefing/21656122-campaigns-let-doctors-help-suffering-and-terminally-ill-die-are-gathering-momentum.

Fletcher, Joseph. *Morals and Medicine*. Boston: Beacon, 1960.

———. *Situation Ethics: The New Morality*. Philadelphia: Westminster, 1968.

Fox, Renee C., and Judith P. Swazey. *Observing Bioethics*. New York: Oxford University Press, 2008.

Frank, Arthur W. *At the Will of the Body: Reflections on Illness*. Boston: Houghton Mifflin, 2002.

———. *The Wounded Storyteller: Body, Ethics and Illness*. 2nd ed. Chicago: University of Chicago Press, 2013.

Gawande, Atul. *Being Mortal: Medicine and What Matters in the End*. New York: Holt, 2014.

———. "The Best Possible Day." *The New York Times*, October 5, 2014. https://www.nytimes.com/2014/10/05/opinion/sunday/the-best-possible-day.html?_r=0.

———. *Complications: A Surgeon's Notes on an Imperfect Science*. New York: Holt, 2002.

Gaylin, Willard. "The Frankenstein Factor." *New England Journal of Medicine* 297 (1976) 665–67.

Gaylin, Willard, et al. "Doctors Must Not Kill." *Journal of the American Medical Association* 259 (1988) 2139–40.

Goldhill, Michael. "How American Health Care Killed My Father." *The Atlantic*, September 2009. https://www.theatlantic.com/magazine/archive/2009/09/how-american-health-care-killed-my-father/307617/.

Gorsuch, Neil M. *The Future of Assisted Suicide and Euthanasia.* Princeton: Princeton University Press, 2006.

Gould, Stephen Jay. "The Median Isn't the Message." https://people.umass.edu/biep540w/pdf/Stephen%20Jay%20Gould.pdf .

Greenawalt, Kent. *Religious Convictions and Political Choice.* New York: Oxford University Press, 1988.

Halifax, Joan. *Being with Dying: Cultivating Compassion and Fearlessness in the Presence of Death.* Boston: Shambhala, 2009.

Hanson, Mark J., and Daniel Callahan, eds. *The Goals of Medicine: The Forgotten Issues in Health Care Reform.* Washington, DC: Georgetown University Press, 1999.

Hardwig, John. "Is There A Duty to Die?" *Hastings Center Report* 27 (1997) 34–42.

Harrelson, Walter. "Decalogue." In *The Westminster Dictionary of Christian Ethics*, edited by James F. Childress and John Macquarrie, 146–47. 2nd ed. Philadelphia: Westminster, 1986.

Harvard Medical School. "A Definition of Irreversible Coma: Report of the Ad Hoc Committee of the Harvard Medical School to Examine the Definition of Brain Death." *Journal of the American Medical Association* 205 (1968) 337–40.

Hedberg, Katrina, and David New. "Oregon's Death with Dignity Act: Twenty Years of Experience to Inform the Debate." *Annals of Internal Medicine* 167 (2017) 579–83.

Hojat, Mohammadreza, et al. "The Devil Is in the Third Year: A Longitudinal Study of Erosion of Empathy in Medical School." *Academic Medicine* 84 (2009) 1182–91.

Hough-Telford, Catherine, et al. "Vaccine Delays, Refusals, and Patient Dismissals: A Survey of Pediatricians." *Pediatrics* 138 (2016) 1–9. https://pediatrics.aappublications.org/content/pediatrics/138/3/e20162127.full.pdf.

Huxley, Aldous. *Brave New World.* New York: Harper, 2005.

Institute of Medicine. *Mitochondrial Replacement Techniques: Ethical, Social, and Policy Considerations.* Washington, DC: National Academies Press, 2016.

———. *Relieving Pain in America: A Blueprint for Transforming Prevention, Care, Education, and Research.* Washington, DC: National Academies Press, 2011.

James, William. "The Moral Equivalent of War." In *War and Morality*, edited by Richard A. Wasserstrom, 4–14. Belmont, CA: Wadsworth, 1970.

Jefferson, Thomas. "Follow Truth (Quotation)." https://www.monticello.org/site/jefferson/follow-truth-quotation.

Jennings, Tom, prod. *Frontline*, Season 33, episode 6, "Being Mortal." Aired February 10, 2015, on OPB. https://www.pbs.org/wgbh/frontline/film/being-mortal.

John Paul II. *Evangelium Vitae* [*The Gospel of Life*]. http://w2.vatican.va/content/john-paul-ii/en/encyclicals/documents/hf_jp-ii_enc_25031995_evangelium-vitae.html.

Jonas, Hans. "The Right to Die." *Hastings Center Report* 8 (1978) 31–36.

Jones, Robert P. *Liberalism's Troubled Search for Equality: Religion and Cultural Bias in the Oregon Physician-Assisted Suicide Debates.* Notre Dame, IN: University of Notre Dame Press, 2007.

Jonsen, Albert R. *The Birth of Bioethics.* New York: Oxford University Press, 1998.

———. *The New Medicine and the Old Ethics*. Cambridge: Harvard University Press, 1990.

Jonsen, Albert R., and Stephen Toulmin. *The Abuse of Casuistry: A History of Moral Reasoning.* Berkeley: University of California Press, 1998.

Kahn, Michael W. "What Would Osler Do?: Learning from 'Difficult' Patients." *New England Journal of Medicine* 361 (2009) 442–43.

Kalanithi, Paul. *When Breath Becomes Air.* New York: Random House, 2016.

Kass, Leon R. "Averting One's Eyes or Facing the Music?: On Dignity in Death." *Hastings Center Studies* 2 (1974) 67–80.

Keller, Eric J. "Is Medicine a Choice or a Calling?" *KevinMD*, June 7, 2013. https://www.kevinmd.com/blog/2013/06/medicine-choice-calling.html.

Kierkegaard, Soren. "At a Graveside." In *Three Discourses on Imagined Occasions*, edited by Howard V. Hong and Edna V. Hong, 69–102. Princeton: Princeton University Press, 1993.

———. *Works of Love*. Translated by Howard V. Hong and Edna V. Hong. New York: Harper Perennial, 2009.

King, Martin Luther, Jr. "I've Been to the Mountaintop." http://kingencyclopedia.stanford.edu/encyclopedia/documentsentry/ive_been_to_the_mountaintop/.

Kliever, Lonnie D., ed. *Dax's Case: Essays in Medical Ethics and Human Meaning.* Dallas: Southern Methodist University Press, 1989.

Kullberg, Patricia. *On the Ragged Edge of Medicine: Doctoring Among the Dispossessed.* Corvallis, OR: Oregon State University Press, 2017.

Lakoff, George, and Mark Johnson. *Metaphors We Live By.* Chicago: University of Chicago Press, 1980.

Leder, Drew. *The Absent Body.* Chicago: University of Chicago Press, 1990.

Lee, Lisa M., et al. "Teaching Bioethics." *Hastings Center Report* 44 (2014) 10–11.

Lemmon, E. J. "Moral Dilemmas." *The Philosophical Review* 70 (1962) 139–58.

Lewis, C. S. *The Four Loves.* New York: Harcourt Brace, 1988.

———. *A Grief Observed.* New York: Harper Collins, 1996.

Lewontin, Richard C. "The Confusion over Cloning." *New York Review of Books* 44 (October 23, 1997) 18–23.

Macklin, Ruth. "The New Conservatives in Bioethics: Who Are They and What Do They Seek?" *Hastings Center Report* 36 (2006) 34–43.

Madison, James. "A Memorial and Remonstrance Against Religious Assessments." In *The Sacred Rights of Conscience: Selected Readings on Religious Liberty and Church-State Relations in the American Founding*, edited by Daniel L. Dreisbach and Mark David Hall, 309–13. Indianapolis: Liberty Fund, 2009.

———. "A Proclamation." In *The Sacred Rights of Conscience: Selected Readings on Religious Liberty and Church-State Relations in the American Founding*, edited by Daniel L. Dreisbach and Mark David Hall, 458–59. Indianapolis: Liberty Fund, 2009.

———. "Speech in the First Congress Introducing Amendments to the U.S. Constitution." In *The Sacred Rights of Conscience: Selected Readings on Religious Liberty and Church-State Relations in the American Founding*, edited by Daniel L. Dreisbach and Mark David Hall, 418–25. Indianapolis: Liberty Fund, 2009.

Marco, Tony, et al. "Portland Train Stabbings: FBI Looking into Possible Hate Crime Charges." *CNN News*, May 28, 2017. https://www.cnn.com/2017/05/26/us/portland-train-stabbing/index.html.

Marrott, Robert L. "Witnesses, Law of." In *Encyclopedia of Mormonism*, edited by Daniel H. Ludlow, 1569–70. New York: Macmillan, 1992. https://eom.byu.edu/index.php/Witnesses,_Law_of.

Martin, Emily. *The Woman in the Body: A Cultural Analysis of Reproduction*. Boston: Beacon, 1987.

May, William F. "Corrective Vision: The Role of Applied Ethics." *Reflections* 4 (1997) 1–3.

———. *The Physician's Covenant: Images of the Healer in Medical Ethics*. 2nd ed. Louisville: Westminster John Knox, 2001.

———. *Testing the Medical Covenant: Active Euthanasia and Health Care Reform*. Grand Rapids: Eerdmans, 1996.

McCleod, Carolyn. "Trust." In *Stanford Encyclopedia of Philosophy*. http://plato.stanford.edu/entries/trust/.

McCormick, Richard A. "Abortion: Rules for Debate." *America* 139 (1978) 26–30.

———. "Physician Assisted Suicide: Flight from Compassion." *The Christian Century* 108 (1992) 1132–34.

McDermott, Walsh. "Evaluating the Physician and His Technology." In *Doing Better and Feeling Worse: Health in the United States*, edited by John H. Knowles, 135–57. New York: Norton, 1977.

McDermott, Walsh, and David E. Rogers. "Technology's Consort." *American Journal of Medicine* 74 (1983) 353–58.

McKenny, Gerald P. *To Relieve the Human Condition: Bioethics, Technology, and the Body*. Albany, NY: State University of New York Press, 1997.

Medstar Good Samaritan Hospital. "Mission, Vision and Values." http://www.medstargoodsam.org/our-hospital/mission-vision-and-values/#q={}.

Meilaender, Gilbert. *Body, Soul, and Bioethics*. Notre Dame, IN: University of Notre Dame Press, 1995.

Messikomer, Carla M., et al. "The Presence and Influence of Religion in American Bioethics." *Perspectives in Biology and Medicine* 44 (2001) 485–508.

Mill, John Stuart. "On Liberty." In *The English Philosophers: From Bacon to Mill*, edited by Edwin A. Burtt, 949–1041. New York: The Modern Library, 1939.

———. "Utilitarianism." In *Mill: Utilitarianism*, edited by Samuel Gorovitz, 11–42. Indianapolis: Bobbs-Merrill, 1971.

Miller, Donald G. "Some Observations on the New Testament Concept of Witness." *The Asbury Theological Journal* 43 (1988) 55–71.

Miller, Franklin G., et al. "Dealing with Dolly: Inside the National Bioethics Advisory Commission." *Health Affairs* 17 (1998) 264–67.

Miller, Richard G. *Friends and Other Strangers: Studies in Religion, Ethics, and Culture*. New York: Columbia University Press, 2016.

Montgomery, Kathryn. "Narrative." In *Bioethics*, edited by Bruce Jennings, 2138–41. 4th ed. New York: Macmillan, 2014.

Moreno, Jonathan D. "The End of the Great Bioethics Compromise." *Hastings Center Report* 35 (2005) 14–15.

Murphy, Timothy F. "In Defense of Irreligious Bioethics." *American Journal of Bioethics* 12 (2012) 3–10.

National Academy of Medicine. *Physician-Assisted Death: Scanning the Landscape*. Washington, DC: National Academies Press, 2018.

National Bioethics Advisory Commission. *Cloning Human Beings.* Vol. 1. Rockville, MD: Government Printing Office, 1997.

Niebuhr, H. Richard. *Christ and Culture.* New York: Harper & Row, 1951.

———. *The Responsible Self: An Essay in Christian Moral Philosophy.* San Francisco: Harper & Row, 1963.

Niebuhr, Reinhold. *An Interpretation of Christian Ethics.* New York: Knopf, 1997.

———. "Why the Christian Church Is Not Pacifist." In *War and Christian Ethics,* edited by Arthur Holmes, 301–13. Grand Rapids: Baker, 1975.

Nuland, Sherwin. *How We Die: Reflections on Life's Final Chapter.* New York: Knopf, 1993.

———. *The Wisdom of the Body.* New York: Knopf, 1997.

Nussbaum, Martha. *Liberty of Conscience: In Defense of America's Tradition of Religious Equality.* New York: Basic, 2008.

Obama, Barack. "Obama's Commencement Address at Notre Dame." *The New York Times,* May 17, 2009. https://www.nytimes.com/2009/05/17/us/politics/17text-obama.html.

———. "Obama's Health Care Speech to Congress." *The New York Times,* September 9, 2009. http://www.nytimes.com/2009/09/10/us/politics/10obama.text.html.

Ofri, Danielle. "Not on the Doctor's Checklist, but Touch Matters." *The New York Times,* August 3, 2010. https://www.nytimes.com/2010/08/03/health/03case.html.

Oregon Health Authority, Public Health Division. "Oregon Death with Dignity Act: 2017 Data Summary." http://www.oregon.gov/oha/PH/PROVIDERPARTNERRESOURCES/EVALUATIONRESEARCH/DEATHWITHDIGNITYACT/Documents/year20.pdf.

Osler, Sir William. "Aequanimitas." In *Aequanimitas, With Other Addresses to Medical Students, Nurses and Practitioners of Medicine,* 1–13. Philadelphia: Blakiston & Son. http://www.medicalarchives.jhmi.edu/osler/aeqtable.htm

———. "The Master Word in Medicine." https://profiles.nlm.nih.gov/ps/access/GFBBVV.pdf.

Otterman, Sharon. "In Hospices and Homes, Music Therapy Offers End-of-Life Grace Note." *The New York Times,* January 16, 2018. https://www.nytimes.com/2018/01/15/nyregion/music-therapy-nursing-home-hospice.html.

Outka, Gene. *Agape: An Ethical Analysis.* New Haven, CT: Yale University Press, 1972.

Parsi, Kayhan, and Myles N. Sheehan, eds. *Healing as Vocation: A Medical Professionalism Primer.* New York: Rowman & Littlefield, 2006.

Peabody, Francis. "The Care of the Patient." *Journal of the American Medical Association* 88 (1927) 877–82.

Pew Research Center. "America's Changing Religious Landscape." http://assets.pewresearch.org/wp-content/uploads/sites/11/2015/05/RLS-08-26-full-report.pdf.

Pope, Thaddeus Mason. "Medical Aid in Dying: When Legal Safeguards Become Burdensome Obstacles." *The ASCO Post,* December 25, 2017. http://www.ascopost.com/issues/december-25-2017/medical-aid-in-dying-when-legal-safeguards-become-burdensome-obstacles/.

Presidential Commission for the Study of Bioethical Issues. *Bioethics for Every Generation: Education and Deliberation in Health, Science, and Technology.* Washington, DC: Presidential Commission, 2016. https://bioethicsarchive.georgetown.edu/pcsbi/sites/default/files/PCSBI_Bioethics-Deliberation_0.pdf.

President's Commission for the Study of Ethical Problems in Medicine and Biomedical and Behavioral Research. *Splicing Life: A Report on the Social and Ethical Issues of Genetic Engineering with Human Beings.* Washington, DC: President's Commission, 1982.

Prothero, Stephen. *Religious Literacy: What Every American Needs to Know—and Doesn't.* New York: HarperCollins, 2007.

Quill, Timothy E. "Physician-Assisted Death in the United States: Are the Existing 'Last Resorts' Enough?" *Hastings Center Report* 38 (2008) 17–22.

Ragosta, John. *Religious Freedom: Jefferson's Legacy, America's Creed.* Charlottesville: University of Virginia Press, 2013.

Ramsey, Paul. "Ethics and Chronic Illness." Lecture presented at the Hastings Center, Garrison, NY, June 1987.

———. *Fabricated Man: The Ethics of Genetic Control.* New Haven, CT: Yale University Press, 1970.

———. "The Indignity of 'Death with Dignity.'" In *On Moral Medicine: Theological Perspectives in Medical Ethics,* edited by Stephen E. Lammers and Allen Verhey, 209–22. 2nd ed. Grand Rapids: Eerdmans, 1998.

———. *The Patient as Person: Explorations in Medical Ethics.* New Haven, CT: Yale University Press, 1970.

Rasinski, Kenneth A., et al. "A Sense of Calling and Primary Care Physicians' Satisfaction in Treating Smoking, Alcoholism, and Obesity." *Archives of Internal Medicine* 172 (2012) 1423–24.

Rawls, John. *Political Liberalism.* New York: Columbia University Press, 1993.

Reich, Warren T. "Speaking of Suffering: A Moral Account of Compassion." *Soundings* 72 (1989) 83–108.

Rheinstein, Max, ed. *Max Weber on Law in Economy and Society.* Cambridge: Harvard University Press, 1954.

Rhoades, D. R., et al. "Speaking and Interruptions during Primary Care Office Visits." *Family Medicine* 33 (2001) 528–32.

Ridley, Aaron. *Beginning Bioethics: A Text with Integrated Readings.* New York: St. Martin's Press, 1998.

"The Right to Die." *The Economist* 415 (June 27, 2015) 9–10. http://www.economist.com/news/leaders/21656182-doctors-should-be-allowed-help-suffering-and-terminally-ill-die-when-they-choose.

Rorty, Richard. *Philosophy and Social Hope.* New York: Penguin, 1999.

———. "Religion in the Public Square: A Reconsideration." *Journal of Religious Ethics* 31 (2003) 141–49.

Rosenthal, David I., and Abraham Verghese. "Meaning and the Nature of Physicians' Work." *New England Journal of Medicine* 375 (2016) 1813–15.

Royal College of Physicians of London. *Doctors in Society: Medical Professionalism in a Changing World.* London: Royal College of Physicians, 2005.

Ruff, Jeffrey C., and Jeremy Barris. "The Sound of One House Clapping: The Unmannerly Doctor as Zen Rhetorician." In *House and Philosophy: Everybody Lies,* edited by Henry Jacoby, 84–97. Hoboken, NJ: Wiley & Sons, 2009.

Sanders, Lisa. *Every Patient Tells a Story: Medical Mysteries and the Art of Diagnosis.* New York: Broadway, 2009.

Savulescu, Julian. "Conscientious Objection in Medicine." *BMJ* 332 (2006) 294.

Schenck, David, and Larry R. Churchill. *Healers: Extraordinary Clinicians at Work.* New York: Oxford University Press, 2012.

Schneiderman, Lawrence J., et al. "Medical Futility: Response to Critiques." *Annals of Internal Medicine* 125 (1996) 669–74.

Schroeder, Steven A. "We Can Do Better: Improving the Health of the American People." *New England Journal of Medicine* 357 (2007) 1221–28.

Senecal, Jo McElroy. "Bearing Witness." *The New York Times*. March 25, 2015. https://opinionator.blogs.nytimes.com/2015/03/25/bearing-witness/.

Shakespeare, William. *Hamlet, Prince of Denmark*. In *The Complete Plays of William Shakespeare*, 788–821. New York: Chatham River, 1984.

Shapiro, Harold T., et al. "The Confusion over Cloning: An Exchange." *New York Review of Books* 45 (March 5, 1998) 46.

Shorb, John. "Medicine as Vocation: Interview with Daniel Sulmasy." *Church Health Reader*, September 15, 2010. http://chreader.org/medicine-vocation/.

Smith, David H. "On Paul Ramsey: A Covenant-Centered Ethic for Medicine." In *Theological Voices in Medical Ethics*, edited by Allen Verhey and Stephen E. Lammers, 7–29. Grand Rapids: Eerdmans, 1993.

Stahl, Ronit Y., and Ezekiel J. Emanuel. "Physicians, Not Conscripts—Conscientious Objection in Health Care." *New England Journal of Medicine* 376 (2017) 1380–85.

Stark, Michael D., and Grace Stark. "Physicians Without Chests: On the Call to End Conscientious Objection in Medicine." *The Public Discourse*, June 2017. http://www.thepublicdiscourse.com/2017/06/19567/.

Sulmasy, Daniel P. *The Healer's Calling: A Spirituality for Physicians and Other Health Care Professionals*. Mahwah, NJ: Paulist, 1997.

Sweet, Victoria. *God's Hotel: A Doctor, A Hospital, and a Pilgrimage to the Heart of Medicine*. New York: Riverhead, 2012.

Thernstrom, Melanie. *The Pain Chronicles: Cures, Myths, Mysteries, Prayers, Diaries, Brain Scans, Healings, and the Science of Suffering*. New York: Farrar, Straus and Giroux, 2010.

Thomson, Judith Jarvis. "A Defense of Abortion." In *The Problem of Abortion*, edited by Joel Feinberg, 121–39. Belmont, CA: Wadsworth, 1973.

Tolstoy, Leo. *The Death of Ivan Ilyich and Confession*. Translated by Peter Carson. New York: Norton, 2014.

Toulmin, Stephen. "How Medicine Saved the Life of Ethics." *Perspectives in Biology and Medicine* 25 (1982) 736–50.

———. "The Tyranny of Principles." *Hastings Center Report* 11 (1981) 31–39.

United States Conference of Catholic Bishops. *Ethical and Religious Directives of Catholic Health Care Services*. 5th ed. http://www.usccb.org/issues-and-action/human-life-and-dignity/health-care/upload/Ethical-Religious-Directives-Catholic-Health-Care-Services-fifth-edition-2009.pdf.

Veatch, Robert M. *The Basics of Bioethics*. 3rd ed. New York: Pearson Education, 2012.

———. *Hippocratic, Religious, and Secular Medical Ethics: The Points of Conflict*. Washington, DC: Georgetown University Press, 2012.

Verghese, Abraham. "The Calling." *New England Journal of Medicine* 352 (2005) 843–44.

———. "Culture Shock: Patient as Icon, Icon as Patient." *New England Journal of Medicine* 359 (2008) 2748–51.

———. "How Tech Can Turn Doctors into Clerical Workers." *The New York Times*, May 16, 2018. https://www.nytimes.com/interactive/2018/05/16/magazine/health-issue-what-we-lose-with-data-driven-medicine.html.

———. "Treat the Patient, Not the CT Scan." *The New York Times*, February 27, 2011. http://www.nytimes.com/2011/02/27/opinion/27verghese.html?_r=0.

Verhey, Allen. "'Playing God' and Invoking a Perspective." *Journal of Medicine and Philosophy* 20 (1995) 347–64.

———. *Reading the Bible in the Strange World of Medicine.* Grand Rapids: Eerdmans, 2003.

Walters, LeRoy. "Religion and the Renaissance of Medical Ethics in the United States: 1965–1975." In *Theology and Bioethics: Exploring the Foundations and Frontiers*, edited by Earl E. Shelp, 3–16. Dordrecht, the Netherlands: Reidel, 1985.

Walzer, Michael. *Interpretation and Social Criticism.* Cambridge: Harvard University Press, 1987.

———. "Political Action: The Problem of Dirty Hands." *Philosophy & Public Affairs* 2 (1973) 160–80.

Washington, George. "Farewell Address." In *The Sacred Rights of Conscience: Selected Readings on Religious Liberty and Church-State Relations in the American Founding*, edited by Daniel L. Dreisbach and Mark David Hall, 468–70. Indianapolis: Liberty Fund, 2009.

Weber, Max. "Politics as a Vocation." In *From Max Weber: Essays in Sociology*, edited by H. H. Gerth and C. Wright Mills, 77–128. New York: Oxford University Press, 1958.

———. *The Protestant Ethic and the Spirit of Capitalism.* Translated by Talcott Parsons. New York: Scribner, 1958.

———. "Science as a Vocation." In *From Max Weber: Essays in Sociology*, edited by H. H. Gerth and C. Wright Mills, 129–56. New York: Oxford University Press, 1958.

———. "The Social Psychology of the World's Religions." In *From Max Weber: Essays in Sociology*, edited by H. H. Gerth and C. Wright Mills, 267–301. New York: Oxford University Press, 1958.

White, Lynn, Jr. "The Historical Roots of Our Ecologic Crisis." *Science* 155 (1967) 1203–7.

Wicclair, Mark R. *Conscientious Objection in Health Care: An Ethical Analysis.* New York: Cambridge University Press, 2011.

Wynia, Matthew. "The Birth of Medical Professionalism: Professionalism and the Role of Professional Associations." In *Healing as Vocation: A Medical Professionalism Primer*, edited by Kayhan Parsi and Myles N. Sheehan, 23–34. New York: Rowman & Littlefield, 2006.

Index of Topics and Names

12031329R00199

Made in the USA
Monee, IL
20 September 2019